Hepatology and Transplant Hepatology

Jawad Ahmad, MD, FRCP

Hepatology and Transplant Hepatology

A Case Based Approach

With Contributions by
Shahid M. Malik MD, Assistant Professor of Medicine, Division of Gastroenterology, Hepatology & Nutrition, University of Pittsburgh School of Medicine, Pittsburgh, PA

James S. Park, MD, CNSC, Assistant Professor of Medicine, Division of Liver Diseases, Mount Sinai Liver Cancer Program, Recanati-Miller Transplantation Institute, Mount Sinai School of Medicine, New York, NY

David A. Sass, MD, Associate Professor of Medicine and Surgery, Associate Chief, Division of Gastroenterology and Hepatology, Drexel University College of Medicine, Philadelphia, PA

Springer

Jawad Ahmad, MD, FRCP
Associate Professor of Medicine
Division of Liver Diseases
Recanati-Miller Transplantation Institute
Mount Sinai School of Medicine
NewYork, NY
USA
jawad.ahmad@mountsinai.org

ISBN 978-1-4419-7084-8 e-ISBN 978-1-4419-7085-5
DOI 10.1007/978-1-4419-7085-5
Springer New York Dordrecht Heidelberg London

Library of Congress Control Number: 2010937227

Printed on acid-free paper

Springer is part of Springer Science+Business Media (www.springer.com)

Preface

Over the last few decades, hepatology and transplant hepatology have emerged as individual disciplines, separate from gastroenterology, and this has been recognized by the American Board of Internal Medicine who have offered a transplant hepatology board examination since 2006. In the USA and Europe, there are increasing numbers of specialists who consider themselves exclusively as hepatologists, and even among this group there is differentiation into nontransplant and transplant hepatology.

Many textbooks of medicine are an excellent reference source but are difficult to read. For students and trainees, a basic understanding of epidemiology and pathogenesis of disease entities are important but management of a specific clinical condition mirrors the real world (and many examination situations). A patient rarely presents with acute hepatitis B or with primary sclerosing cholangitis but is much more likely to present with an acute hepatitis or abnormal liver enzymes. Similarly, patients after liver transplantation present with symptoms or abnormal blood tests or imaging rather than a specific diagnosis. The way to approach such patients is the idea behind this book.

Each case is based on real examples but I have changed some of the demographics to protect patient confidentiality. The first page is a description of the case with pertinent history, physical and laboratory findings followed by a series of questions. The second page is an image or laboratory test which helps to clinch the diagnosis and the third page is a discussion of the case which answers the questions and provides a differential diagnosis where appropriate and several references.

The book is separated into three sections: general hepatology, advanced liver disease, and transplant hepatology. The first section deals mainly with outpatient cases such as abnormal liver tests or imaging. I have deliberately focused on the latter two sections as these are the type of clinical scenarios seen in the transplant hepatology board exam and are the type of cases encountered in the inpatient setting in many large hospitals. The majority of cases pertain to patients presenting acutely to the emergency room or are examples of everyday consults you might see on the inpatient service. The transplant cases are a mixture of the more common conditions that are encountered by transplant hepatologists. Some of the cases are straight-forward and some are more difficult but all the cases illustrate an important teaching point. I hope I have included a breadth of cases that will appeal to students, residents, and fellows, as well as physician extenders and nursing staff involved in the care of patients with liver disease.

For the genesis and all the way through the production of this text, I am indebted to many colleagues and trainees. There are far too many to individually name but I would be amiss if I did not mention all the liver and gastroenterology specialists at the Royal Free Hospital in London who first fostered my interest in hepatology and transplant medicine as a medical student and as a house officer. My consultants/attending staff in the UK and the USA always afforded me the opportunity to manage patients under their care with a degree of independence that enabled critical thinking. As an attending physician in the USA, I have been humbled to interact with many residents and fellows who have taken my occasional caustic nature on rounds (based on the British medical student teaching system!) with good humor and I hope I have influenced them positively as I was influenced by all my teachers. My colleagues at the University of Pittsburgh including Drs. Shaikh and Rabinovitz, and my co-authors Drs. Sass, Malik, and Park, deserve special mention, as do all the gastroenterology fellows at the University of Pittsburgh over the last 10 years, the most recent hepatology fellows at Mount Sinai School of Medicine, and the staff at the Veterans Affairs Pittsburgh Healthcare System, specifically Kathy Downey CRNP. I am sure you will recognize some of the cases.

Finally, I would like to acknowledge my parents, Gulzar and Iftikhar, for their wisdom; my children, Leila, Noor, and Aryia, for their enthusiasm; and my wife, Mary, for her tolerancc. This book is dedicated to them all.

New York, NY
May 2010

Jawad Ahmad, MD, FRCP

Contents

Table of Normal Laboratory Parameters

Component	Ref range
Prothrombin time (PT)	11.5–15.5 seconds
INR	0.9–1.3
Glucose-BLD	65–99 mg/dl
Sodium-BLD	135–145 mEq/l (mmol/l)
Potassium-BLD	3.5–5.0 mEq/l (mmol/l)
Carbon dioxide-BLD	22.0–32.0 mEq/l (mmol/l)
Urea nitrogen-BLD	11–25 mg/dl
Albumin, BLD	3.4–5.2 g/dl
Alkaline phosphatase, (ALP) BLD	30–110 iu/l
Creatinine-serum (creat)	0.7–1.2 mg/dl
Total Protein-BLD	6.0–8.3 g/dl
ALT (SGPT)	10–53 iu/l
AST (SGOT)	10–50 iu/l
LDH-BLD	100–220 iu/l
Uric acid-BLD	4.0–9.0 mg/dl
Gamma GTP-BLD (GGT or GGTP)	10–54 iu/l
Calcium, BLD	8.5–11.0 mg/dl
Bilirubin total (Tbili)	0.1–1.2 mg/dl
Bilirubin direct	0.0–0.8 mg/dl
White blood cell	4.5–11.0 × $10^3/\mu l$
Hemoglobin (Hb)	13.9–16.3 g/dl
Hematocrit	42.0–52.0%
Platelet	150–450 × $10^3/\mu l$
Iron, serum	50–200 mcg/dl
TIBC	250–400 mcg/dl
Transferrin saturation	15–50%
Alpha fetoprotein (AFP)	0.0–9.0 ng/ml
TSH	0.34–5.60 miu/l
Alpha-1-antitrypsin	83–199 mg/dl
Ceruloplasmin	16–40 mg/dl
Ferritin	30–400 ng/ml
Prograf (FK) level	4–16 ng/ml

Component	Ref range
Cyclosporine level	150–250 ng/ml
Cholesterol	<200 mg/dl
LDL-cholesterol	<130 mg/dl
HDL-cholesterol	30–75 mg/dl
Triglyceride	40–175 mg/dl
CEA	<2.5 ng/ml
CA19-9	<40 iu/ml
Lactate	0.3–2.3 mEq/l
Ammonia (NH3)	11–35 μmol/l
HbA1c	3.8–5.0%
ANA	<1:40
SMA	<1:40
AMA	<10 iu/ml (<1:40)
M2	<1:40
IgG	700–1,600 mg/dl
IgM	40–230 mg/dl
IgA	70–400 mg/dl
Troponin-I	<0.4 ng/ml
CPK	60–300 ng/ml
Phosphate	0.8–1.5 mmol/l
Urine	
Specific gravity	1.003–1.040
pH	4.6–8.0
Na	10–40 mEq/l
K	<8 mEq/l
Cl	<8 mEq/l
Protein	1–15 mg/dl
Osmolality	80–1300 mOsm/l
Blood gas	
Arterial pH	7.35–7.45
$PaCO_2$	35–45 mmHg
HCO_3	22–26 mEq/l
O_2 sat	96–100%
PaO_2	85–100 mmHg
BE	−2 to +2 mmol/l

Part I
General Hepatology

Cases 1–26

Case 1

A 51-year-old Caucasian man presents to your outpatient clinic with abnormal liver enzymes for several years. He is accompanied by his wife. He is asymptomatic without evidence of jaundice, fever or chills, weight loss. He has no past medical history and is on no prescribed medication. He denies any over the counter or herbal medicines. He does not drink significantly (once or twice a year) but smokes a packet of cigarettes a day and works as a salesman. He is happily married with grown up children. There is no history of intravenous drug use or cocaine. His father had Hodgkin's lymphoma.

Review of symptoms is negative except for some shortness of breath on exertion and nonproductive cough.

Physical exam reveals normal vitals, weight 232 pounds, height 72 inches.

There is no scleral icterus or spider nevi. Heart and lungs are normal. Abdomen reveals a smooth liver felt 3 cm below the right costal margin. There is no splenomegaly, ascites, or ankle edema.

Laboratory Parameters

Tbili 0.5 mg/dl
AST 88 iu/l
ALT 108 iu/l
ALP 455 iu/l
GGTP 495 iu/l

Normal renal function and hemogram

Questions

1. What is the differential diagnosis?
2. What test(s) should you order?
3. What treatment options (if any) are required?

J. Ahmad, *Hepatology and Transplant Hepatology: A Case Based Approach*,
DOI 10.1007/978-1-4419-7085-5_1, © Springer Science+Business Media, LLC 2011

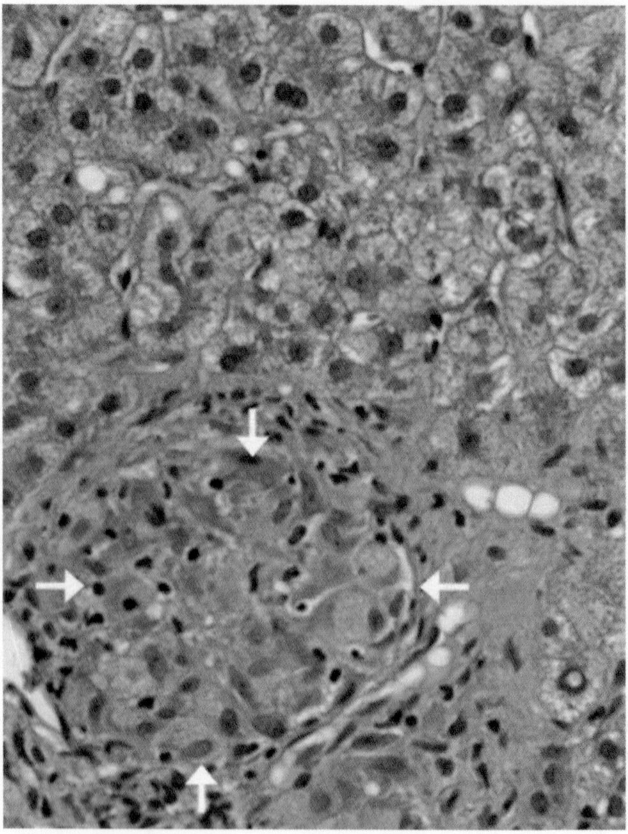

Fig. 1.1 Liver biopsy H&E ×250

Answer: Hepatic Sarcoid

The liver enzyme abnormalities in this case show mildly elevated transaminases but significantly elevated cholestatic enzymes. The elevated GGT implies that the high ALP is from the liver but ALP isoenzymes could be ordered to confirm this but are rarely necessary. The bilirubin is normal and cholestatic liver disease means an elevated ALP, not necessarily jaundice. Cholestatic disease can be classified as intra- or extra-hepatic, the latter typically from biliary obstruction.

The first test required in this situation is an imaging study to determine if the biliary tree is dilated which would imply biliary obstruction. Ultrasound or CAT scan would be reasonable but MRI has the added benefit of MRCP to obtain a cholangiogram. One of the differential diagnoses is primary sclerosing cholangitis (PSC). This inflammatory disease of the biliary tree may not cause biliary ductal dilation and hence can be missed by USS or CT. A good quality MRI with MRCP will typically show PSC changes (although can still miss early PSC or small duct PSC).

Laboratory tests should include the usual panel of viral and metabolic tests. Autoimmune blood work is important in this case to look for primary biliary cirrhosis (PBC) (which typically affects middle-aged women) as well as overlap conditions such as autoimmune cholangiopathy. An elevated antimitochondrial antibody (or the M2 fraction) is almost diagnostic for PBC.

If blood work and imaging is unhelpful then liver biopsy is usually required. The diagnostic possibilities if biliary obstruction is ruled out are myriad but include several medications, PBC (which can be AMA negative in a few percent of cases), autoimmune cholangiopathy, cholestatic viral hepatitis (hepatitis C and B can cause this but typically after liver transplantation), and essentially any process that can cause infiltration of the liver including fatty liver, amyloid, sarcoid, lymphoma, and metastatic disease. Granulomatous hepatitis is a diagnosis of exclusion where the liver is infiltrated by granulomas. This can be seen in PBC but also in TB and with a variety of bacterial and fungal infections, hence the need to exclude these entities before making a diagnosis.

This patient had a serum ACE level twice the upper limit of normal and had had a chest X-ray several months ago that demonstrated hilar prominence. His liver biopsy confirmed granulomas. He was started on steroids by his lung specialist with some improvement in his liver enzymes.

Hepatic sarcoid is typically an indolent disease that has to be differentiated from causes of granulomatous hepatitis. Blood work ruled out infection and the lung involvement confirmed sarcoid. Isolated hepatic sarcoid can occur and anecdotally can be treated with steroids but this is of no proven benefit. Similarly, ursodeoxycholic acid can be used with improvement in liver enzymes but it is unclear whether this improves survival. Most patients with hepatic sarcoid do well with just periodic assessment.

References

1. Pratt DS, Kaplan MM. Evaluation of abnormal liver-enzyme results in asymptomatic patients. N Engl J Med 2000;342:1266–71.
2. Drebber U, Kasper HU, Ratering J, et al. Hepatic granulomas: histological and molecular pathological approach to differential diagnosis – a study of 442 cases. Liver Int 2008;28:828–34.

Case 2

A 41-year-old female presents to the emergency room with right lower quadrant pain. She denies fever or chills and has had no change in urine or stool color. She has noticed some burning in the urine.

Her past medical history is significant for hypertension and she takes metoprolol. There is also a history of an anxiety type disorder and she undergoes regular counseling.

She takes some herbal supplements although she does not recall all their names.

She is married with two young children.

On examination, her vital signs are stable except for mild tachycardia. She has mild tenderness in the right lower quadrant without peritoneal signs. Her bowel sounds are present and she has no ascites. Extremities are without edema.

Laboratory Parameters Show

WBC 5.7 × 10^3/μl
Hemoglobin 13.4 g/dl
Tbili 0.7 mg/dl
AST 24 iu/l
ALT 21 iu/l
Creatinine 0.7 mg/dl
Alpha-fetoprotein (AFP) 2 ng/ml

There is concern for appendicitis and a CT scan is obtained which shows a normal appendix but a lesion is seen in the liver. The ER resident has already told her that she is concerned about a malignancy.

Questions

1. What are the diagnostic considerations?
2. What are the next appropriate tests?
3. Is a liver biopsy appropriate?

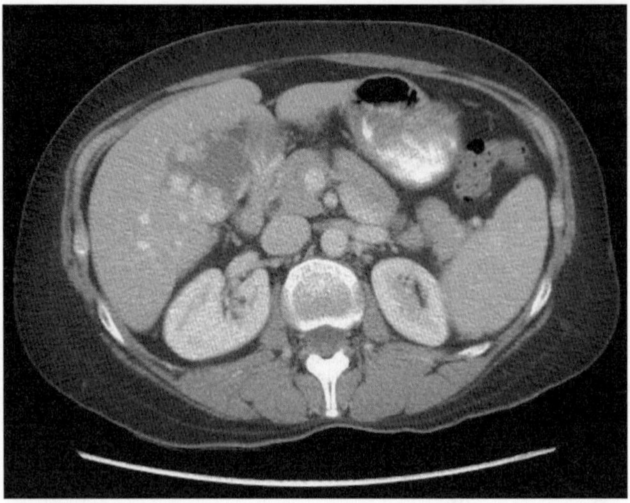

Fig. 2.1 CT scan

Answer: Hepatic Hemagioma

The differential diagnosis in a patient presenting with a liver lesion really depends on the clinical situation. It is helpful to know if the patient has underlying chronic liver disease as most hepatocellular carcinoma (HCC) occurs in the setting of chronic liver disease. This patient had no known history of liver disease and no risk factors for viral hepatitis, and her liver enzymes were found to be normal. She was incidentally found to have a lesion in the liver with a normal AFP. I would caution against using AFP as a screening test for HCC but in this case it was reassuring. Problems would have arisen if the AFP was marginally elevated and patients have undergone inadvisable biopsies in this situation. In this case, the CT scan was diagnostic for hemangioma with classic peripheral nodular enhancement in the early phase of contrast, followed by a filling in during the late phase (data not shown) which can persist for several minutes and lesions can remain hyperdense. Other imaging modalities can be used to diagnose hemangiomas with high accuracy. MRI usually shows a smooth homogeneous mass that has distinct borders and has low signal intensity on T1 images and hyperintensity on T2 images. Gadolinium enhancement produces a similar picture as contrast-enhanced CT. A tagged red cell scan (Technetium-99m) is another effective way for diagnosing hemangiomas but ultrasound is less accurate and a lesion suspected of being a hemangioma should be confirmed with other imaging modalities, especially in a patient with underlying liver disease or cirrhosis.

Hepatic hemangiomas are the most common benign hepatic lesion tumors with a prevalence of up to 15–20%. They can range in size with any lesion over 5 cm defined as a giant hemangioma. They are typically solitary, more common in women (suggesting a role for female sex hormones, particularly as they can enlarge during pregnancy); more common in the right lobe and can be associated with hemangiomas in other organs.

Most lesions are asymptomatic and stable over time. They are noted during imaging for an unrelated reason and if symptoms occur they usually consist of dull pain or a feeling of fullness in the upper abdomen but acute pain can be the result of thrombosis or bleeding into the tumor and can cause fever and abnormal liver enzymes.

Management should consist of reassurance for small lesions (<1–2 cm). Giant hemangiomas can be followed but there are no guidelines as to the frequency and no treatment is required even for very large lesions in the absence of symptoms.

Surgery can be employed for large symptomatic lesions and transplant is an option in selected cases with unresectable lesions. Acute bleeding can be managed with arterial embolization.

References

1. Tait N, Richardson AJ, Muguti G, et al. Hepatic cavernous haemangioma: a 10 year review. Aust N Z J Surg 1992;62:521.
2. Gandolfi L, Leo P, Solmi L, et al. Natural history of hepatic haemangiomas: clinical and ultrasound study. Gut 1991;32:677.
3. Popescu I, Ciurea S, Brasoveanu V, et al. Liver hemangioma revisited: current surgical indications, technical aspects, results. Hepatogastroenterology 2001;48:770.

Case 3

A 19-year-old man is sent to your outpatient office by the local university health clinic for evaluation of abnormal liver enzymes. He is essentially asymptomatic but complains of occasional itching. His appetite is good and his weight has been stable. He denies abdominal pain, fever, chills, and change in urine or stool color. He has no other medical problems and is not taking any prescribed medications but does take several protein supplements and vitamins. He is an offensive lineman on the university football team.

He has undergone cholecystectomy when he was 17 for cholecystitis although no records are available. He recalls being jaundiced at that time but he made a full recovery.

He denies any substance abuse and denies significant alcohol.

His family history is significant for hypertension in his mother and father but there is no history of liver disease or cancer.

On exam, he looks well. Vital signs show height 76 in., weight 305 pounds. His blood pressure and pulse are normal.

There is no scleral icterus and his cardiovascular, respiratory, and abdominal exams are all normal.

Laboratory Studies

Hb 14.7 g/dl
Platelets 125,000/μl
INR 1.3
Tbili 1.8 mg/dl
AST 68 iu/l
ALT 85 iu/l
ALP 265 iu/l
GGT 187 iu/l
Albumin 3.8 g/dl
Creatinine 1.4 mg/dl

Ultrasound of the right upper quadrant is normal

Questions

1. What is the next best test?
2. Are there any other blood tests that are necessary?
3. Is this a treatable condition?
4. Is there a risk of cancer in this condition?

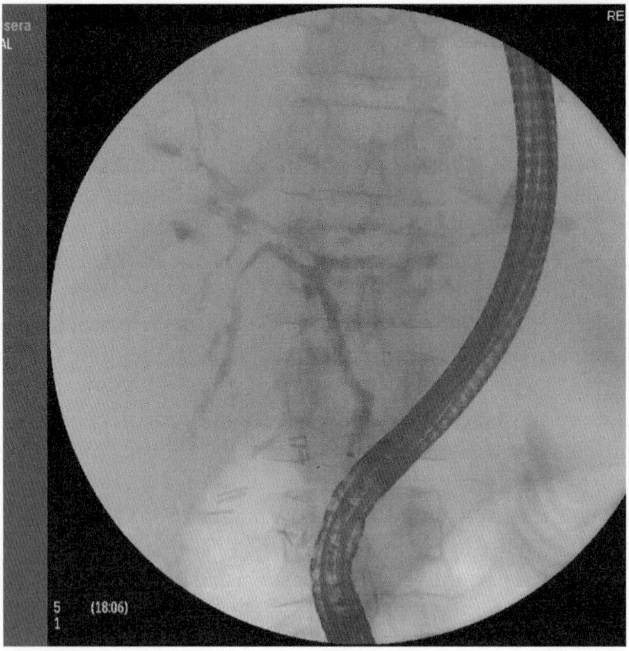

Fig. 3.1 ERCP image

Answer: Primary Sclerosing Cholangitis (PSC)

This is a fairly typical presentation for PSC. A young person (usually male) sent for essentially asymptomatic elevation of liver enzymes. The pattern is predominantly cholestatic although the transaminases are also mildly elevated. About two-thirds of PSC patients will have underlying inflammatory bowel disease (mainly ulcerative colitis but occasionally Crohn's disease), and this can also be silent.

The differential diagnosis here is the same as in Case 1. The negative ultrasound should not dismiss biliary problems and I typically would get an MRI/MRCP in this situation since the ducts may be diseased and yet not dilated. This patient was too big for the MRI machine.

The laboratory tests are incomplete since I would check an antimitochondrial antibody level (or M2) and serum IgM to look for PBC although this is unlikely in a young man. The other important blood test is an IgG4 level. A small subset of PSC patients has autoimmune disease (in the spectrum of autoimmune pancreatitis that can affect the biliary tree) and are responsive to steroids. In that sense, this could be a treatable disease. Typical PSC does not respond to drug treatment although many patients are placed on ursodeoxycholic acid (ursodiol). This can make liver enzymes to improve but does not alter the natural history of the disease. A recent study has suggested that high-dose ursodiol (28–30 mg/kg) may be harmful to PSC patients and I do not use this dose.

The patient went on to have an ERCP since he could not get an MRI, and the cholangiogram shows the typical beading and stricturing of PSC with involvement of both the intra- and extra-hepatic biliary tree. A liver biopsy is not necessary for the diagnosis and the classic onion skinning of the bile ducts mentioned in textbooks is rarely seen.

The ultimate treatment for PSC is liver transplant and long-term outcomes are excellent. This patient already has a low platelet count and likely has portal hypertension. Many PSC patients have well-maintained liver synthetic function and have a low model for end-stage liver disease (MELD) score. They may be good candidates for live donor liver transplant (although this patient's size will be a problem) but can get listed with a MELD exception if they have documented episodes of cholangitis. This patient's cholecystectomy 2 years ago was probably not cholecystitis but cholangitis given the fact he was jaundiced.

Cholangiocarcinoma is a risk in PSC patients with several natural history studies suggesting a lifetime incidence of 10–15%. It is somewhat ironic that this patient is a football player since Walter Payton, the Chicago Bears running back in the 1980s (I am showing my age) tragically died of cholangiocarcinoma in the setting of PSC which had remained undiagnosed throughout his football career.

References

1. Angulo P, Lindor KD. Primary sclerosing cholangitis. Hepatology 1999;30:325.
2. Mendes FD, Jorgensen R, Keach J, et al. Elevated serum IgG4 concentration in patients with primary sclerosing cholangitis. Am J Gastroenterol 2006;101:2070.
3. Lindor KD, Kowdley KV, Luketic VA, et al. High-dose ursodeoxycholic acid for the treatment of primary sclerosing cholangitis. Hepatology 2009;50:808.

Case 4

A 51-year-old African American lady is referred to you for evaluation of hepatomegaly noted by her family physician. He had sent her for abdominal imaging but she has not yet had this performed. She describes several years of abdominal discomfort, not related to meals and worsening abdominal distension. Several family members have had similar problems and one died of a stroke.

She is seeing a renal physician for chronic renal failure and is due to start hemodialysis next week.

She denies any over the counter medications but takes a calcium channel blocker for hypertension.

She does not smoke, drink, or abuse drugs.

She is married with three grown up children.

Exam demonstrates a well-looking patient, BP 140/90, and anicteric sclerae. She has a soft ejection systolic murmur and an early diastolic murmur. Her abdomen is markedly distended but nontender. Liver is felt in the right lower quadrant and there is some dullness in the flanks. She has some mild peripheral edema.

Laboratory Studies

Hb 11.7 g/dl
Platelets 174,000/μl
INR 1.1
Tbili 0.3 mg/dl
AST 17 iu/l
ALT 11 iu/l
ALP 153 iu/l
Albumin 2.7 g/dl
Creatinine 3.4 mg/dl

Questions

1. What is the genetic basis of this disease?
2. Apart from abdominal imaging, consideration should be given for imaging of which two other organs?

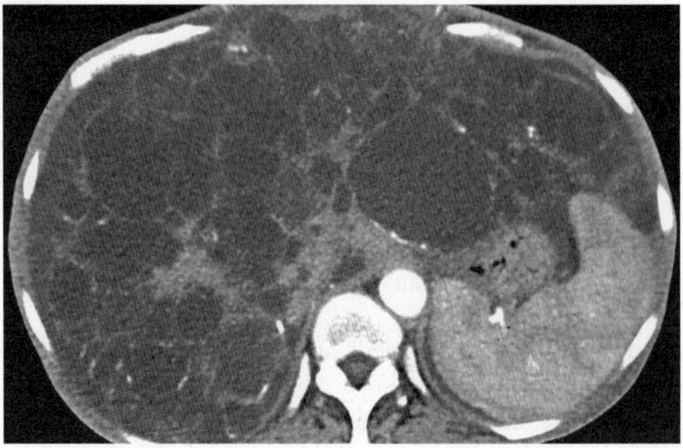

Fig. 4.1 CT scan abdomen

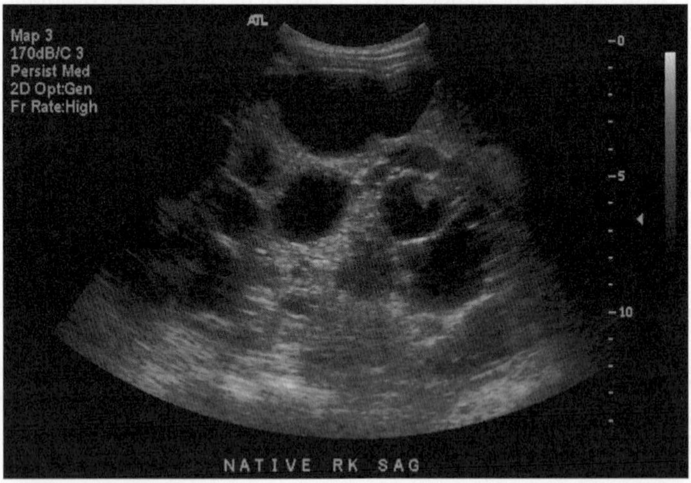

Fig. 4.2 Renal ultrasound

Answer: Autosomal Dominant Polycystic Kidney Disease with Liver Involvement

The renal failure, family history, and abdominal exam give the diagnosis away. The CT scan confirms a massively enlarged liver with multiple cysts as does the renal ultrasound of the right kidney.

The diagnosis must be autosomal dominant polycystic kidney disease (ADPKD) since there is renal involvement rather than the less common autosomal dominant polycystic liver disease which is not associated with kidney involvement or cerebral aneurysms. Autosomal recessive polycystic kidney disease is always associated with liver involvement, but is a disease of children and is much less common than ADPKD.

ADPKD has an incidence of between 0.1 and 0.2% of live births and several genetic defects have been identified, mainly located on chromosome 16. The clinical presentation is variable depending on the genetic mutation and some patients will be asymptomatic and not require any renal replacement therapy.

Hepatic involvement increases with age, and massive cysts appear more commonly in women, particularly those who are multiparous, suggesting a role for estrogen/progesterone. Most patients remain asymptomatic without hepatic dysfunction. However, rarely cysts may rupture and become infected presenting with acute symptoms.

Indication for surgical/radiological intervention includes severe, constant symptoms, and wasting. Options available range from percutaneous drainage, resection (or fenestration) in selected cases, and liver transplantation. Occasionally, the liver involvement is so massive that liver transplantation is required to enable enough room for kidney transplantation. Outcome after liver transplantation is good in several series.

Other extra-renal manifestations of ADPKD include cardiac valvular abnormalities (perhaps explaining this patient's early diastolic murmur suggestive of aortic incompetence), and cerebral aneurysms, with an incidence as high as 10%. However, screening is only recommended in patients with a prior rupture or family history of rupture since the natural history of small aneurysms (less than 7 mm) is good and there is some risk of the imaging study causing worsening renal function (administration of gadolinium during MR imaging is associated with nephrogenic systemic fibrosis).

References

1. Newman KD, Torres VE, Rakela J, et al. Preliminary experience with a combined hepatic resection–fenestration procedure. Ann Surg 1990;212:30–7.
2. Kirchner GI, Rifai K, Cantz T, et al. Outcome and quality of life in patients with polycystic liver disease after liver or combined liver–kidney transplantation. Liver Transpl 2006;12:1268–77.

Case 5

A 50-year-old lady presents to your outpatient office having been referred from her primary care provider for abnormal liver enzymes. She describes several weeks of some nonspecific symptoms including flu-like symptoms with fatigue and myalgias but no fever or chills. Her past medical history is significant for hypertension controlled on medication. She has also had breast reduction surgery and a hysterectomy.

She is a married lady with one child. She works in a law firm. She denies smoking, alcohol use, intravenous drug use, or cocaine use. She has had no remote blood transfusions.

Her older sister has been treated for hepatitis C and has had thyroid problems but there is no other family history.

Exam reveals a well-looking lady, weight 142 pounds, stable vital signs, no stigmata of chronic liver disease, and completely unremarkable abdomen.

Laboratory Studies

Hb 11.9 g/dl
Platelets 217,000/μl
WBC 9.5 × 10^3/μl
INR 1.1
Tbili 0.8 mg/dl
AST 617 iu/l
ALT 1,301 iu/l
ALP 185 iu/l
GGT 265 iu/l
Albumin 3.7 g/dl
Total protein 8.5 g/dl
Creatinine 0.7 mg/dl

Ultrasound abdomen
Normal sized liver but markedly heterogeneous echo pattern. No biliary dilation.

Questions

1. What other tests are required to make a *definitive* diagnosis?
2. Is a liver biopsy necessary?

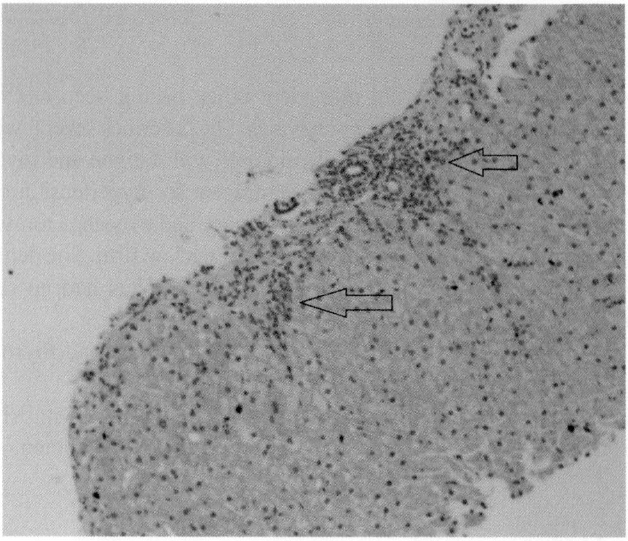

Fig. 5.1 Liver biopsy H&E ×100

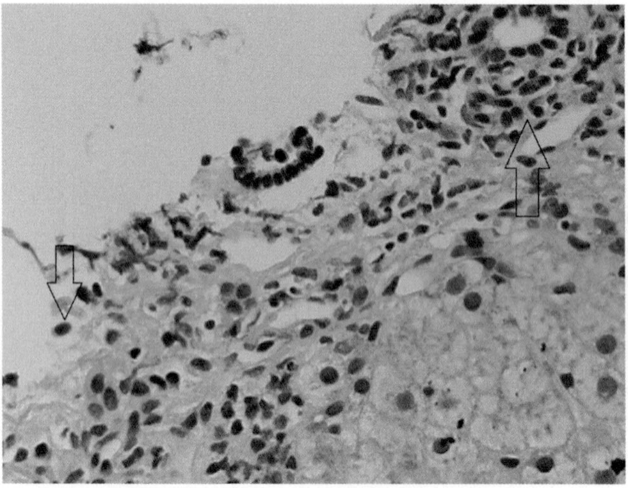

Fig. 5.2 Liver biopsy H&E ×250

Answer: Autoimmune Hepatitis

This middle-aged lady presents with minimal symptoms except for fatigue and markedly elevated transaminases. The differential diagnosis includes viral hepatitis (although she has no real risk factors), toxic- or drug-induced injury, and autoimmune disease.

The initial work-up would include viral hepatitis serology and autoimmune markers including antinuclear antibody (ANA), smooth muscle antibody (SMA), and quantitative immunoglobulins.

Autoimmune hepatitis (AIH) is a disease of unknown etiology, much more common in women, with a variable clinical presentation from asymptomatic patients, sometimes debilitating symptoms, and fulminant hepatic failure. Extrahepatic manifestations are common and include hemolytic anemia, idiopathic thrombocytopenic purpura, type 1 diabetes, thyroid disease, celiac disease (CD), and ulcerative colitis.

The liver biopsies show an inflammatory infiltrate in the portal tracts (arrowed) which is made up of lymphocytes and plasma cells (the cells with eccentrically placed nuclei – Fig. 5.2, left arrow). The infiltrate invades the sharply demarcated hepatocyte boundary (limiting plate) surrounding the portal tract and spills into the surrounding lobule (periportal infiltrate) which is termed piecemeal necrosis or interface hepatitis. In this patient, the biopsy was taken several weeks after treatment and the inflammatory infiltrate has likely improved. The trichrome stain showed architectural distortion of the hepatic lobule with bridging fibrosis.

The diagnosis of AIH can be difficult and used to be based on a complex scoring system developed by the International Autoimmune Hepatitis Group (IAIHG). This has been simplified for routine clinical practice and involves Laboratory Studies. A biopsy is not absolutely essential since a probable diagnosis can be made without histology. The scoring system is as follows:

Autoantibodies	One point if the ANA or SMA are 1:40
	Two points if the ANA or SMA are ≥1:80
IgG	One point if the IgG is greater than the upper limit of normal
	Two points if the IgG is >1.10 times the upper limit of normal
Liver histology	One point if the histological features are compatible with AIH
	Two points if the histological features are typical of AIH
Exclude HCV/HBV	Two points if viral hepatitis has been excluded

A probable diagnosis of AIH is made if the total points are 6 while a definite diagnosis is made if the total points are ≥7.

AIH is treated with immunosuppression. The American Association for the Study of Liver Disease (AASLD) guidelines suggest:

Prednisone in combination with azathioprine or a higher dose of prednisone alone is the appropriate treatment for severe AIH in adults.

Prednisone in combination with azathioprine is the preferred initial treatment because of its lower frequency of side effects.

All patients treated with prednisone alone or in combination with azathioprine must be monitored for the development of drug-related side effects.

This patient responded quickly to oral prednisone and was started on azathioprine after several weeks as a steroid sparing agent. Her liver enzymes normalized and her symptoms improved.

References

1. Krawitt EL. Autoimmune hepatitis. N Engl J Med 2006;354:54.
2. Hennes EM, Zeniya M, Czaja AJ, et al. Simplified criteria for the diagnosis of autoimmune hepatitis. Hepatology 2008;48:169–76.
3. Czaja AJ, Freese DK. Diagnosis and treatment of autoimmune hepatitis. Hepatology 2002;36:479.

Case 6

A 53-year-old Caucasian woman is referred to the liver clinic for evaluation of abnormal LFTs. She presents with a 3-month history of diarrhea with 10–12 loose bowel movements per day. There is no associated abdominal pain or hematochezia. There is an associated 10 pound weight loss. There is no recent travel history, sick contacts, fevers, chills, nausea, vomiting, or new medications.

Physical exam showed a 5′3″, 100 lb woman. No jaundice, no pallor, no cutaneous stigmata of chronic liver disease, no hepatosplenomegaly, edema, or ascites.

Lab Parameters

Total bilirubin 0.5 mg/dl
AST 124 iu/l
ALT 117 iu/l
ALP 130 iu/l
Albumin 2.2 g/dl

Hemogram was normal

Prior work-up by outside gastroenterologist was as follows:

Stool studies: negative for enteric pathogens and parasites
Colonoscopy with random biopsies: normal
Abdominal ultrasound: normal appearing liver and a small gallbladder polyp
Serologies for hepatitis A, B, C: negative
Autoimmune serologies: ANA, SMA, LKM, AMA: negative
Normal ferritin, ceruloplasmin, and α1-antitrypsin levels

Questions

1. What is the likely diagnosis?
2. What diagnostic testing should be ordered?
3. What is the pathophysiology of abnormal LFTs in this disease?
4. What is the role of a liver biopsy?

Anti-gliadin antibody > 167 (normal range < 20).
Anti-endomysial antibody > 221 (normal range < 20).

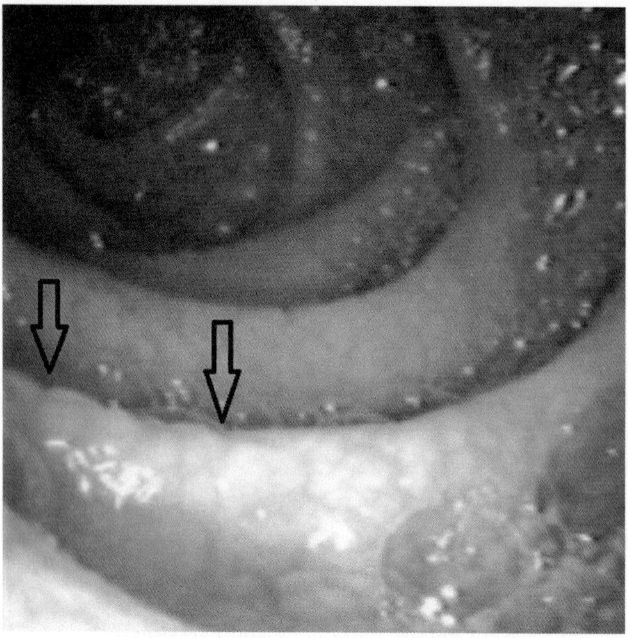

Fig. 6.1 Endoscopic image

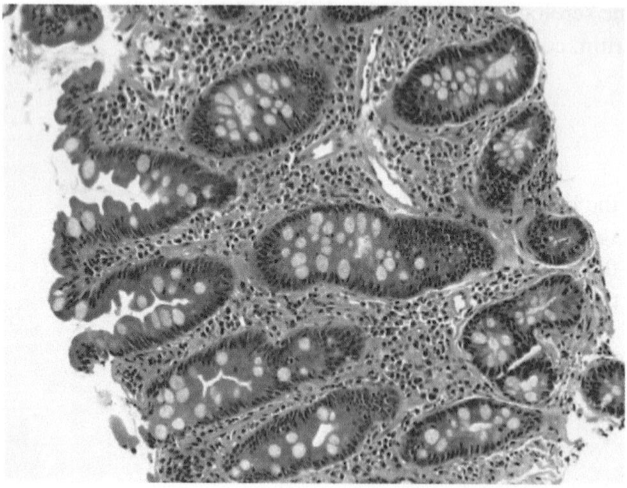

Fig. 6.2 ×100 Magnification

Answer: Celiac Disease (CD)

Mild elevation in transaminases may be seen in nonhepatic diseases, e.g., thyroid disease (hypo- and hyperthyroidism), muscle disorders (myositis and rhabdomyolysis), and adrenal insufficiency. It may also be seen in patients with CD (gluten-sensitive enteropathy).

The clinical clues for a diagnosis of CD may be the presence of an iron deficiency anemia, chronic diarrhea, and hypoalbuminemia. Liver blood test abnormalities affect patients with classic CD or may be the sole presentation of atypical CD.

A diagnosis can be made by obtaining CD antibodies and a confirmatory small bowel biopsy can be performed.

The endoscopic image (Fig. 6.1) shows the classic scalloped duodenal mucosa and the histology shows villous atrophy and intraepithelial lymphocytes in the duodenal mucosa.

The mechanisms underlying liver injury in CD are poorly understood. There is increased intestinal permeability in CD which may facilitate the entry of toxins, antigens, and inflammatory substances into the portal circulation, and these mediators may have a role in the liver involvement in CD. Alternatively, there may be a pathogenic role for the humoral-mediated immune responses in the liver injury.

A gluten-free diet leads to normalization of serum transaminases in 75–95% of patients, usually within 1 year of good adherence to the diet. For those whose liver enzymes remain elevated despite a gluten-free diet, a liver biopsy can be performed to further assess for etiology. Most will have nonspecific findings on biopsy.

References

1. Rubio-Tapia A, Murray JA. The liver in celiac disease. Hepatology 2007;46:1650–58.
2. Novacek G, Miehsler W, Wrba F, et al. Prevalence and clinical importance of hypertransaminasemia in celiac disease. Eur J Gastroenterol Hepatol 1999;11:283–8.

Case 7

A 29-year-old female presents with a 1 year history of recurrent epigastric and substernal chest pain, lasting from 1 to 8 hours, associated with some nausea and sweating. She was initially treated for GERD without relief. One attack was associated with jaundice and leukocytosis, prompting an ER visit. Ultrasound showed a normal gallbladder, no cholelithiasis, and a dilated extra-hepatic common bile duct. She was later seen in the outpatient GI office.

Physical examination revealed a thin young woman with no jaundice, no cutaneous stigmata of liver disease, and normal abdominal examination.

Lab Parameters

Tbili 0.5 mg/dl
AST 52 iu/l
ALT 67 iu/l
ALP 51 iu/l
GGTP 57 iu/l
Albumin 4.9 g/dl

An abdominal CT scan (Fig. 7.1) was obtained to further clarify the finding seen on prior ultrasound. There was a fusiform dilation of the common bile duct (yellow arrowhead) measuring 26 mm, with prompt tapering at the pancreatic head.

Questions

1. What diagnostic procedure should be performed next?
2. What is the diagnosis and classification of this disease?
3. How should the patient be managed?

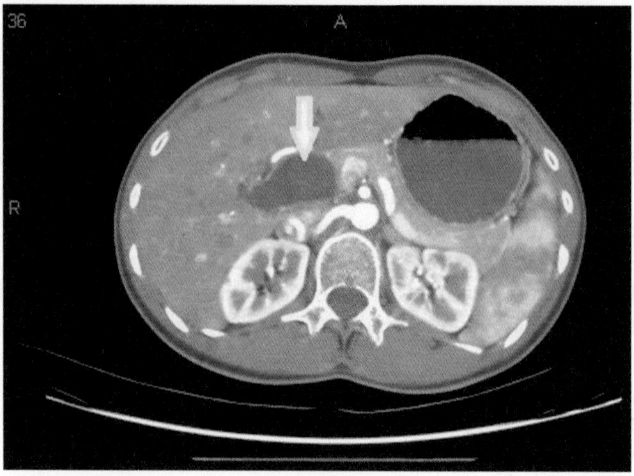

Fig. 7.1 CT abdomen scan

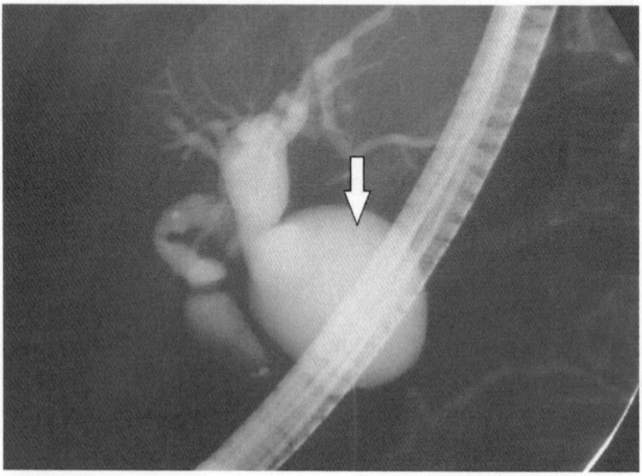

Fig. 7.2 Cholangiogram

Answer: Choledochal Cyst

This patient needs an ERCP. The cholangiogram (Fig. 7.2) shows a large type 1b choledochal cyst (black arrow). There was a 2 cm common bile duct stricture below the cyst and an anomalous pancreaticobiliary junction (APBJ). Bile duct brushings were negative for malignancy.

Choledochal cysts are cystic dilations occurring singly or in multiples throughout the bile ducts.

The classification scheme is known as the Todani classification:

Type I (a, b, and c): extra-hepatic bile duct alone
Type II: diverticulum of the extra-hepatic bile duct
Type III: choledochocele (involving intraduodenal duct)
Type IV: multiple intra- and extra-hepatic cysts
Type V: Caroli's disease

The pathologic features of the cyst are variable, ranging from normal bile duct epithelium to carcinoma. Seventy percent of patients have an APBJ which may be a significant factor for the development of malignancy in the cyst. A long (>2 cm) common channel is thought to be responsible for a free reflux of pancreatic enzymes and choledochal cyst formation.

A diagnosis of choledochal cyst should be considered when a dilated portion of the bile ducts or ampulla is identified, especially in the absence of an overt obstruction. An ERCP can demonstrate cystic dilation of the bile duct, exclude overt obstruction, delineate the presence of an APBJ, and demonstrate stones or a malignancy in the cyst.

Surgical excision is usually recommended to decrease the risk of malignant degeneration. This patient underwent a cholecystectomy, cyst excision, and biliary reconstruction with a Roux-en-Y hepaticojejunostomy.

References

1. Todani T, Watanabe Y, Narusue M, et al. Congenital bile duct cysts: classification, operative procedures, and review of 37 cases including cancer arising from choledochal cyst. Am J Surg 1977;134:263–9.
2. Singham J, Yoshida EM, Scudamore CH. Choledochal cysts: classification and pathogenesis. Can J Surg 2009;52:434–40.

Case 8

A 20-year-old Indian college student is admitted with acute severe hepatitis. He was in his usual state of health until his recent trip back home to India to attend a family function. While there, about 6 weeks prior to this admission, he developed a febrile illness with a temperature to 103°F associated with nonbloody diarrhea of about ten bowel movements per day. He consulted with a physician in India and testing for malaria was negative. This illness resolved after about 5 days. Several of his relatives and friends had similar symptomatology.

Since returning to the USA, he has complained of a 1 week history of anorexia, weakness, and lower abdominal discomfort. He has experienced a 10 lb weight loss during this period. He has noted some yellowing of his eyes. He denies any skin rash, arthralgias, or pruritus. He has taken no new prescribed or over the counter medications, no history of acetaminophen use. He is not sexually active, and denies alcohol or recreational drug use. There is no family history of liver disease.

Physical examination revealed a young, jaundiced patient with no cutaneous stigmata of chronic liver disease. He was awake, alert, orientated ×3 with no encephalopathy or evidence of asterixis. Abdominal exam revealed mild right upper quadrant tenderness with no hepatosplenomegaly or ascites. There were no skin rashes.

Lab Tests on Admission

Total bilirubin 21.8 mg/dl
ALT 4,872 iu/l
AST 6,432 iu/l
ALP 190 iu/l
GGTP 65 iu/l
Albumin 3.4 g/dl
Total protein 6.9 g/dl

INR 3.0

Questions

1. What is the differential diagnosis?
2. What would be the appropriate lab testing?
3. Does this patient have fulminant hepatic failure?

Lab Results

Hepatitis A IgM: negative
Hepatitis B surface Ag and core IgM: negative
Hepatitis C Ab and HCV RNA: negative
CMV IgM: negative
HSV IgM: negative
EBV IgM and Monospot: negative

ANA: negative
SMA: negative
LKM: negative
Serum IgG: 1,450 mg/dl (normal: <1,560)

Acetaminophen level: undetectable

Ceruloplasmin: 40 mg/dl

Urine drug screen: negative

Hepatitis E IgM (+)

Answer: Acute Hepatitis E

The differential diagnosis for patients presenting with acute severe hepatitis with marked hepatocellular liver injury include:

Acute viral hepatitis (hepatitis A, B, rarely C, E, EBV, CMV, HSV)
Acute autoimmune hepatitis
Ischemic hepatitis (shock liver)
Acute hepatitis due to a dose-related or idiosyncratic drug reaction
Toxic ingestion (e.g., acetaminophen)
Acute Wilson's disease

Hepatitis E is endemic in many developing countries where it causes substantial morbidity. It is rarely seen in industrialized countries, and largely confined to travelers returning from endemic countries, as was the case in this patient. Patients with unexplained hepatitis should be tested for hepatitis E, whatever their age or travel history.

The virus is spread primarily by the fecal-oral route and is associated with both sporadic infections and epidemics in areas with poor sanitation and weak public-health infrastructures. The antibody response to hepatitis E infection follows a conventional course with specific IgM usually detectable at the onset of symptoms or deranged liver function. IgG reaches a peak shortly thereafter. Much like hepatitis A, hepatitis E is usually a self-limited acute infection, very rarely progressing to fulminant hepatic failure. There is no chronic form of the disease and cirrhosis is not part of the natural history.

Although this patient had severe hepatitis with evidence of hepatic synthetic dysfunction, he did not meet the criteria for fulminant hepatic failure as he had no evidence of encephalopathy.

Reference

1. Dalton HR Bendall R, Ijaz S, et al. Hepatitis E: an emerging infection in developed countries. Lancet Infect Dis 2008;8:698–709.

Case 9

A 43-year-old lady presents to your clinic for a second opinion having been diagnosed with liver cancer.

She has a history of chronic hepatitis C but a liver biopsy within the last year demonstrated mild inflammation and stage I fibrosis and she elected to defer treatment. She has been essentially well but had experienced some dyspepsia for a few days a month ago and underwent an upper GI endoscopy that was normal and a CT scan was ordered. The scan was reported as showing a hypervascular lesion in the left lobe and an AFP level was mildly elevated at 26 ng/ml (normal range 5–20).

She does not drink alcohol or smoke and likely acquired hepatitis C through a blood transfusion at the time of an ectopic pregnancy as a teenager which required a hysterectomy. She has been on hormone replacement therapy as a result.

She is married and works as a secretary.

She denies any prescribed or over the counter medications.

On exam she is very anxious. Vitals show BP 140/90 and pulse is 100 beats per minute. Her sclerae are anicteric and her abdomen is soft without masses.

Laboratory Studies

Hb 13.0 g/dl
Platelets 252,000/μl
INR 1.1
WBC 5.9 × 10^3/μl
Tbili 0.3 mg/dl
AST 40 iu/l
ALT 46 iu/l
ALP 87 iu/l
Albumin 3.5 g/dl
Creatinine 0.6 mg/dl
HCV RNA 300,000 iu/ml
CT scan as shown

Questions

1. What further work-up is required?
2. Is a liver biopsy indicated?

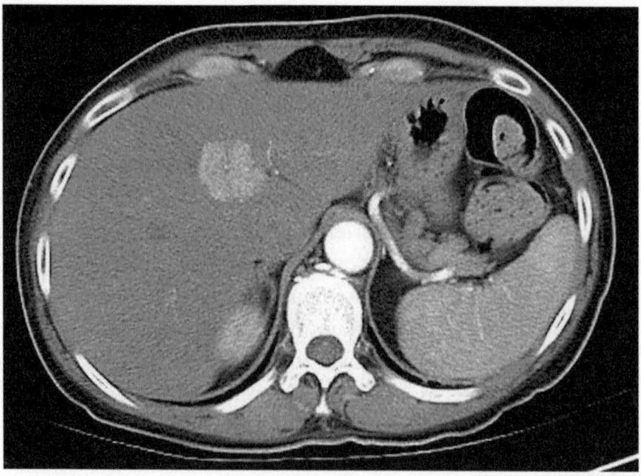

Fig. 9.1 CT scan

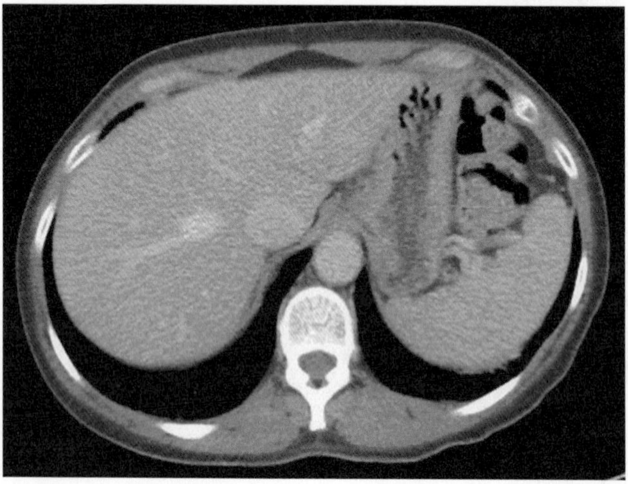

Fig. 9.2 CT scan

Answer: Focal Nodular Hyperplasia

The differential diagnosis in a patient presenting with a contrast-enhancing liver mass really depends on the clinical situation. In patients with cirrhosis or chronic hepatitis B infection, one should be vigilant about hepatocellular carcinoma (HCC). In females with no obvious liver disease, hepatic adenoma (HA), hemangioma, or focal nodular hyperplasia (FNH) should be considered in the differential diagnosis. In this case, she has hepatitis C but minimal fibrosis so should not be at risk for hepatocellular carcinoma (HCC). The liver enzymes are mildly elevated as is the AFP, not unusual in patients with chronic hepatitis C. The CT scan (Figs. 9.1 and 9.2) shows a mass measuring 3.1 cm in segment 4 of the liver. The mass demonstrates a lobular contour with arterial enhancement which equilibrates on delayed images. Closer examination of Fig. 9.1 shows a thin linear vascular scar within the mass-characteristic of FNH.

FNH is another lesion that is typically detected incidentally on imaging. Ultrasound lacks accuracy in making a definitive diagnosis as FNH has similar characteristics to adenoma or HCC. A triphasic CT scan that is properly timed is very sensitive for FNH but lacks high specificity as the fibrolamellar variant of HCC can have a central scar (which is only seen in a third of FNH lesions). Technetium sulfur colloid scanning is a good test for FNH since most lesions contain Kupffer cells which will take up the colloid (as opposed to adenomas which will not). MRI can also be used to make a diagnosis of FNH if gadolinium enhanced since the lesion will rapidly enhance and then become isointense on delayed images while the central scar will enhance later as the contrast agent takes longer to get into its fibrous center.

FNH is a common benign hepatic tumor which is thought to result from an aberrant hyperplastic response to the excess perfusion from the anomalous arteries that are seen in these lesions, although a similar response can be seen in FNHs that are supplied by branches of the portal vein. There is an association with other congenital vascular lesions such as hemangiomas and hereditary hemorrhagic telangiectasia.

Lesions are usually single and smaller than 5 cm and are more common in women. Unlike HAs, there does not appear to be an association with female sex hormones although there are reports of FNH being more common in women who use the oral contraceptive pill and occasionally enlarging during pregnancy.

Patients with FNH need reassurance and liver biopsy is generally not required (particularly as the histology can be variable). Surgery is rarely required for very symptomatic or rapidly enlarging lesions.

References

1. Wanless IR, Mawdsley C, Adams R. On the pathogenesis of focal nodular hyperplasia of the liver. Hepatology 1985;5:1194.
2. Shamsi K, De Schepper A, Degryse H, Deckers F. Focal nodular hyperplasia of the liver: radiologic findings. Abdom Imaging 1993;18:32.

3. Scalori A, Tavani A, Gallus S, et al. Oral contraceptives and the risk of focal nodular hyperplasia of the liver: a case-control study. Am J Obstet Gynecol 2002;186:195.

Case 10

A healthy 55-year-old woman is referred for evaluation of persistently elevated blood AST level over a period of 8 months. She completely denies any symptoms and does not recall any episodes of jaundice in the past. Her only history is hyperlipidemia and mitral valve prolapse. She takes no medications. There is no personal or family history of jaundice, skeletal muscle, thyroid or hemolytic disorders. There was also no history of alcohol or drug use.

Table 10.1 Trend of LFT's

Date	Total bili	AST	ALT	ALP	GGT	Albumin
Month 1	0.4	427	28	109	27	4.2
Month 3	0.2	363	30	95	10	3.7
Month 6	0.2	368	37	122	11	3.8
Month 7	0.3	399	37	130	12	4.1
Month 8	0.3	427	24	123	16	4.3

Note: normal AST: 15–37 iu/l

Physical examination was unremarkable.

Prior work-up included a normal abdominal CT scan and negative serologies for viral, autoimmune, and genetic/metabolic liver diseases.

Questions

1. What are some of the diagnostic considerations?
2. What confirmatory test can be ordered to establish the diagnosis?

LDH CPK Aldolase TSH	All normal

Plasma electrophoresis:
immunoglobulin-complexed AST

Answer: Macro-AST

Aspartate aminotransferase (AST) is an enzyme in the gluconeogenic pathway that facilitates the synthesis of glucose from noncarbohydrate sources. It catalyzes the reaction of oxaloacetate to malate. AST is found in both the mitochondria and cytosol in a number of different organs, including liver, heart, skeletal muscle, kidney, brain, pancreas, and blood.

AST, which may be cytoplasmic or mitochondrial, is a well-known enzyme found in clinically significant amounts in the tissue of liver, skeletal muscle, heart, and, to a lesser extent, erythrocytes. These were excluded by testing for LDH, CPK, aldolase, and TSH; none of which were shown to be abnormal.

Electrophoresis testing confirmed that the patient had an immunoglobulin-complexed AST. This macromolecule presumably caused a persistent increase in measured AST activity. The majority of *macro-AST* cases have been described in asymptomatic individuals and can be diagnosed by the way of exclusion chromatography, electrophoresis, and activation assays with pyridoxal 5-phosphate.

Recognition of this entity may obviate the need for more invasive investigations to which patients may be unnecessarily subjected. Being a benign condition, patients can be reassured that no specific treatment is required.

References

1. Litin SC, O'Brien JF, Pruett S, et al. Macroenzyme as a cause of unexplained elevation of aspartate aminotransferase. Mayo Clin Proc 1987;62:681.
2. Trimester S, Douglas DD. Development of macro-aspartate aminotransferase in a patient undergoing specific allergen injection immunotherapy. Am J Gastroenterol 2005;100:243–5.

Case 11

A 35-year-old South Asian male is sent to his primary care physician upon insistence of his wife for a "routine check-up." The patient generally feels well although he does complain of some mild fatigue. He has no significant medical or surgical history and takes no medications, prescription, or otherwise. He is married to a physician and has a healthy 4-year-old daughter. The patient is originally from Bangalore, India but has been in the USA for the last 9 years. He works fulltime as a software engineer and admits to a sedentary lifestyle. He does not drink or smoke and has no history of high-risk behavior. Family history is positive for diabetes in his mother and older sister.

Physical exam is notable for a healthy appearing male with a BMI of 33.1 kg/m^2. His blood pressure is 142/88. He has truncal obesity and a smooth liver that is palpable 3.5 cm below his right costal margin. He has no peripheral edema or stigmata to suggest chronic liver disease.

Laboratory Data Are Notable for

Fasting glucose of 98 mg/dl
Tbili 0.7 mg/dl
AST 62 iu/l
ALT 109 iu/l
AP 72 iu/l
GGTP 55 iu/l

Albumin 4.5 mg/dl

LDL 99 mg/dl
HDL 30 mg/dl
TG 250 mg/dl

Serologies for Hepatitis A indicate previous exposure
Testing for Hepatitis B and C is negative
ANA 1:160 (homogenous)
Remainder of chronic liver disease work-up negative

Questions

1. What is the differential diagnosis of the abnormal liver tests?
2. What additional testing if any would you recommend?
3. What treatment if any would you recommend?

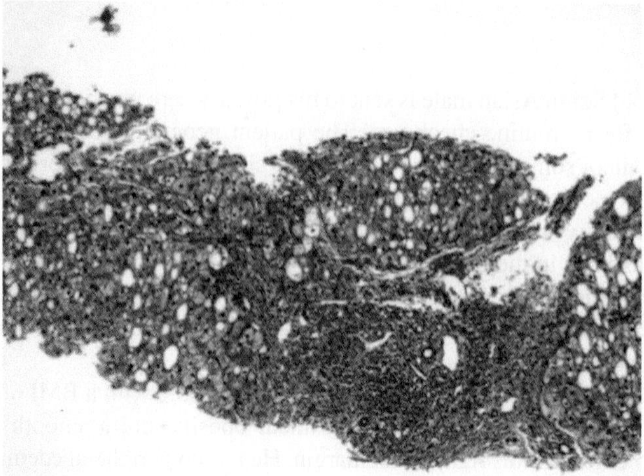

Fig. 11.1 Low power trichrome ×100

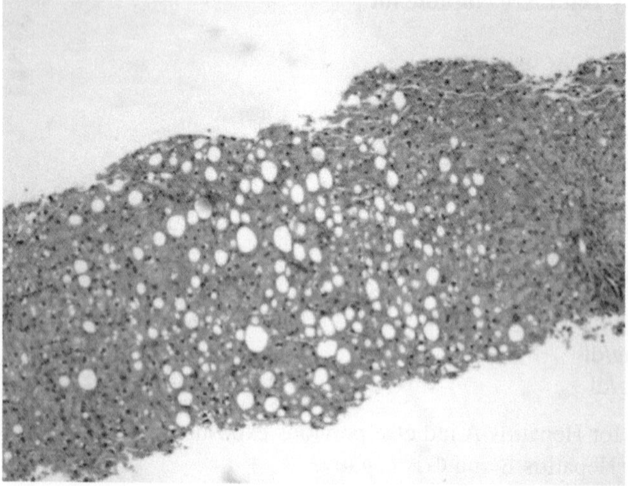

Fig. 11.2 Low power liver biopsy H&E ×100

Answer: Nonalcoholic Steatohepatitis

Nonalcoholic fatty liver disease (NAFLD) is now considered the most common cause of chronic liver disease in the Western world. It is a clinicohistopathologic diagnosis. Although it is now recognized that fatty liver can occur concomitantly with other liver diseases, in its purest form its diagnosis still requires the exclusion of underlying viral disease and alcohol. Most studies exclude patients who consume more than 40 g of alcohol per week (clinical parameters may be slightly more liberal). It consists of a spectrum of diseases ranging from bland (without inflammation) steatosis at one end, nonalcoholic steatohepatitis (NASH) in the middle, and end-stage liver disease at the other.

The presentation of this gentleman is very typical for NASH and underlines the significant challenges associated with the disease. As with many forms of chronic liver disease, most patients with NAFLD present without signs or symptoms. The most common presentation is mild abnormalities in liver function tests noted during a work-up yearly health physical or as surveillance in patients on antihyperlipidemic agents.

Although liver function tests are typically the first screening test for liver disease, many times, as presented here, there is a poor correlation between enzyme abnormalities and degree of liver dysfunction. This patient has mild elevations in liver enzymes but has severe steatosis and inflammation and early cirrhosis. The trichrome stain (Fig. 11.1) reveals early cirrhosis with bridging fibrosis and early nodule formation. Steatosis (the fat does not take up the stain) and a few scattered inflammatory cells are seen in Fig. 11.2. A majority of patients with NASH will have *some* degree of elevation in liver function tests, as opposed to patients with bland steatosis in which only 20% of patients have abnormalities. The AST/ALT ratio (AAR) in NASH is typically less than 1. This is opposite to what is classically seen in acute alcoholic hepatitis where the ratio is usually above 2.

Given the poor correlation of liver enzymes with liver injury, at present liver biopsy is the best diagnostic tool for confirming the diagnosis of NAFLD. It is also the most sensitive and specific means of providing important prognostic information. There are no guidelines or recommendations regarding which patients should be biopsied. Controversy exists to the necessity of biopsy in all patients suspected of fatty liver disease. Those against routine biopsy point to several factors including overall good prognosis in a majority of patients with fatty liver disease, a current lack of effective therapy, and costs and risks associated with liver biopsy. Histologically, the disease is characterized by macrovesicular hepatic steatosis and is indistinguishable from alcoholic liver injury.

The exact incidence and prevalence of NAFLD remains unknown. It is estimated that NAFLD affects between 20 and 40% of the Western world, with the Asian and Pacific regions being less affected. The majority of cases occur in people between the ages of 40–60 years, but it is becoming increasingly prevalent in the pediatric population. Although initially thought to be a disease primarily of females, NAFLD is now known to affect both sexes equally. Ethnic differences seem to play a role in the prevalence of fatty liver in the USA with Hispanic people more affected than white people. There is some evidence to suggest that African Americans are less susceptible to the progressive form of the disease.

The incidence and prevalence of NASH is much more difficult to ascertain because of the necessity of biopsy (as opposed to transabdominal imaging) in order to make the diagnosis. Data suggest that approximately 3% of individuals from developed countries have NASH. Patients who have NASH progress 9–20% of the time to cirrhosis, and up to one-third of these patients will die from complications of liver failure or require liver transplantation. It is expected that cirrhosis secondary to NASH will become the primary indication for LT in the next 10 years, superseding HCV.

Although the pathophysiology of primary NAFLD is not yet fully understood, the most widely held hypothesis implicates insulin resistance as the key mechanism leading to the accumulation of excessive triglyceride accumulation in the liver and subsequent development of hepatic steatosis. Once steatosis is present, some have proposed a "second-hit" or additional oxidative injury, which is required to manifest the necroinflammatory component seen in steatohepatitis.

Almost all treatment modalities for patients with NAFLD are targeted at steps in the proposed pathogenesis of the disease and focus primarily on reducing risk factors of the metabolic syndrome. Steatosis alone probably does not warrant treatment as it is felt to have a relatively benign course. Even in patients with NASH, there are only disease-oriented outcome data. Since NASH has the potential to progress to cirrhosis in a significant number of patients, treatment may be considered in those with more advanced disease on biopsy. Several treatments improve liver enzyme abnormalities, radiographic findings, and histological disease progression, the most recent of these being pioglitazone and vitamin E. However, there are no data that demonstrate improvements in morbidity or mortality. Effective treatment options are desperately needed to prevent future disease-related morbidity and mortality.

The patient in this case was instructed to lose weight through a combination of diet and exercise and in addition was started on 800 u of vitamin E daily. At 3-month follow-up, he had managed to lose 6 pounds and there was mild improvement in his liver function tests.

References

1. Aithal GP, Thomas JA, Kaye PV, et al. Randomized, placebo-controlled trial of pioglitazone in nondiabetic subjects with nonalcoholic steatohepatitis. Gastroenterology 2008;135:1176–84.
2. Chalasani NP, Sanyal AJ, Kowdley KV, et al. Pioglitazone versus vitamin E versus placebo for the treatment of non-diabetic patients with non-alcoholic steatohepatitis: PIVENS trial design. Contemp Clin Trials 2009;30:88–96.

Case 12

A 36-year-old Caucasian female presents with a constellation of symptoms. Two weeks prior to admission, she developed muscle aches, fatigue, and general malaise. A week later she began to develop intermittent fevers, chills, sore throat, rhinorrhea, and congestion. She was placed on a 7-day course of amoxicillin for presumed upper respiratory infection, but her symptoms persisted. She also reports anorexia, nausea, and mild abdominal discomfort. She has also noticed darkening of her urine and pale colored stools. She eventually was sent to the hospital when she developed what she described as a "swollen neck." One month prior to the onset of her symptoms, the patient was prescribed an oral contraceptive to better regulate her menses and help with facial acne. She discontinued the medication 1 week into her illness. The patient has a medical history significant for asthma, depression, and anxiety. Her medications include duloxetine, clonazepam, montelukast sodium, and albuterol. The patient is a fulltime nursing student. She is originally from Canada but moved to the USA 3 months ago. She currently lives in a dormitory with other nursing students. She is single and is not currently sexually active. She drinks only on "special occasions." She does not smoke or use any illicit drug use. Her father died at 47 of a myocardial infarction. Her mother is 52 and has multiple sclerosis.

On exam, she is febrile to 102.5°F, pulse is 100, BP 130/72, her saturations are 94% on room air; BMI is 20.2 kg/m^2. She is awake and alert, but appears tired and lethargic. Her sclerae are icteric. She has some mild visible facial edema. Oropharynx reveals moderately erythematous tonsils without exudates. She has palpable tender submandibular, cervical, and posterior auricular lymphadenopathy. The largest lymph node is ~2 cm. Heart and lungs are normal. Abdomen is soft, but diffusely tender. Her liver is palpable 7 cm below the costal margin and her spleen is easily palpable just to the left of the umbilicus. She has no lower extremity edema and no rash. There are no focal neurological deficits. She has no other stigmata of chronic liver disease.

Laboratory Data

Electrolytes and renal function normal
WBC 7,000K with 7% atypical lymphocytes
Hemoglobin 10 g/dl with normal MCV
Platelets 150 × 10^3/μl
Tbili 5.7 mg/dl (Conj 4.4 mg/dl)
AST 280 iu/l
ALT 280 iu/l
AP 885 iu/l
GGTP 402 iu/l
LDH 614 iu/l
Amylase and lipase normal

Hepatitis A, B, and C viral serologies negative
ANA 1:40 (homogenous); smooth muscle Ab negative, IgG 1,750 mg/dl
AMA negative
Ceruloplasmin, Alpha one antitrypsin level normal

Questions

1. What is the differential diagnosis?
2. Would you recommend any additional testing?
3. What treatment if any would you recommend?

Monospot +
EBV IgG Ab68 u/ml
EBV IgM Ab > 160

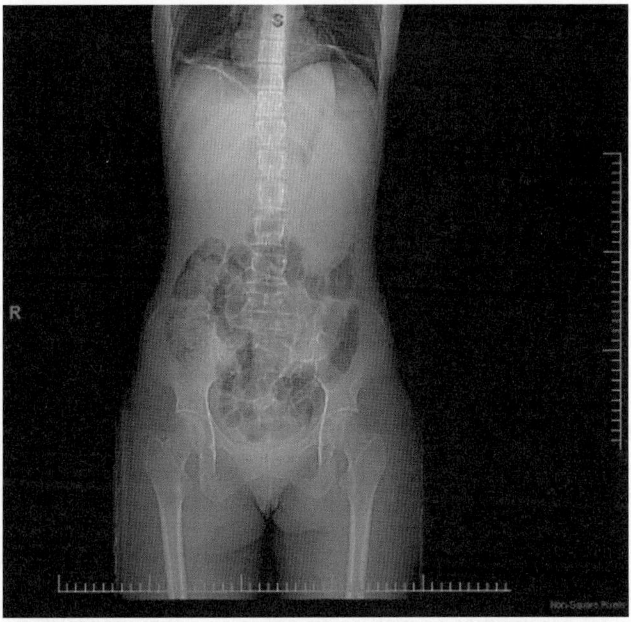

Fig. 12.1 CT scan scout image

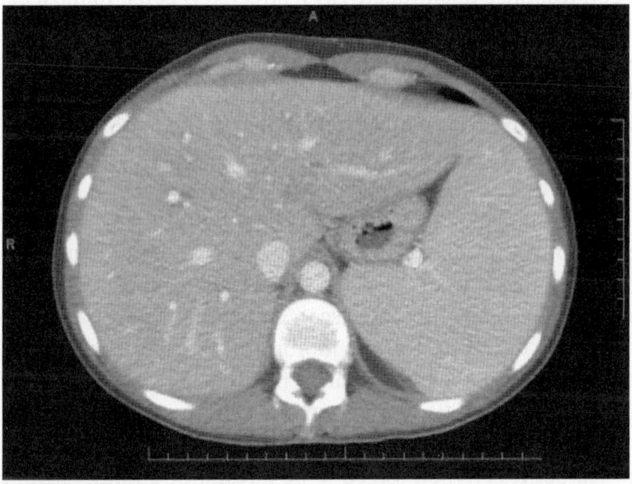

Fig. 12.2 CT scan abdomen

Answer: EBV Hepatitis

The constellation of symptoms including: fever, malaise, fatigue, sore throat in addition to exam findings of palpable bilateral cervical lymphadenopathy, hepatosplenomegaly, and laboratory findings including atypical lymphocytes, and elevated liver function tests all make infectious mononucleosis the likely diagnosis in this case. Other atypical viral hepatitis such as CMV is also possible. Hepatitis A, B, and C typically will not present with this degree of lymphadenopathy or splenomegaly as demonstrated in the imaging.

In addition, a CT scan of the neck was performed revealing extensive bilateral adenopathy with enlarged tonsillar and submandibular glands; largest measuring 2.2 × 1.9 cm.

Epstein–Barr virus (EBV) is part of the herpes virus family. It is most commonly transmitted by oropharyngeal secretions, hence the term "kissing disease." Transmission by blood transfusion and from transplanted organ in a previously seronegative recipient has also been reported. It is the primary causative agent of infectious mononucleosis. More than 90% of the world's population carries EBV as a life-long, latent infection of B lymphocytes, and it is associated with the development of B-cell lymphomas, T-cell lymphomas, Hodgkin's lymphoma, and nasopharyngeal carcinomas as well as an aggressive lymphoproliferative disorder in transplant recipients. A majority of infections are subclinical, and patients never seek medical attention. The clinical illness when apparent is the result of an intense cytotoxic T-cell response to eliminate EBV-infected B cells. In most cases, primary EBV infection in children is asymptomatic with seroconversion. When primary infection occurs in adolescents or adulthood, it presents with the classic triad of fever, oropharyngitis, and bilateral lymphadenitis.

Reactivation of disease is not a prominent issue with EBV, in contrast to other common herpesviruses, but it has been associated with an aggressive lymphoproliferative disorder in transplant recipients.

Elevated liver function tests are very common and are seen in 90% of cases, while severe cholestasis and jaundice are seen in less than 5% of patients. Splenomegaly is reported in up to 60% of cases, hepatomegaly is not as common. Although not seen in this particular case, a commonly seen complication (in up to 80%) of cases is the development of a morbilliform rash following the administration of ampicillin and, to a lesser extent, penicillin.

Severe cholestatic hepatitis like the one seen in this case presentation is a rare complication of EBV infection. The mechanism for the obstructive component is not well known, but it is hypothesized to be a result of a mildly swollen bile duct. Hepatitis owing to primary EBV infection is usually mild and self-limited, although a handful of cases of acute liver failure have been reported, primarily in immunocompromised hosts.

An evaluation of infectious mononucleosis has demonstrated that the virus does not infect hepatocytes, biliary epithelium, or vascular endothelium, but rather it is the infiltration of CD8 T cells that lead to indirect hepatocyte damage.

The diagnosis of EBV infection is made by appropriate clinical symptoms, laboratory findings, and a positive IgM antibody against EBV capsid antigen (EBV VCA-IgM) and heterophil antibody tests. The EBV-specific serology is a confirmative diagnostic tool, but can be negative initially in patients who have been ill for only a few days at the time of their first visit. However, within 1–2 weeks, antibodies to EBV-specific antigen appear at the expected titers. The serology of anti-VCA-IgM generally persists for about 1–2 months. The original serologic test for infectious mononucleosis, the Paul-Bunnell heterophil antibody test, is specific, but insensitive during the first week of illness. The false-negative rate is as high as 25% in the first week. The primary acute EBV infection is associated with VCA-IgM, VCA-IgG, and absent EBV nuclear antigen antibodies.

Treatment for infectious mononucleosis hepatitis is usually supportive as the illness is generally self-limiting. Steroids and antiviral medications have been utilized to treat the cases of severe infectious mononucleosis hepatitis. Acyclovir has not been shown to be efficacious for the treatment of severe EBV hepatitis.

This patient was seen in follow-up in the medicine clinic 3 months later. Her symptoms had completely resolved, she had returned to school and a check of her liver function tests revealed complete normalization.

References

1. Crum NF. Epstein–Barr virus hepatitis: case series and review. South Med J 2006;99:544–7.
2. Méndez-Sánchez N, Aguilar-Domínguez C, Chávez-Tapia NC, et al. Hepatic manifestations of Epstein–Barr viral infection. Ann Hepatol 2005;4:205–9.
3. Shaukat A, Tsai HT, Rutherford R, et al. Epstein–Barr virus induced hepatitis: an important cause of cholestasis. Hepatol Res 2005;33:24–6.

Case 13

A 29-year-old Caucasian female presents with a 2-week history of periodic fever, headache, and abdominal pain. The patient was admitted several days into her illness. She had blood work drawn and an infectious work-up which was unrevealing and was discharged home on no medications, with a presumptive diagnosis of a "viral illness." She returned with persistent symptoms. She has a past medical history significant for endometriosis, fibromyalgia, depression, and anxiety. She underwent an appendectomy 7 years ago, and 3 years ago she underwent a total abdominal hysterectomy with bilateral salpo-ophorectomy. She takes escitalopram oxalate for her depression/anxiety and is on estrogen replacement therapy. She has not been on any recent antibiotics. She has taken occasional ibuprofen and acetaminophen for her present illness, but nothing in excess. The patient is married and lives with her husband and two young children. She works as a receptionist at a veterinary clinic. She has no history of alcohol abuse, smoking, tattoos, or blood transfusions.

On physical exam, her temperature is 100.4°F, the remainder of her vital signs are normal; BMI is 26 kg/m^2. She is laying in bed holding her head. She is awake and alert. Neurological exam is normal with no findings suggestive of meningeal involvement. Cardiac and pulmonary exams are normal. Her abdomen is soft and without tenderness. Bowel sounds are normal and active. There is no appreciable hepatomegaly, spleen tip was palpable in Traube's space. There is no peripheral edema or palpable adenopathy. She has no stigmata to suggest chronic liver disease.

Laboratory Data

Electrolytes and renal function normal
WBC is 10K with 29% neutrophils (44–77) and 66% lymphocytes (13–44) with 13% atypical lymphocytes

Remainder of hemogram is normal

Tbili 0.8 mg/dl
AST 153 iu/l
ALT 272 iu/l
AP 189 iu/l
GGTP 220 iu/l
LDH 447 iu/l

Questions

1. What additional testing if any would you recommend?
2. What treatment if any would you recommend?

Serological work-up
Monospot negative
EBV IgG 80
EBV IgM negative
CMV IgG Ab UD
CMV IgM Ab+
6-month follow-up
LFTs normalize
CMV IgM negative and CMV IgG Ab+ at 55

Liver Biopsy

Liver biopsy revealing portal, lobular, and sinusoidal lymphocytosis
Minimal fibrosis and steatosis

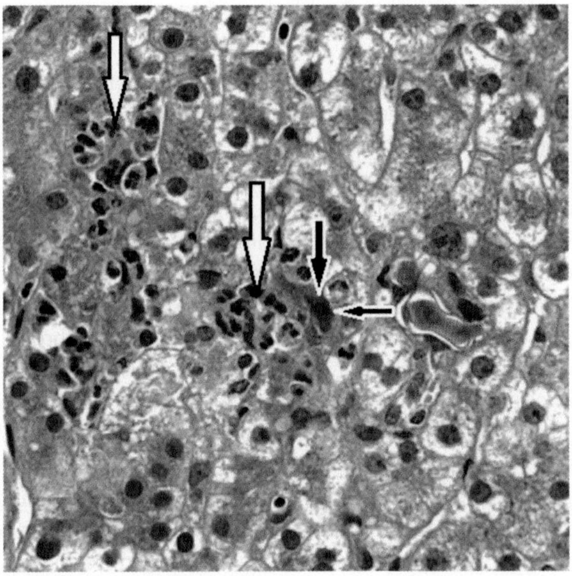

Fig. 13.1 H&E original magnification × 600

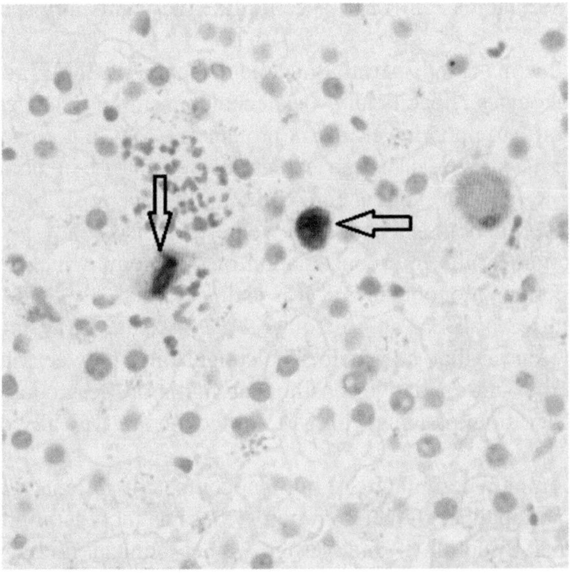

Fig. 13.2 Immunohistochemical stain (*black arrows*)

Answer: Acute Cytomegalovirus Hepatitis

Although an unusual cause of hepatitis in an immunocompromised host, this patient's age, protracted fever, cephalgia, splenomegaly, atypical lymphocytosis, moderately elevated liver function tests, and elevated LDH all suggest an active cytomegalovirus (CMV) infection.

The proportion of humans with evidence of prior CMV infection varies throughout the world, with seroprevalence rates ranging between 40 and 100% of the adult population. Seroprevalence generally correlates inversely with a country's socioeconomic development, with highest rates observed in developing countries throughout Africa and Asia. Although CMV infection is very common throughout the world, clinical illness is only seen in a small number of patients. Because of improved socioeconomic circumstances and awareness of hygiene, CMV seroprevalence has declined in industrialized countries. This theoretically may increase the incidence of clinical disease.

The greatest risk of CMV infection is seen in those who are immunocompromised (such as post-transplant patients) and fetuses during the intrauterine period. Transmission of infection can occur via multiple routes including: sex, close contact, blood or tissue exposure, occupational (working with infants and children), and perinatal.

The diagnosis of acute CMV is considered probable with the detection of CMV-specific IgM antibodies (suggesting recent seroconversion) and the observation of at least a fourfold increase in CMV-specific IgG titers in paired specimens at least 2–4 weeks apart.

CMV antigenemia assays permit the rapid detection of CMV proteins in peripheral blood leukocytes. Specifically, the technique employs tagged monocolonal antibodies specific to pp65 lower matrix protein of CMV in peripheral blood polymorphonuclear leukocytes. Though extensively evaluated in immunosuppressed patients, the role of CMV antigenemia assay in the diagnosis of CMV disease in immunocompetent patients has not been well established.

CMV infection results in a constellation of symptoms which resembles EBV-associated infectious mononucleosis. It is estimated that 79% of infectious mononucleosis is caused by EBV and the other 21% by acute CMV infection. Several important differences that may help in distinguishing between the two are that lymphadenopathy and exudative tonsillopharyngitis are less common in patients with CMV. In addition, patients with CMV infection are typically older than those with EBV.

The most common complaints of immunocompetent patients with CMV infection are fever and malaise. Other common symptoms include: night sweats, headache, abdominal discomfort, and vertigo. Other clinical findings may include palpable splenomegaly and mild leukocytosis with relative lymphocytosis. In one study involving 22 "outpatients" diagnosed with acute CMV infection, all 22 had mild to moderate elevations in AST and ALT with nearly 60% having an elevated GGT as well. LDH was elevated in all 20 patients in whom it was checked.

A study has been conducted to compare patients having CMV hepatitis with those of hepatitis A, B, and C. Patients with CMV hepatitis were much more likely to be febrile and have fever of longer duration and less likely to be icteric. Cervical lymphadenopathy and splenomegaly were frequent. The mean peak value of transaminases levels was statistically lower in CMV hepatitis than hepatitis A, B, and C. The ratio of ALT/LDH was significantly lower in acute CMV versus A, B, and C. The number of peripheral white blood cells and lymphocytes increased much more in patients with CMV. Although atypical lymphocytes appeared in all, the frequency was higher in CMV.

Histological features include: mononuclear cell infiltrating the portal areas, along with giant cells, microscopic granulomas, and a few foci of necrosis. "Owl's eye" are rare but when present are more frequent within the bile duct epithelium. The first image (Fig. 13.1) shows neutrophilic microabscesses (white arrows) with CMV inclusion (double arrow). The second image (Fig. 13.2) confirms CMV on immunohistochemical stain.

In solid-organ transplantation, the risk of developing clinically significant CMV infection depends primarily on the CMV serostatus of the donor and recipient. Seronegative recipients of an allograft from a seropositive donor are at greatest risk and without effective prophylaxis, up to 75% will develop CMV disease. Hepatitis is the most common organ-specific complication of CMV infection following liver transplantation.

Among patients with symptomatic CMV infection, especially the mononucleosis syndrome, the illness is generally self-limited, with complete recovery over a period of days to weeks. Antiviral therapy is not usually indicated. The patient presented here was seen in follow-up in the liver clinic 8 weeks after discharge, her symptoms had all resolved and her liver tests had normalized. Serologies indicated seroconversion with the loss of IgM antibodies and + IgG.

CMV should be high on the differential of a feverish illness with malaise and headache accompanied by mild-to-moderate hepatitis.

References

1. Just-Nübling G, Korn S, Ludwig B, et al. Primary cytomegalovirus infection in an outpatient setting – laboratory markers and clinical aspects. Infection 2003;31:318–23.
2. Kanno A, Abe M, Yamada M, et al. Clinical and histological features of cytomegalovirus hepatitis in previously healthy adults. Liver Int 2008;17:129–32.

Case 14

A 20-year-old white female with no significant past medical history presents to her primary care physician with complaints of intermittent RUQ pain for 3 months. The patient states she gets intermittent attacks of abdominal pain once every 2–3 weeks. The episodes are severe in nature and cause her significant distress. She does get some associated nausea with the pain but denies emesis. The episodes are not consistently related to food. At the visit to her PCP's office she is complaining of pain. The patient lives with her parents and two siblings all of whom are in good health. She is sexually active in a monogamous relationship and states she uses protection "most of the time." She works as a waitress at a local restaurant and is applying to nursing school. She has two tattoos, the first obtained 2 years ago. She denies any history of illicit drugs. She does admit to "getting drunk" on weekends with her friends.

Exam reveals a healthy appearing young female in moderate distress complaining of abdominal pain. She is afebrile and vital signs are stable; BMI is 22.4 kg/m^2. Lungs and heart exam are normal. Abdomen is soft, she is mildly tender diffusely but no Murphy's sign is elicited. Her liver edge is 2 cm and palpable and slightly tender. There is no splenomegaly. Extremities are normal. There is no palpable adenopathy. She has mild palmar erythema. Laboratory tests are drawn revealing:

No previous laboratory tests available for review

Tbili 0.6 mg/dl
AST 110 iu/l
ALT 190 iu/l
AP 418 iu/l
GGTP 507 iu/l

Amylase/lipase are normal
CBC, electrolytes, and renal function are normal

A RUQ US is obtained revealing a normal liver and gallbladder but the common bile duct is measured at 7.5 mm.

The patient undergoes an ERCP, limited evaluation of the esophagus, and stomach is normal. The ampulla appears normal. Cholangiogram reveals a mildly dilated CBD at approximately 8 mm. The intrahepatic ducts are normal. No filling defects are seen. A sphincterotomy is performed for presumed sphincter dysfunction.

The patient is seen in follow-up 2 weeks later. Her abdominal pain is somewhat improved although she continues to have "attacks" of pain, albeit less frequent. A HIDA scan is ordered and her gallbladder ejection fraction is 28%.

The patient is referred to general surgery and undergoes an uneventful laparoscopic cholecystectomy. Pathology from the gallbladder reveals chronic cholecystitis without stones. Intraoperatively, the liver is reported to be grossly normal.

The patient is sent to the liver clinic 3 months after her cholecystectomy, her painful attacks have subsided; however, she continues to have elevated liver function tests.

Tbili 0.2 mg/dl
AST 78 iu/l
ALT 78 iu/l
AP 199 iu/l
GGTP 355 iu/l

Electrolytes, hemogram, and kidney function all remain normal
Total protein 8.7 g/dl, albumin 4.2 g/dl

Serological work-up
Additional Laboratory Data
IgG 1,940 mg/dl (751–1,560); serum IgA and IgM normal
ANA + 1:640 (centromere pattern)
p-ANCA (Anti-Neutrophilic Cytoplasmic Ab) 80 (normal < 20)
SMA 12 EU (normal < 20)
Liver Kidney Microsomal Ab < 40
Anti M2-Mitochondrial Ab 3 (normal < 20)

MRI/MRCP is performed and is completely normal with the CBD measured at 0.6 cm

Questions

1. What is the differential diagnosis?
2. What additional testing if any would you recommend?
3. What treatment if any would you recommend?

Liver Biopsy

Dense inflammatory infiltrate of lymphocytes and plasma cells
Interface hepatitis, proliferation of bile ducts, and lymphocytic cholangitis
Portal and periportal fibrosis

Answer: Autoimmune Cholangitis

This is a challenging case. The patient initially presented with intermittent right upper quadrant pain and elevated liver function tests. The list of conditions which present with acute onset of pain (not related to hepatomegaly) and elevated liver tests is relatively short and include: biliary obstruction (stone, sludge, sphincter dysfunction, and tumor) and hepatic abscess.

Proceeding first to ERCP was very reasonable in this case, with the primary concern being type I sphincter of Oddi dysfunction (intermittent pain, elevated liver tests, and dilated bile duct) although this diagnosis is typically reserved for patients who have had previous cholecsytectomy. The patient had some improvement in symptoms and a mild decline in liver function tests. Her symptoms post-ERCP, however, were still somewhat consistent with a biliary process, and the decision was made to proceed with cholecystectomy. Her painful attacks subsided, yet her enzymes remain elevated weeks afterwards pointing toward intrinsic liver disease. The pattern of elevation in her enzymes, autoimmune serologies, and eventually biopsy findings were consistent with a diagnosis of autoimmune cholangitis (AIC).

AIC is a chronic liver disease of unknown etiology that has cholestatic clinical, laboratory and/or histological changes typically in the setting of positive ANA with or without SMA in the absence of antimitochondrial antibodies (AMA). Its place in the spectrum of autoimmune liver disease is still debated and has been variously categorized as a variant of primary biliary cirrhosis (PBC) or autoimmune hepatitis (AIH) or a hybrid of both, although some experts suspect it is a distinct disease entity.

Patients with AIC are distinguished from patients with PBC by having higher serum levels of AST and a lower concentration of serum immunoglobulins. Its cholestatic features and inconsistent response to corticosteroid therapy have distanced it from AIH. In a study of 20 patients diagnosed prospectively with AIC, patients had clinical features which seem to resemble a combination of type 1 AIH and PBC. Like the aforementioned conditions, there is a predominance to affect females, but it differs in that those patients with AIC have higher serum AST and bilirubin levels, greater occurrence of ANA and/or SMA, absence of AMA, higher modified score for AIH, and a lower serum immunoglobulin M concentration. Similarly, patients differed from type I AIH by having lower serum AST, immunoglobulin G levels, higher serum alkaline phosphatase, and lower modified score for AIH.

Histological features of AIC seem to be a composite of histological patterns seen in PBC, AIH, and PSC including: destructive cholangitis, isolated granuloma, ductopenia, portal lymphoplasmacytic infiltrate, portal fibrosis, fibrous obliterative cholangitis, and biliary obstructive features.

Case reports and series suggest that patients with AIC respond poorly to therapy with corticosteroid regimens and ursodeoxycholic acid. In one study, only one of eight patients treated with corticosteroids satisfied clinical, biochemical, and histological criteria for remission.

This particular patient had significant improvement in enzymes on combination of steroids and azathioprine; however, she was unable to tolerate the medication because of multiple side effects including alopecia and severe headaches. The patient was switched to mycophenolate mofetil and her liver tests have completely normalized. Repeat liver biopsy (done 1 year after initial) shows significant improvement in both inflammation and fibrosis.

References

1. Czaja AJ, Carpenter HA, Santrach PJ, et al. Autoimmune cholangitis within the spectrum of autoimmune liver disease. Hepatology 2000;31:1231–8.
2. Czaja AJ, Bayraktar Y. Non-classical phenotypes of autoimmune hepatitis and advances in diagnosis and treatment. World J Gastroenterol 2009; 15: 2314–28.

Case 15

A 26-year-old female was referred by her primary doctor for evaluation of a liver mass which was found incidentally during the work-up of persistent cough and chest pain. Her past medical history included generalized anxiety disorder and mitral valve prolapse. There was no past history of liver disease. She is sexually active and takes oral birth control.

The patient's chest X-ray 2 months ago showed a possible shadow in the left lung field which after extensive work-up was diagnosed as a granuloma from prior histoplasmosis. During this work-up, she underwent a CT scan of the abdomen that demonstrated a 3.4 cm mass in the left lateral segment of the liver. An MRI scan with gadolinium was performed.

Laboratory Parameters Showed

WBC 6.0×10^3/ul
Hemoglobin 12.0 g/dl
Tbili 0.9 mg/dl
AST 19 u/l
ALT 17 u/l
Creatinine 0.7 mg/dl
AFP 6 ng/ml

Questions

1. What are the diagnostic considerations?
2. What are the next appropriate tests?

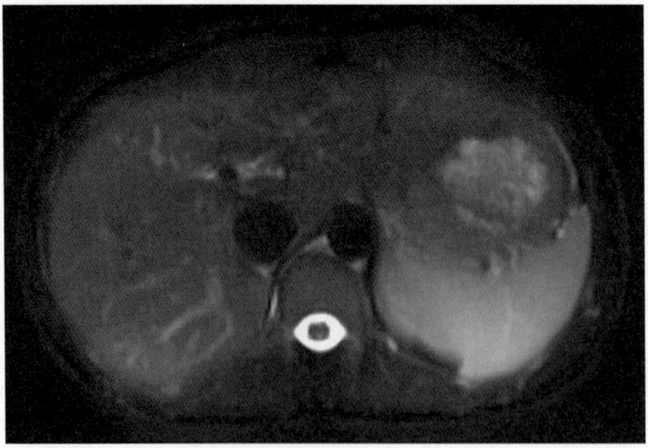

Fig. 15.1 MRI T2 weighted image

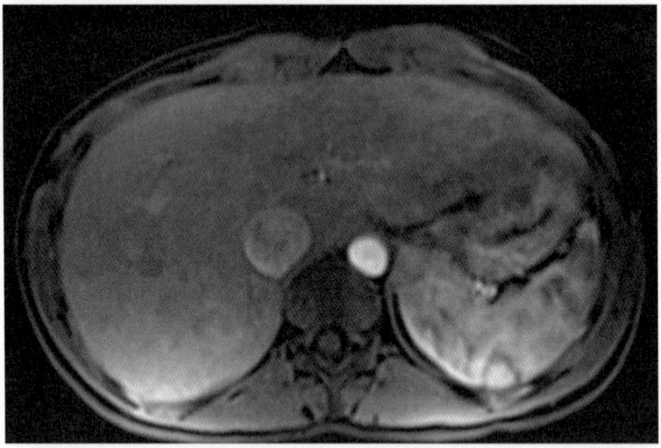

Fig. 15.2 T1 weighted image

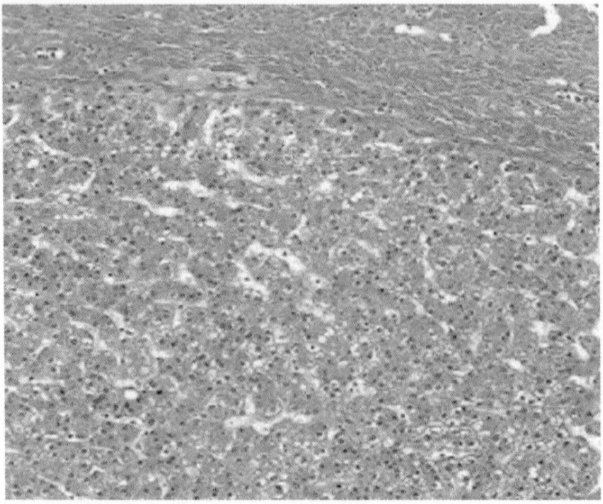

Fig. 15.3 Liver biopsy H&E stain ×100

Answer: Hepatic Adenoma (HA)

As stated in the other cases with a liver lesion, the differential diagnosis in a patient presenting with a contrast-enhancing liver mass is dependent on the clinical presentation and if there is underlying cirrhosis. In young females with no evidence of liver disease, HA, hemangioma, or FNH should be considered in the differential diagnosis for an enhancing lesion. In this case, she has no known history and risk factors for chronic liver disease.

HA is a hepatic neoplasm that occurs most often in young females of reproductive age. They are usually single lesions in the right lobe but can range widely in size.

The relationship of HA with oral contraception (OCP) is based on the dramatic increase in their incidence since the 1960s which coincides with the rise in OCP use. Multiple studies have shown a direct correlation between the development of HA and the length and total dose of female hormone treatment. The causal relationship is strengthened by the regression of HA with discontinuation of OCPs, and their increase in size during pregnancy and subsequent decrease in the months after delivery.

Men are not immune from the development of HA as they can also be seen in body-builders using anabolic steroids and in patients with glycogen storage diseases who are typically male.

Most patients are asymptomatic with normal liver function. Large adenomas may cause abdominal discomfort and occasionally HAs may rupture and bleed into the peritoneal cavity which presents with peritoneal signs and shock. Unlike other benign lesions, there appears to be a risk of malignant transformation with HAs which has been quantified at about 10% which is likely an overestimate.

Multiphasic CT scan or gadolinium-enhanced MRI is best to identify and characterize a HA with the main difficulty being differentiation from FNH. If an enhancing central scar is seen, the diagnosis of FNH can be made. Contrast CT characteristically shows peripheral enhancement during the early phase and then centripetal flow during the portal venous phase. MRI images (Figs. 15.1 and 15.2) are more variable but can be definitive if the lesion shows enhancement on T2 weighted images that increase after gadolinium is given.

As shown in the pathology slide (Fig. 15.3), HAs are composed of sheets of cells closely resembling normal hepatocytes that are arranged in plates separated by sinusoids. The cells are larger than normal and contain glycogen and lipid, and are arranged in a pattern that is notable for the absence of bile ducts and portal tracts, helping to distinguish HA from normal liver and FNH. Percutaneous liver biopsy or fine needle aspiration is rarely necessary particularly because of the risk of bleeding.

Management is controversial with some recommendations based on the presence of symptoms and the size of the lesion. Surgical resection is suggested for large lesions (>5 cm) and patients with symptoms, and acute bleeding is an indication for emergent resection. Patients with known adenomas should likely avoid pregnancy and stop OCPs.

References

1. Grazioli L, Federle MP, Brancatelli G, et al. Hepatic adenomas: imaging and pathologic findings. Radiographics 2001;21:877.
2. Rooks JB, Ory HW, Ishak KG, et al. Epidemiology of hepatocellular adenoma. The role of oral contraceptive use. JAMA 1979;242:644.
3. Ault GT, Wren SM, Ralls PW, et al. Selective management of hepatic adenomas. Am Surg 1996;62:825.

Case 16

A 50-year-old man with hepatitis C, genotype 1a infection, presents to your liver clinic with dyspnea on exertion, nonproductive cough, and nonpruritic rash on both upper extremities.

The patient has been on a 48-week course of pegylated interferon α2a and ribavirin treatment. He has completed 42 weeks of treatment and his HCV viral load was undetectable (<600 iu/ml) at week 12 of treatment.

He denies fever or chills and his appetite is good although he has lost a few pounds during the treatment. He is otherwise well and is keen to complete treatment. He has not required any growth factor support. He is not taking any other medications.

His physical examination is remarkable for lungs with diffuse inspiratory crepitus and arms with multiple, violaceous, nonbalancing papules measuring 1–3 cm in diameter. His abdomen is soft and nontender.

Laboratory Parameters

Hb 12.1 g/dl
WBC 6.1 × 10^3/ul
Platelet 390 × 10^3/ul
PT 13 seconds
Tbili 0.7 mg/dl
AST 40 u/l
ALT 14 u/l
Creatinine 1.0 mg/dl
HCV viral load < 600 iu/ml

Questions

1. What is the diagnosis?
2. What are the next appropriate tests?
3. Is this a reversible condition?

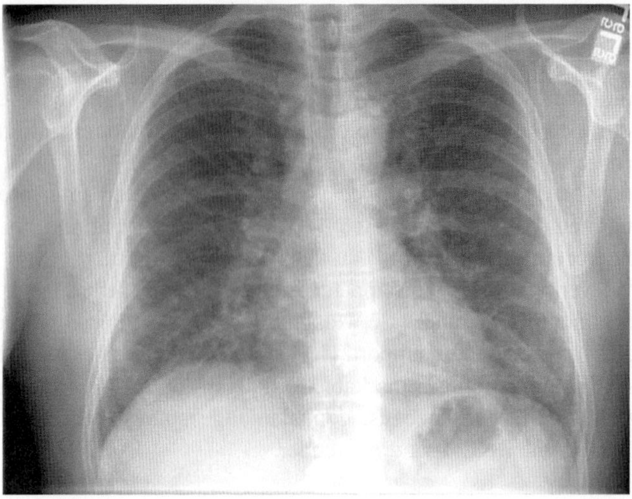

Fig. 16.1 Chest X-ray

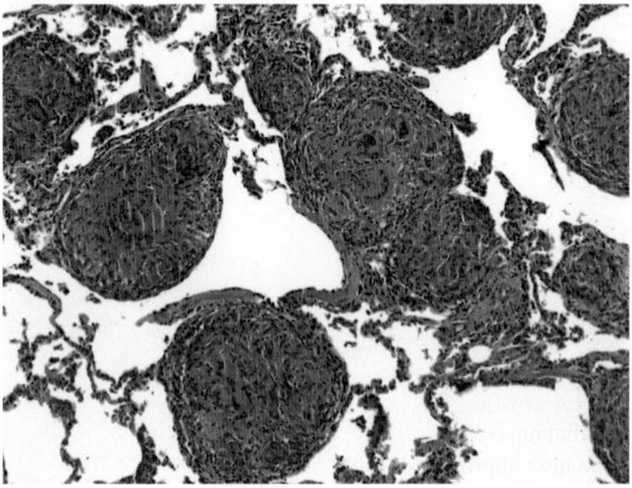

Fig. 16.2 Lung biopsy (H&E stain)

Answer: Interferon-Induced Sarcoidosis

Alpha interferon (and ribavirin) has been the only treatment for chronic HCV for almost 20 years. The mechanism of action is complicated but it has marked immunomodulatory effects and many reports have been published associating interferon therapy with the induction of autoimmune phenomena. There are many case reports of interferon inducing sarcoidosis. Chronic HCV has several extra-hepatic manifestations but sarcoidosis is not one of them. The most common organs involved in interferon-induced sarcoidosis are the lungs and skin but I myself have seen hepatic sarcoid on patients treated with pegylated interferon. The clinical presentation of interferon-induced sarcoidosis is insidious and can be confused with common constitutional side effects of these drugs. The mean time of onset of disease is little less than a year so it commonly occurs toward the end of therapy. Typically the sarcoidosis resolves after cessation of interferon therapy but in those with persistent disease, oral corticosteroid induces rapid resolution of symptoms.

It can be difficult to diagnose sarcoidosis in patients on treatment for HCV but a chest X-ray is a reasonable first test as pneumonitis has been described with HCV treatment. In patients with a normal chest X-ray but persistent symptoms, a chest CT scan would not be unreasonable. In this case, the chest X-ray (Fig. 16.1) demonstrates bilateral hilar lymphadenopathy. Biopsy was obtained confirming noncaseating granulomas. In addition, a serum angiotensin-converting enzyme (ACE) level is worth checking and will often be elevated.

In patients with hepatic sarcoid, the diagnosis is even more difficult since a rise in liver enzymes is not uncommon during treatment, even cholestatic enzymes. The serum ACE level may be helpful in this situation but occasionally liver biopsy is required. Most HCV experts would recommend continuing treatment even if liver enzymes rise but I typically will get concerned if the ALT or AST reaches 350–400 iu/l (from a baseline of 2–3× the upper limit of normal), or the cholestatic enzymes get beyond 2× the upper limit of normal, irrespective of the viral load, and I have a low threshold for getting a biopsy.

References

1. Cogrel O, Doutre MS, Marliere V, Beylot-Barry M, Couzigou P, Beylot C. Cutaneous sarcoidosis during interferon alfa and ribavirin treatment of hepatitis C virus infection: two cases. Br J Dermatol 2002;146:320–4.
2. Hoffmann RM, Jung MC, Motz R, et al. Sarcoidosis associated with interferon-alpha therapy for chronic hepatitis C. J Hepatol 1998;28:1058–63.
3. Adla M, Downey KK, Ahmad J. Hepatic sarcoidosis associated with pegylated interferon alfa therapy for chronic hepatitis C: case report and review of literature. Dig Dis Sci 2008;53:2810–2.

Case 17

A 51-year-old Caucasian lady is referred to your outpatient clinic for elevated liver enzymes. She complains of some fatigue which she puts down to looking after her elderly mother.

She denies abdominal pain or fever. Her bowels move normally and she denies weight loss. There has been no change in urine or stool color.

Her past medical history is significant for hypertension, hyperlipidemia, and hypothyroidism. She denies prior surgery.

Her current medications include metoprolol, simvastatin, and levothyroxine. She also takes a baby aspirin daily. She does not smoke or use alcohol. She is married with grown children.

Her family history is significant for thyroid disease in her mother and sister but no liver disease or cancer.

Physical exam reveals normal vitals, weight 212 pounds, height 67 in.

There is no scleral icterus but she has palmar erythema and several spider nevi. Heart and lungs are normal. Abdomen reveals an obese abdomen with an enlarged liver felt 6 cm below the right costal margin. There is no splenomegaly, ascites, or ankle edema.

Laboratory Parameters

Hb 11.8 g/dl
Platelets 99,000/μl
INR 1.3
Creatine 0.9 mg/dl
Tbili 1.5 mg/dl
AST 48 iu/l
ALT 44 iu/l
ALP 289 iu/l
GGTP 168 iu/l
Albumin 2.8 g/dl
AMA positive 1:640
Total cholesterol 387 mg/dl
Ultrasound shows an echogenic liver

Questions

1. Is she at risk for coronary atherosclerosis?
2. Should she be treated with lipid lowering agents?

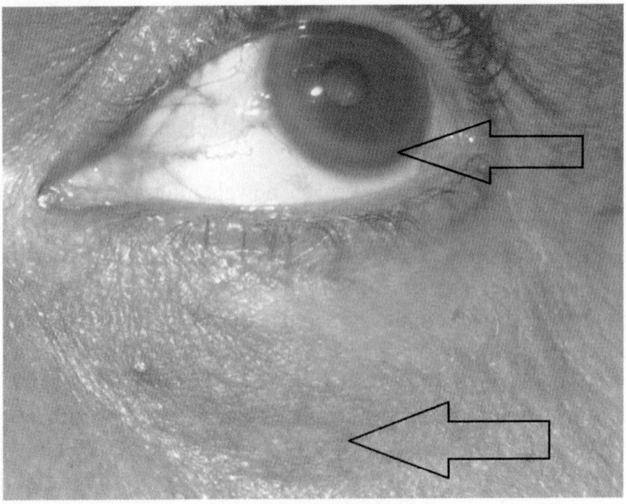

Fig. 17.1

Answer: Hypercholesterolemia in Patient with Primary Biliary Cirrhosis (PBC)

This lady has cirrhosis from PBC. She has cholestatic liver enzymes, no biliary obstruction on imaging, a positive AMA, and symptoms that fit with PBC. Contrary to popular belief among residents and fellows, pruritus is not the most common symptom, occurring only in one-third of patients at presentation, but rather fatigue, which is seen in up to half of patients. It typically presents in the fourth to sixth decade and is seen almost exclusively in women.

Striking hepatic enlargement is often found, occasionally in asymptomatic patients. Hepatomegaly becomes more common as the disease progresses and is eventually found in approximately 70% of cases. Xanthelasmas occur around the periorbital folds (as seen in the image together with corneal arcus, Fig. 17.1) and are relatively common, occurring in approximately 10% of patients. Xanthomas are less common and correlate with total plasma cholesterol levels. They develop on the elbows, palms, soles, buttocks, knees, back, and chest and are usually seen in patients with plasma cholesterol levels above 600 mg/dl (15.6 mmol/l).

AMA is the serologic hallmark of PBC. They are present in about 95% of patients with PBC and most assays are 95% sensitive and 98% specific for PBC.

Treatment is with ursodiol at 13–15 mg/kg which has shown a survival benefit in PBC in those who have a biochemical response.

Serum lipids can be very elevated in PBC, with total cholesterol levels often in the 300–400 mg/dl range and may exceed 1,000 mg/dl (26 mmol/l) in patients with xanthomas. However, the composition of cholesterol can include striking elevations of high-density lipoproteins (HDL) which may explain why patients with PBC, despite striking hypercholesterolemia, are not at increased risk of death from atherosclerosis. There does not appear to be any correlation between the total cholesterol and the total bilirubin level.

Data on drug therapy for hypercholesterolemia in PBC are limited and there is a risk of increased toxicity with statin drugs since they are excreted in bile. Since the risk of adverse coronary events does not seem to be elevated, these drugs likely should be avoided. Plasmapheresis can be used to treat xanthomatous neuropathy and symptomatic xanthomas that occur on the palms.

References

1. Kaplan MM. Primary biliary cirrhosis. N Engl J Med 2005;353:1261.
2. Long RG, Scheuer PJ. Sherlock presentation and course of asymptomatic primary biliary cirrhosis. Gastroenterology 1977;72(6):1204–7.
3. Solaymani-Dodaran M, Aithal GP, Card T, et al. Risk of cardiovascular and cerebrovascular events in primary biliary cirrhosis: a population-based cohort study. Am J Gastroenterol 2008;103:2784.

Case 18

A 48-year-old female presents to the emergency room with several weeks of painless jaundice and poorly controlled blood sugar. She denies abdominal pain or fever but has had some nausea and has lost a few pounds in weight. Her urine has become darker although she denies pale stool. She has noticed some itching.

Her past medical history is significant for chronic HCV which has never been treated due to her poorly controlled diabetes. She has genotype 1 disease with a recent low viral load. She also has hypertension but denies coronary artery disease.

Her current medications include insulin, amlodipine, and an antihistamine which was started a few days ago by her primary care doctor. She had been taking lisinopril and a thiazide diuretic previously but these were stopped when she became jaundiced. She denies any over the counter medications or herbal supplements.

She does not smoke or drink. She is married and lives with her husband and teenage daughter. There is no family history of liver disease.

Her review of systems is otherwise negative.

On exam she looks well but is obviously jaundiced. Vital signs show weight 213 pounds, BP 150/80, pulse 92, and she is afebrile.

She has scleral icterus but no palmar erythema or spider nevi.

Heart and lungs are normal.

A liver edge is palpable but her abdomen is otherwise normal. There is a trace of ankle edema.

Laboratory Studies

Hb 10.6 g/dl
Platelets 313,000/μl
WBC 6.3×10^3/μl
INR 1.0
Creatinine 0.7 mg/dl
Tbili 12.1 mg/dl
Direct bili 7.8 mg/dl
AST 323 iu/l
ALT 452 iu/l
GGTP 1,042 iu/l
ALP 383 iu/l
Albumin 3.9 g/dl
Blood glucose 354 mg/dl
Ferritin 1,257 ng/ml
Transferrin saturation 43%
ANA negative
AMA negative
SMA 1:320

Questions

1. What other tests are required?
2. What are the possible etiologies of her liver enzyme abnormalities?

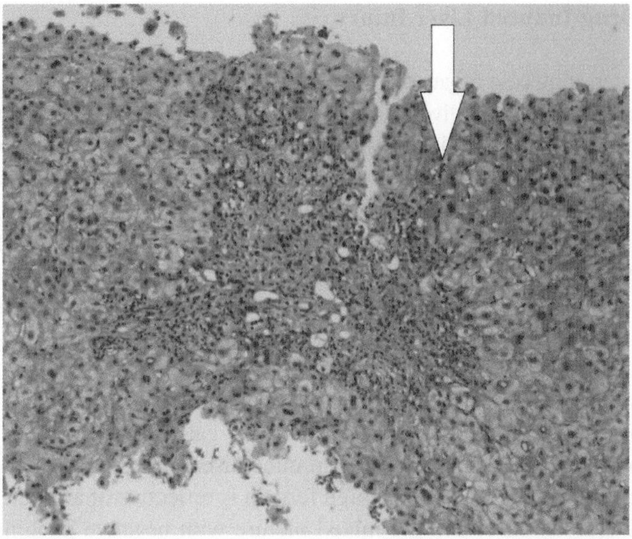

Fig. 18.1 Liver biopsy H&E ×100

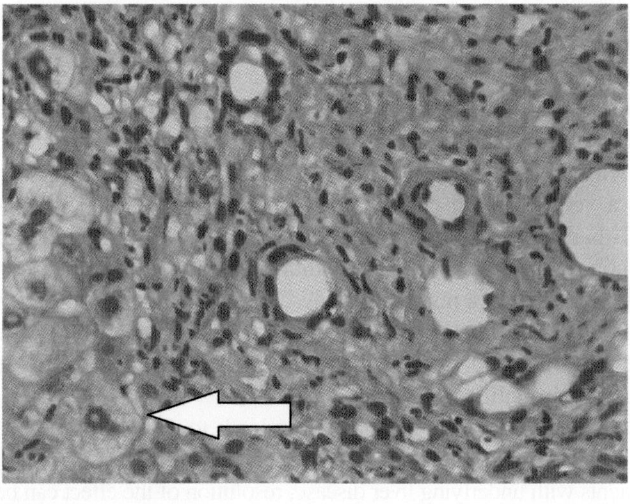

Fig. 18.2 Liver biopsy H&E ×250

Answer: Drug-Induced Liver Injury

This is an interesting case of jaundice and a mixed picture of liver enzyme abnormalities in someone with underlying liver disease from hepatitis C. She does not appear to have cirrhosis but the differential diagnosis is really whether this is related to her hepatitis C or perhaps she has some other process in addition. She has had this for several weeks and her exam is relatively benign except for jaundice. Hepatitis C can cause an aggressive cholestatic disease but this is typically in immunosuppressed patients and is associated with a high viral load which is not the case here. She could have developed HCC even if she does not have cirrhosis but this is very uncommon in hepatitis C (as opposed to hepatitis B where HCC can develop in patients with minimal fibrosis).

Perhaps she has biliary obstruction from stones or cancer. Hence, abdominal imaging is necessary. She in fact had an ultrasound that was normal and an MRI/MRCP that showed a normal biliary tree without gallstones.

The blood work argues against autoimmune disease (despite the mildly elevated SMA which is nonspecific) and the high ferritin is reflective of an acute phase reaction. The insidious onset and the mixed picture with negative imaging and blood work make a liver biopsy necessary. Even without the biopsy, a drug-induced reaction has to be considered.

The biopsy shows hepatocytic cholestasis (Fig. 18.1) with feathery degeneration (Fig. 18.2). The portal tract in Fig. 18.1 shows mild edema and a mixed inflammatory infiltrate (without a significant number of plasma cells), but no significant interface hepatitis. There is moderate lobular activity with foci of parenchymal necrosis. The trichrome stain showed only mild portal fibrosis. These findings could be seen with biliary obstruction but the negative imaging makes this most consistent with drug-induced liver injury (DILI).

DILI is a very common entity, accounting for up to 10% of all adverse drug reactions. It is the most common cause of acute liver failure in the USA, and the most common reason for medication withdrawal by the FDA.

It can be classified in a number of ways, either by the pattern of enzyme abnormalities, histology, or mechanism (direct versus idiosyncratic). In general, if there is jaundice and elevation of transaminases, the prognosis is worse than isolated transaminase abnormalities (Hy's law).

Typically, withdrawal of the causative drug leads to reversal of the injury but there can be progressive disease leading to fibrosis or cirrhosis, despite discontinuation of the drug. In patients with underlying liver disease, resolution of the effect can be prolonged.

In this case, the offending drug was probably lisinopril since ACE inhibitors as a class can cause cholestatic injury. However, a quick glance at any drug book such as the PDR (physician's desk reference) in the USA will tell you that virtually any drug can cause liver test abnormalities.

Reference

1. Lee WM. Drug-induced hepatotoxicity. N Engl J Med 2003;349:474.

Case 19

A 55-year-old lady is referred for a percutaneous liver biopsy in order to stage hepatitis C-induced liver disease. A prior imaging study showed no evidence of cirrhosis or portal hypertension. The biopsy is performed by a fellow under your supervision. Ultrasound is used to identify a suitable site in the right flank and no vessels or biliary radicles are seen. The biopsy is carried out using a Menghini needle with suction and a 2 cm core is obtained with a single pass and no immediate complications are noted. The patient is discharged home and asked to follow-up in the liver clinic the following week. Two days later, the patient returns to the hospital with a chief complaint of melena for 12 h. She denies hematemesis but does report mild abdominal pain. She denies taking any medication.

She has no other relevant medical history.

Her exam is notable for a BP of 110/60, pulse 104, and she is afebrile. There is no palmar erythema, sclera icterus, or spider nevi. Abdomen demonstrates mild epigastric tenderness but bowel sounds are heard. Liver and spleen are impalpable.

The patient is admitted to hospital and an upper endoscopy is performed.

Initial Laboratory Parameters Show

WBC 9×10^3/ul
Hemoglobin 11 g/dl (baseline 12 g/dl)
Platelet 205×10^3/ul
Protime 13 s
Tbili 1.9 mg/dl (baseline 0.5 mg/dl)
AST 105 iu/l (baseline 43 iu/l)
ALT 107 iu/l (baseline 35 iu/l)
Creatinine 1.0 mg/dl

Questions

1. What does the endoscopy show?
2. What are the next appropriate tests?

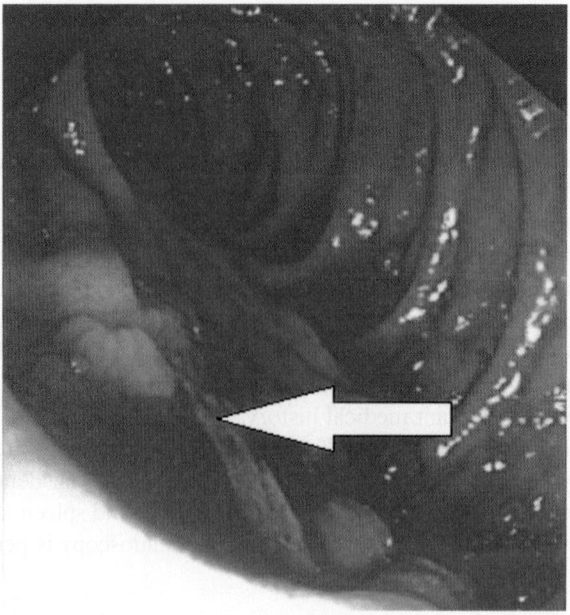

Fig. 19.1 Endoscopy

Answer: Hemobilia as a Complication of Liver Biopsy

This lady has very likely developed a complication from her liver biopsy. She does not appear to have cirrhosis and was well up until shortly after the biopsy. She could have another non-liver cause of bleeding but the rise in liver enzymes and bilirubin strongly suggest bleeding from the liver or biliary tree (hemobilia).

Despite patient trepidation, liver biopsy is a very safe procedure in experienced hands with a mortality rate of 1 in 10,000 and a rate of complications requiring hospitalization of 2–3%. The morbidity and mortality rates are highest in patients with a malignant lesion or if there is a bleeding diathesis.

The most common complication is pain (25–30%) and rarely requires intervention except for analgesics. Severe pain warrants further investigation.

Significant intraperitoneal bleeding occurs in less than 1% of biopsies and is usually apparent within a few hours. Hence the recommendation to monitor vital signs in patients after a biopsy for 2–4 hours. If significant bleeding is suspected, the patient should be resuscitated and imaging is typically indicated. Management will depend on location and severity but angiography and then surgery if necessary is the usual algorithm.

Bleeding can be intraperitoneal, intrahepatic, or hemobilia, the latter being the least common.

Other complications include bile peritonitis, perforation of colon or pneumothorax, and infection usually from transient bacteremia.

Hemobilia classically presents with the triad of gastrointestinal bleeding, biliary pain, and jaundice. The bleeding can be arterial or venous (particularly if portal hypertension is present) and can be acute but usually delayed. Apart from liver biopsy, hemobilia can also be seen with any intervention in the liver such as TIPS, arterial chemoembolization, percutaneous biliary drainage, or with tumors or abscesses in the liver or from hepatic artery aneurysms.

The diagnosis is made at endoscopy if blood is seen coming from the papilla as noted in this case (Fig. 19.1, arrow) or can be made on imaging, which can be ultrasound, hepatobiliary scintigraphy, CT or MRI or angiogram. Sometimes, a side viewing duodenoscope is useful to visualize the papilla.

Treatment for significant hemobilia after a liver biopsy usually involves angiographic embolization but occasionally surgery is required.

References

1. Bravo AA, Sheth SG, Chopra S. Liver biopsy. N Engl J Med 2001;344:495.
2. Piccinino F, Sagnelli E, Pasquale G, Giusti G. Complications following percutaneous liver biopsy. A multicentre retrospective study on 68,276 biopsies. J Hepatol 1986;2:165.
3. Rockey DC, Caldwell SH, Goodman ZD, et al. Liver biopsy. Hepatology 2009;49:1017.

Case 20

A 48-year-old white female was given a diagnosis of primary biliary cirrhosis (PBC) based on the findings of an intraoperative liver biopsy performed because her liver appeared "abnormal" at the time of a total abdominal hysterectomy 5 years ago. At that time, the patient had mild elevations in liver function tests and was placed on ursodeoxycholic acid. She presents to an outside hospital with a 1 week history of darkening of her urine and lightening of her stools. Three days later she noted her eyes turning yellow. Her review of systems is positive for fatigue and joint pains, but she denies fevers, chills, abdominal pain, rash, or pruritus. Her liver function tests upon admission to the hospital reveal: Tbili 7.2 mg/dl, AST 517 iu/l, ALT 478 iu/l, AP 389 iu/l. The impression on an abdominal CT reads: "significant retroperitoneal lymphadenopathy suspicious for lymphoma." The patient is transferred to your institution for further evaluation. She has a medical history significant for mitral valve repair 2 years ago and is maintained on chronic oral anticoagulation. Other past medical history includes hypertension, osteopenia, and gastroesophageal reflux disease. She underwent a laparoscopic cholecystectomy over 15 years ago. Her outpatient medications include: ursodeoxycholic acid 1,500 mg daily, omeprazole, warfarin, vit-C + D, and metoprolol. She had previously been vaccinated for hepatitis A and B virus when she was diagnosed with PBC. The patient lives with her husband of 16 years and they have one 12-year-old daughter who has type I diabetes. The patient works fulltime on a dairy farm. She has a 20-year smoking history and currently smokes half pack per day. She drinks one to two cans of beer per month. There is no history of blood transfusions or high-risk behavior. The patient's mother is 68 and has COPD and hypothyroidism, her father is 70 and has rheumatoid arthritis.

Physical exam reveals a well-nourished female who is jaundiced but in no distress. She is afebrile with normal vital signs; BMI of 34.6 kg/m^2. She has deep scleral icterus, numerous spider nevi, and marked palmar erythema. There is no palpable lymphadenopathy. Her lungs and heart are normal. Abdomen is soft, nontender, previous surgical scars are well healed. The liver is palpable 4.5 cm below the costal margin and is firm. The spleen tip is palpable. There is no appreciable ascites. There is no peripheral edema. Neurologically she is oriented and there is no asterixis.

Laboratory Studies

Tbili 7.2 mg/dl
AST 500 iu/l
ALT 774 iu/l
AP 336 iu/l
GGTP 388 iu/l
WBC 5,000/μl

Hemoglobin 14 g/dl
Platelets 80,000/μl
INR 1.4
Electrolytes and renal function are normal
ANA 1,280 (centromere),
SMA 86, M2 4.8 (strongly positive), IgG 3,230, IgA 478, IgM 510

Questions

1. What is the differential diagnosis for the elevation in liver function tests?
2. How do you account for the findings on the CT scan?
3. Would you recommend any further testing?
4. What therapy would you recommend?

Liver Biopsy

Background reveals: florid duct lesions, ductopenia. In addition, there is prominent lobular and interface necroinflammatory activity. Portal to portal bridging fibrosis (stage 3/6)

Answer: Primary biliary cirrhosis/autoimmune hepatitis (PBC/AIH) Overlap with Acute Flare

The onset of jaundice and acute elevation in liver function tests speak against the natural history of PBC and more likely indicate some "superimposed" injury on top of the underlying disease. As opposed to AIH, the natural history of PBC is not to flare in this manner. The differential diagnosis includes a drug-induced injury, alcoholic hepatitis, viral hepatitis, and malignancy. The patient's age, sex, pattern of elevation in liver function tests, positive M2, ANA, SMA, IgG, and IgM all point toward a diagnosis of AIH/PBC overlap. The diagnosis was confirmed with liver biopsy.

PBC and AIH are distinct immune-mediated liver diseases with their own clinical, biochemical, and histological features. It is now well established, however, that the diseases can occur simultaneously or consecutively in a syndrome which has been termed PBC/AIH overlap.

The pathophysiological mechanisms of PBC/AIH overlap remain unknown. It may be a unique autoimmune process that has unique effects on both hepatocytes and biliary ducts. Others believe that the disease is a "variant" of either AIH or PBC, hence the term "hepatic variant of PBC." A third theory is that the syndrome results when the two different diseases coexist in the same patient. Although it is a well-recognized entity, diagnostic criteria have not yet been standardized. Czaja proposed that patients who are positive for AMA or M2 and have an autoimmune score compatible with either probable or definite should be classified with overlap. Detailed diagnostic criteria for the PBC/AIH overlap syndrome, known as the Paris criteria, have also been proposed (see Table 20.1).

PBC/AIH overlap is not a rare entity; the prevalence of overlap has been reported in 5–19% of PBC patients and 5–8% of AIH patients. Not surprisingly, as seen in the individual disease entities, a majority of patients (over 85%) with overlap are middle-aged females.

Patients with features of PBC/AIH overlap have been reported to be at a greater risk of developing symptomatic portal hypertension and subsequently having more adverse outcomes (death and/or orthotopic liver transplantation). However, studies have also suggested that when patients with overlap are treated with a combination of immunosuppressive drugs and ursodeoxycholic acid, the 10-year survival rates are excellent. It is imperative therefore in distinguishing the overlap syndrome from PBC or AIH alone because therapeutic options and long-term outcomes may be different between the two groups.

The frequency and clinical importance of lymphadenopathy in PBC has been the subject of considerable interest. While it was previously suggested that lymphadenopathy in PBC is an uncommon phenomenon, recent studies demonstrate it is extremely common. Abdominal lymphadenopathy is seen in up to 88% of patients with PBC (versus around 45% in other causes of cirrhosis). Sampled nodes in PBC patients undergoing liver transplantation have invariably demonstrated benign reactive hyperplasia, as opposed to disseminated malignancy.

The patient in this case was started on steroid therapy in addition to ursodeoxycholic acid. She was seen 2 weeks after discharge with significant improvement in her enzyme levels and symptoms. At 6 weeks, she had near normalization of liver tests, her steroids were tapered, and azathioprine was introduced.

Table 20.1 Paris criteria for overlap syndrome

Requires the presence of at least two of the three accepted criteria for both PBC and AIH
PBC
1. Serum ALP 2× greater than ULN; or serum GGT 5× greater than ULN
2. +AMA or M2
3. Liver biopsy showing florid duct lesions
AIH
1. Serum ALT 5× greater than ULN
2. IgG levels 2× ULN or positive SMA
3. Liver biopsy showing moderate or severe periportal or periseptal lymphocytic piecemeal necrosis

Adapted from Chazouilleres O, Wendum D, Serfaty L, et al. Primary biliary cirrhosis-autoimmune hepatitis overlap syndrome: clinical features and response to therapy. Hepatology 1998;28:296–301

References

1. Blachar A, Federle MP, Brancatelli G. Primary biliary cirrhosis: clinical, pathologic, and helical CT findings in 53 patients. Radiology 2001;220:329–36.
2. Kuiper EM, Zondervan PE, Buuren HR. Paris criteria are effective in diagnosis of primary biliary cirrhosis and autoimmune hepatitis overlap syndrome. Clin Gastroenterol Hepatol 2010;8(6):530–4.
3. Yokokawa J, Saito H, Kanno Y, et al. Overlap of primary biliary cirrhosis and autoimmune hepatitis: characteristics, therapy, and long term outcomes. J Gastroenterol Hepatol 2010;25:376–82.

Case 21

A 37-year-old African American male with a past medical history significant for schizophrenia and seizure disorder is found down in his brother's bathtub. The patient does not respond to verbal stimuli; however, he does withdraw to pain. He is laying in urine and there is blood on the shower wall. The patient's brother calls 911. Upon arrival his temperature is recorded at 96.7°F and the rest of his vital signs are stable, although his breathing is shallow. The patient is intubated on the scene and taken to the emergency room. The patient's prescription medications include valproic acid and seroquel. He is homeless and has been living with his brother for the last 3 weeks. The brother informs paramedics that the patient "smokes like a chimney" and "likes his alcohol." He is not sure if he has ever used illicit drugs. He has no history of tattoos or blood transfusions. He is single and has five children from previous relationships. The patient is currently unemployed. His parents both died in a motor vehicle accident over 25 years ago. The patient's brother is 40 and is in excellent health.

Physical exam is notable for a thin, black male who appears older than his stated age. His BMI is 20.8 kg/m^2. There is a cut on the back of his head which is oozing blood. There are large areas of ecchymoses noted on his back and thighs. His sclerae are nonicteric. His lung sounds are coarse bilaterally. Cardiac exam is normal. His abdomen is scaphoid, there is no appreciable hepatosplenomegaly. He does have some mild clubbing, but no peripheral edema. There are no stigmata of chronic liver disease.

A pan CT scan performed in the ER is normal with no evidence of fracture, injury, or bleed.

Laboratory Data

Sodium 151 mM/l
Potassium 6.3 mM/l
BUN 53 mg/dl
Cr 5.3 mg/dl
Phos 1.8 mg/dl
Calcium 7.4 mg/dl
WBC 19,000/μl
Hb 17 g/dl
Plts 255,000/μl
Tbili 1.1 mg/dl
AST 1,298 iu/l
ALT 390 iu/l
ALP 108 iu/l
GGTP 49 iu/l
INR 1.0

Albumin 3.5 g/dl
CPK 44,590 iu/l
LDH 3,879 u/l
UA: +myoglobin

Questions

1. What is the most likely cause for the elevation in AST/ALT in this case?
2. What Laboratory Studies help clinch the diagnosis?
3. What was the most likely cause for the primary diagnosis in this case?

Answer: Elevated AST/ALT Due to Rhabdomyolysis

Aminotransferases catalyze the conversion of the amino acids alanine and aspartate to alpha-ketoglutarate, providing a source of nitrogen for the urea cycle. Both enzymes are found widely in many tissues, and increased serum levels are a non-specific indicator of disease. Serum concentrations are highest in various hepatic disorders, but increased values are also seen in skeletal muscle, myocardial disease, and hemolysis.

It is important that the clinician be aware that elevated aminotransferases may be caused by disorders other than primary liver. The most common of these are injuries to striated muscle, including muscle myopathies (both subclinical inborn errors and acquired disorders such as polymyositis), seizures, and heavy exercise. Skeletal muscle contains isoenzymes of creatinine kinase, lactate dehydrogenase, AST, and ALT which may be released into the blood following muscle necrosis. AST and ALT may be elevated with muscle injury to variable levels, but can be as high as 10,000 iu and 850 iu/l, respectively.

The patient in this case was diagnosed with rhabdomyolysis, a syndrome characterized by muscle necrosis and the release of intracellular muscle constituents into the circulation. The most common causes include trauma, overexertion, and alcoholism. The illness can range from asymptomatic elevation in serum muscle enzymes to life-threatening cases with lethal electrolyte abnormalities and acute renal failure.

The elevation in transaminases in rhabdomyolysis level is likely almost entirely the result of muscle damage and not liver injury. The evidence for this is that in a majority of cases, the bilirubin, prothrombin time, and GGT are normal. In a study which further supports this theory, 39 runners underwent bloodwork before and after a 246-km continuous race. Post-laboratory values revealed massive elevations in CK, LDH, AST, ALT, but GGT levels showed no difference before and after the race.

The cause of rhabdomyolysis is usually evident as in this case where it was secondary to grand mal seizure and muscle injury in a patient who was "down" for an unknown amount of time. The most common causes of rhabdomyolysis include: trauma, overexertion, and alcoholism. After a fall, individuals may remain on the floor undiscovered for long periods. Ischemic pressure necrosis of muscle may have contributed to the severity of muscle injury in this case.

The classic presentation of rhabdomyolysis includes myalgias, myoglobinuria, and elevated serum muscle enzymes. Elevations in serum aminotransferases are common (one study reported 25% of cases) and can cause confusion if attributed to liver disease. With acute rhabdomyolysis, the AST peak is initially higher than the ALT peak, although as the injury improves, AST and ALT levels become comparable (reflective of the shorter half-life of AST). An elevated ALT in the absence of other evidence of liver disease should lead one to consider muscle injury. This suspicion can be confirmed by an elevated CK and LDH.

The possible presence of rhabdomyolysis should be suspected in any patient who is unable to provide a reliable history with one or more of the following: muscle tenderness, pressure necrosis of skin, signs of trauma or crush injury, blood chemistry abnormalities including hyperkalemia, hyperphosphatemia, and acute renal failure.

Management involves treatment of the underlying cause of the rhabdomyolysis. Aggressive plasma volume expansion is integral. Electrolytes should be carefully monitored for the derangements described.

References

1. Nathwani RA, Pais S, Reynolds TB, et al. Serum alanine aminotransferase in skeletal muscle diseases. Hepatology 2005;41:380–2.
2. Akmal M, Massry SG. Reversible hepatic dysfunction associated with rhabdomyolysis. Am J Nephrol 1990;10:49–52.
3. Skenderi KP, Kavouras SA, Anastasiou CA, et al. Exertional rhabdomyolysis during a 246-km continuous running race. Med Sci Sports Exerc 2006;38:1054–7.

Case 22

A 38-year-old gentleman originally from the West Indies is admitted with new onset jaundice. He has a history of end-stage renal disease secondary to membranoproliferative glomerular nephritis (MPGN). He underwent a cadaveric renal transplant nearly 15 years ago. Within the last year he has developed recurrent kidney disease and is being evaluated for a second kidney transplant. The patient states he was doing well until 2 weeks prior to admission when he began to develop an "upset" stomach with nausea, non-bloody emesis, and anorexia. Over the last 1 week, he noticed his urine darkening and 1 day prior to admission his co-workers noticed yellowing of his eyes, which prompted his admission. On review of systems, he complains of fatigue, malaise, and has lost 12 pounds since the onset of his symptoms. Other notable medical history includes hypertension and gastroesophageal reflux disease. His immunosuppression regimen since his transplant consists of cyclosporine, mycophenolate, and prednisone. His other home medications include: metoprolol, pantoprazole, verapamil, and lisinopril. The patient works as a hospital unit secretary. He is divorced and is living alone and is not currently sexually active. He has one 3-year-old daughter. He does not smoke or drink or use illicit drugs. He did receive blood transfusions during his kidney transplant in 1991 and was maintained on hemodialysis for several years prior to transplant. His mother died of a stroke at the age of 61. His father is 66 and has hypertension and diabetes.

Physical exam reveals a well-developed, well-nourished gentleman, who is comfortable and in no distress. Temperature is 37.4°C, blood pressure 150/98, and heart rate 76 with a BMI of 25.9 kg/m^2. He has scleral icterus. He has no appreciable adenopathy. Heart and lung exams are normal. His abdomen is soft, flat, and nontender. He has a palpable right pelvic kidney. His liver is not enlarged. His spleen is not palpable. There is no appreciable ascites. He has no peripheral edema. There is no palmar erythema or spider angiomas. He is alert and oriented 3×. His neurologic examination is nonfocal. There is no asterixis. He has no bruising.

WBC 14,000 with 88% neutrophils
Hb 10 g/dl, MCV 75 f/U
Platelet 325,000/μl
BUN 69 mg/dl, Cr 5.5 mg/dl
Tbili 8.3 mg/dl; direct 5.7 mg/dl
AST 270 iu/l, ALT 230 iu/l, ALP 150 iu/l, GGT 220 iu/l
Albumin 3.2 g/dl
INR 1.5
NH_3 28 μmol/l
RUQ US: normal liver, no evidence of intra or extra-hepatic ductal dilation

Questions

1. What is the differential diagnosis?
2. What are the risk factors?
3. How could this have potentially been prevented?
4. What are the potential treatment options?

ANA negative
Smooth muscle antibody 34 (weakly positive)
IgG 3,200, IgA 590, IgM 260

Serologies: HBsAg+, sAb−, core+, core IgM+, eAg−, eAb+
Delta negative
DNA 1,429,154,462 iu/ml (3,030,000,000 copies/ml)

HCV Ab negative
HAV total+, IgM negative
CMV IgG+, IgM negative; PCR negative
EBV IgG+, IgM negative; PCR negative

Answer: Acute Hepatitis (HBV), Reactivation in an Immunocompromised Host Leading to Hepatic Failure

The liver function pattern in this case is mixed hepatocellular and cholestatic with marked hyperbilirubinemia. The differential diagnosis is broad and includes acute viral (A, B, and C), given his immunocompromised state viruses like EBV, CMV, and HSV should also be considered; alcoholic hepatitis, autoimmune, cholestatic liver disease (PBC/PSC), sarcoidosis, infiltrating disorders including malignancy; and drug induced injury can always be inserted into the differential of an acute liver injury.

The patient has multiple risk factors for hepatitis B virus (HBV) infection including: hemodialysis, multiple blood transfusions, and surgeries prior to 1992 and his place of birth. The constellation of symptoms seems most consistent with a viral etiology.

Upon further questioning, the patient recalls being told he had hepatitis B in the past, but thought he was "immune." Serologies confirm acute HBV infection or reactivation in the setting of immunosuppression.

Reactivation of HBV is a syndrome marked by abrupt reappearance of HBV DNA in the serum of an individual with inactive or previously resolved HBV infection. Reactivation can be spontaneous, but is most typically seen in scenarios involving depressed states of immune function including: chemotherapy, immunosuppression following organ transplantation, autoimmune conditions and HIV infection. Although a large number of cases of reactivation are subclinical, reactivation can also be severe and result in acute liver failure and death in greater than 10% of cases.

The frequency of reactivation is not well known. A study from China followed 100 patients undergoing chemotherapy for lymphoma for virological, serological, and biochemical evidence of reactivation. Almost one in every two patients who were HBsAg positive developed reactivation. Also noteworthy is that two patients who had evidence of serological resolution (HBsAg negative, HBcore +) developed reactivation with the reappearance of surface antigen. A recent meta-analysis analyzing the role of prophylaxis with lamivudine in preventing reactivation, found the combined rate of reactivation of 13 studies to be 15%.

Given the need for long-term immunosuppression, organ transplantation is a prime setting for the occurrence of reactivation HBV. Reactivation of HBV is almost universal in patients with HBsAg undergoing bone marrow transplantation, as a result of the extreme forms of ablation and immunosuppression utilized. Before the use of antiviral prophylaxis, the rates of HBV reactivation following kidney transplant were as high as 94%. Similarly high rates have been seen in other solid-organ transplants. Liver transplantation is a unique situation and the challenges of reactivation of HBV in this setting will be covered via another case presentation.

All patients undergoing cancer chemotherapy, marked immunosuppressive treatments, organ transplantation should be screened for evidence of previous HBV or ongoing infection.

Persons found to be HBsAg positive should be evaluated and if warranted started on appropriate therapy before starting cancer chemotherapy or immune suppression. Persons found to have inactive HBsAg, or immune tolerant chronic HBV should receive antiviral prophylaxis before starting chemotherapy or immune suppression. Persons found to have anti-HB core without HBsAg should also be considered for antiviral prophylaxis in similar settings. Prophylaxis in general should continue for at least 6 months after stopping chemotherapy or continued indefinitely in the setting of chronic immune suppression.

The patient in this case was started on entecavir upon presentation. Despite a steady decline in HBV DNA, the patient clinically deteriorated over the next several months with worsening renal failure, development of ascites, increasing bilirubin (peak of 30 mg/dl), INR 3.2, and onset of confusion. The patient eventually underwent liver transplantation 10 weeks after initial presentation. Pathological examination of the explant revealed mixed macro- and micronodular cirrhosis consistent with HBV infection; patchy areas of parenchymal extinction with marked cholangiolar proliferation and cholestasis. The patient is currently being maintained on entecavir and hepatitis B immune globulin (HBIG) combination post-transplant. Current serologies are: HBsAg-negative, HBsAb > 250 miu/ml, HBeAg-negative, eAb+; DNA undetectable and normal liver function tests.

References

1. Hoofnagle JH. Reactivation of hepatitis B. Hepatology 2009;49:S156–65.
2. Loomba R, Rowley A, Wesley R, et al. Systematic review: the effect of preventive lamivudine on hepatitis B reactivation during chemotherapy. Ann Intern Med 2008;148:519–28.
3. Lok AS, Liang RH, Chiu EK, et al. Reactivation of hepatitis B virus replication in patients receiving cytotoxic therapy. Report of a prospective study. Gastroenterology 1991;100:182–8.

Case 23

A 47-year-old African American male comes to see you as an outpatient for evaluation of chronic hepatitis C. He was diagnosed several years ago but was afraid of possible complications of treatment and so avoided consultation. He is completely asymptomatic.

His past medical history is significant for hypertension, diet-controlled diabetes, and hypercholesterolemia.

Medications include clonidine, atorvastatin, and milk thistle.

He is married and runs his own printing business.

He used drugs as a teenager and in his early 20s and quit smoking and drinking a few years ago. He occasionally uses marijuana and drinks five to six espresso coffees every day.

There is no family history of liver disease.

The rest of his review of systems is negative.

On exam he looks well and is alert and oriented.
Vital signs show BP 140/80, pulse 68, and he is afebrile. His BMI is 34 kg/m^2.
There is no scleral icterus and no spider nevi.
Heart reveals normal S1 and S2 without added sounds. Chest reveals clear lung fields.
His abdomen is soft and nontender without organomegaly.

Laboratory Studies

Hb 14.9 g/dl
Platelets 307,000/μl
WBC 5.8 × 10^3/μl
INR 1.0
Creatinine 1.4 mg/dl
Tbili 0.7 mg/dl
AST 57 iu/l
ALT 63 iu/l
GGTP 89 iu/l
ALP 76 iu/l
Albumin 4.5 g/dl
HCV RNA 2,000,000 iu/ml
Genotype 1b

Questions

1. Should this patient be treated for hepatitis C now?
2. Does he need a liver biopsy?
3. What factors predict disease progression in this patient?

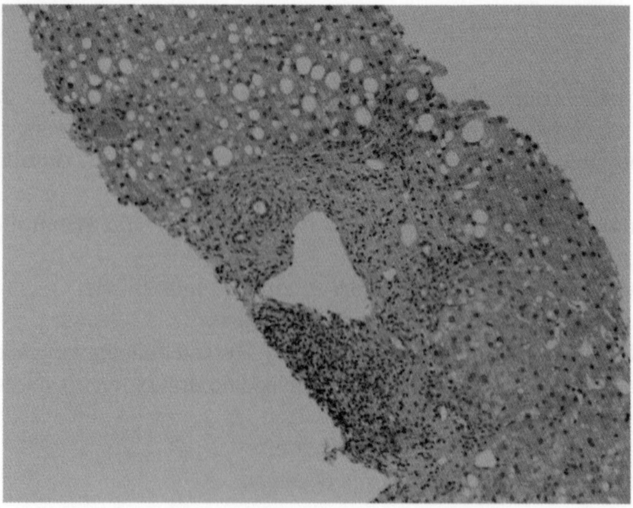

Fig. 23.1 Liver biopsy H&E ×100

Answer: Factors Predictive of Hepatitis C Disease Progression

This is common clinical situation in the outpatient setting: a middle-aged patient with a history of hepatitis C for 20–30 years who now presents completely asymptomatic with mildly elevated liver enzymes.

His exam and liver tests really argue against cirrhosis and yet you cannot be certain. A liver biopsy remains the gold standard for documenting the degree of inflammation and fibrosis in hepatitis C although there are a variety of noninvasive tests that have good predictive power for cirrhosis (and in the case of the Fibroscan, good accuracy for fibrosis).

The question of waiting for treatment relies on probable approval of new direct acting antiviral drugs (DAA), telaprevir, and boceprevir, in 2011. These drugs will be given in combination with the current treatment of pegylated interferon and ribavirin, and will significantly increase the current sustained viral response rate of about 40–50% in genotype 1 patients.

Some patients insist on treatment irrespective of the severity of disease and it would be very reasonable to proceed in this patient since he has elevated liver enzymes and viremia. However, he has several factors predictive of poor response to treatment, including his genotype, obesity, viral load, and his ethnicity.

In this patient, we elected to proceed with a liver biopsy (Fig. 23.1) which I suspect most practitioners would agree with. The debate over whether to biopsy or not really depends on your preference as an argument can be made that if you want to treat everyone with viremia and without contra-indications, a biopsy is not needed.

The liver biopsy shows evidence of a mixed inflammatory infiltrate in the portal tract but also a significant amount of steatosis, which was not surprising given the patient's obesity and metabolic syndrome. The trichrome stain showed portal fibrosis which would indicate mild-to-moderate disease and I personally would wait to treat this patient until DAA are available as his chance of response is probably less than 20%.

Factors that predict disease progression (as opposed to probability of response to interferon-based treatment) include:

Genetic Factors
Older age at acquisition
Coinfection with HIV
Metabolic syndrome and hepatic steatosis
Alcohol
Race – African Americans may have slower disease progression
Use of marijuana
Coffee consumption

Route of acquisition – drug use may be less severe than a blood transfusion (presumably because of the viral inoculum)
Immunosuppression
Amount of inflammation and fibrosis on biopsy

If this patient can stop using marijuana and lose weight to improve his metabolic syndrome and steatosis, he has other factors which would suggest that he is at lower risk of progression and can afford to defer treatment (although there is data that hepatitis C disease progression can accelerate with age).

References

1. Everhart JE, Lok AS, Kim HY, et al. Weight-related effects on disease progression in the hepatitis C antiviral long-term treatment against cirrhosis trial. Gastroenterology. 2009;137:549–57.
2. Wiley TE, Brown J, Chan J. Hepatitis C infection in African Americans: its natural history and histological progression. Am J Gastroenterol 2002;97:700–6.
3. Freedman ND, Everhart JE, Lindsay KL, et al. Coffee intake is associated with lower rates of liver disease progression in chronic hepatitis C. Hepatology 2009;50:1360–9.
4. Yano M, Kumada H, Kage M, et al. The long-term pathological evolution of chronic hepatitis C. Hepatology 1996;23:1334–40.

Case 24

A 21-year-old lady is referred to your outpatient office by her PCP for evaluation of abnormal liver enzymes. She is accompanied by her mother. She denies fever, chills, or abdominal pain, and has had no change in urine or stool color. Her appetite is good and her weight is stable. She denies GI bleeding or ascites.

Her past medical history is essentially unremarkable.

She takes no medications and denies herbal supplements.

She is living at home with her mother. She drinks and smokes occasionally and experimented with drugs 2–3 years ago. She did not finish high school and has several brushes with the local police force for disorderly behavior at the supermarket where she works. Her mother states that her divorce from the patient's father when she was only 14 affected her greatly as prior to this she was a model student.

There is no family history of liver disease.

The rest of her review of systems is negative.

On exam she looks well but looks nervous and uncomfortable but occasionally smiles at her mother. She is alert and oriented without asterixis.

Vital signs show BP 120/70, pulse 78 regular, and she is afebrile. Weight is 120 pounds.

There is no scleral icterus and no spider nevi.

Heart reveals normal S1 and S2 without added sounds. Chest reveals clear lung fields.

Her abdomen is soft and nontender. Her liver and spleen are impalpable. She has no ankle edema.

Laboratory Studies

Hb 11.6 g/dl
Platelets 153,000/μl
WBC 4.6 × 10^3/μl
INR 1.2
Creat 1.0 mg/dl
Tbili 2.1 mg/dl
AST 89 iu/l
ALT 47 iu/l
GGTP 67 iu/l
ALP 41 iu/l
Albumin 3.2 g/dl

Questions

1. What is the diagnosis?
2. How is the diagnosis confirmed?
3. What is the treatment for this condition?
4. How do you monitor response to treatment?

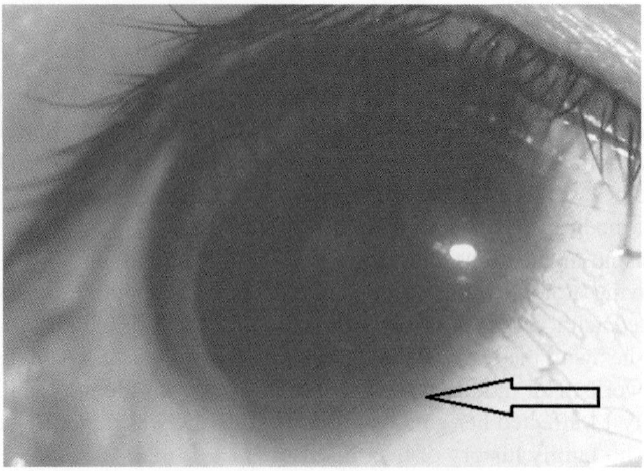

Fig. 24.1

Answer: Wilson Disease

Wilson disease (WD) is one of the favorite diagnoses of medical students due to the variety of clinical presentations (running the entire spectrum from abnormal liver tests to fulminant liver failure) and the Kayser–Fleischer (KF) ring. The images above show the brownish rings that are caused by deposition of granular deposits of copper in Descemet's membrane in the cornea. They are easily seen during a slit-light exam but occasionally can be seen with the naked eye. KF rings are seen in 50–90% of WD patients, with higher figures in those with neurological symptoms. The liver injury in WD is thought to be due to excess copper which facilitates the generation of free radicals that injure the liver. Excess copper leaks into the blood stream and accumulates in and damages other tissues and organs leading to a multisystem disease.

This lady presents with liver enzyme abnormalities that are typical for WD – mildly elevated AST and ALT (with AST higher), a low ALP (which is a good clue in patients presenting with acute liver failure who otherwise have very elevated transaminases), and mildly elevated bilirubin. She appears to be asymptomatic but her personality, odd affect, and difficulties at school and work point toward neuropsychiatric disease, which is seen in up to one-third of patients.

WD is an autosomal recessive disease and the genetic defect involves the copper transporting P-type ATPase (ATP7B) which impairs the formation of ceruloplasmin from apoceruloplasmin, a step that requires copper incorporation in the liver. This leads to a low circulating ceruloplasmin level.

The diagnosis of WD is essentially based on an appropriate clinical setting and laboratory tests, although there is no single test that clinches the diagnosis. The patient is usually a child or young adult (up to age 40) with abnormal liver enzymes and/or neuropsychiatric disease. Most patients have a KF ring. A low serum ceruloplasmin level (<20 mg/dl) is helpful, and a very low level (<5 mg/dl) in the setting of a KF ring is diagnostic. It should be remembered that a low ceruloplasmin level can be seen in other conditions including protein losing enteropathy, nephrotic syndrome, and advanced liver disease or cirrhosis from other causes.

Serum copper is usually decreased in WD but is not easy to measure and/or interpret the results due to the presence of ceruloplasmin and nonceruloplasmin-bound copper.

Twenty-four-hour urinary copper excretion is a useful test for the diagnosis of WD and for monitoring response to therapy. A level of >100 mcg (>1.6 μmol) is usual, and a level of >40 mcg should prompt further investigation.

Liver biopsy can be helpful in making a diagnosis but histology is similar to AIH and NASH, and a positive copper stain can be seen in other cholestatic diseases. A quantitative hepatic copper level of >250 mcg of copper per gram of dry weight (normal < 50 mcg/g of dry weight) is probably diagnostic.

Because of multiple mutations genetic testing is not always possible. However, haplotype linkage analysis may be useful for screening first-degree relatives if there is a specific mutation that can be identified.

Treatment should be for life and involves removing excess copper and then preventing reaccumulation. Copper chelation agents that are used include D-penicillamine, trientine, and zinc (which is used mainly as maintenance). Therapy is monitored by assessing 24 h urinary copper excretion which should be high for the first few months (>2,000 mcg) and then fall to lower levels (200–500 mcg) once excess copper has been removed.

References

1. Roberts EA, Schilsky ML. A practice guideline on Wilson disease. Hepatology 2003;37:1475.
2. Roberts EA, Schilsky ML. Diagnosis and treatment of Wilson disease: an update. Hepatology 2008;47:2089.

Case 25

A 44-year-lady is sent to your outpatient clinic by her primary care provider with a chief complaint of intermittent right upper quadrant pain for 3 months. She denies fever, chills, nausea, or diarrhea. Her liver enzymes are mild elevated.

Her past medical history is remarkable for hypertension and hyperlipidemia for which she takes lisinopril and simvastatin.

She is a married lady and comes to the appointment with her husband. She works in the local hospital as a phlebotomist. She is originally from Egypt and came to the USA 10 years ago. She does not smoke or drink.

Her family history is significant for her father dying of hepatocellular carcinoma (HCC) from cirrhosis secondary to hepatitis C.

On exam she looks anxious and her vital signs show a BMI 27 kg/m^2, BP 135/85, pulse 96, and she is afebrile.

There is no scleral icterus, palmar erythema, or spider nevi.

Her cardiovascular and respiratory systems are normal.

Her abdomen is soft and nontender. There is no ascites. The liver is enlarged felt 5 cm below the right costal margin. The spleen is impalpable.

Laboratory Parameters Show

WBC 8.1 × 10^3/ul
Hemoglobin 12 g/dl
Platelet 197,000/μl
INR 1.1
Tbili 1.8 mg/dl
AST 52 iu/l
ALT 57 iu/l
Creatinine 1.0 mg/dl

Questions

1. What is/are the next appropriate investigations?
2. How is this condition managed?

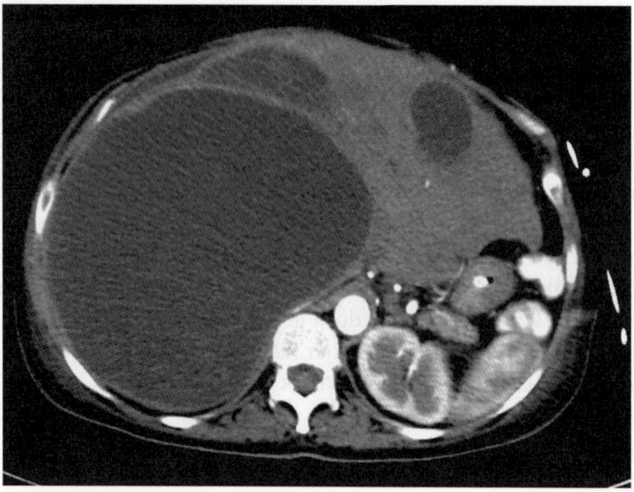

Fig. 25.1 CT of the abdomen

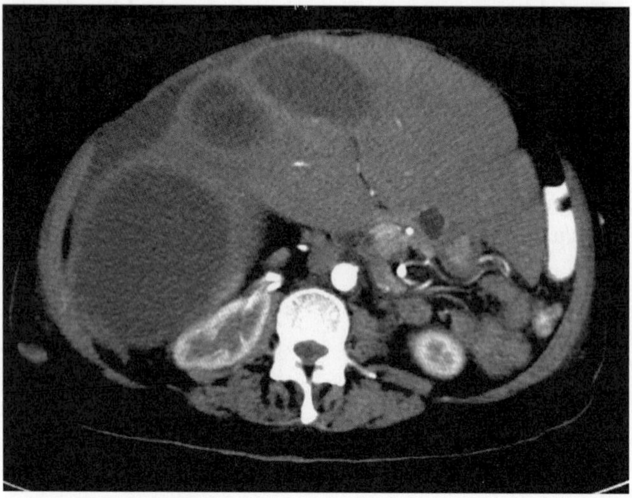

Fig. 25.2 CT of the abdomen

Answer: Echinococcal (Hydatid) Cysts in the Liver

This lady presents with several months of right upper quadrant discomfort and mildly elevated transaminases. The CT scan shows several lesions in the liver that have the density of fluid, hence they are cysts. The largest is 15–20 cm in the right lobe but the liver does not look cirrhotic and there is no ascites or portal hypertension. She is anxious because of her father who died of liver cancer and she is concerned she has something similar. The clue in this case is her ethnicity.

Echinococcal disease is caused by infection with the tapeworm *Echinococcus*. There are several species of *Echinococcus* that can produce infection in humans but *Echinococcus granulosus* typically leads to hepatic cysts. The disease is endemic in several areas of the world including South America, the Middle East, and parts of Sub-Saharan Africa and China, with a prevalence of up to 10–12% in rural areas. Canines are typically the definitive host of the parasite and humans are accidental hosts, infected through contact with infected feces.

The cyst itself is the fully developed metacestode of *E. granulosus* and is filled with fluid that is produced by the inner germinative layer of the cyst. Secondary cysts (brood capsules) bud off internally from this layer, and depending on the presence or absence of protoscolices (adult forms), they are either fertile or infertile.

The primary infection with *E. granulosus* is acquired typically in childhood and is asymptomatic for many years. Symptoms such as pain present when cysts enlarge due to a mass effect. The right lobe is usually affected. More severe symptoms can occur if the cyst presses on the biliary tree or hepatic vasculature or if the cyst ruptures or is secondarily infected.

The diagnosis is made on an appropriate clinical presentation and the presence of a positive *E. granulosus* antibody. Percutaneous aspiration is reserved for situations where the diagnosis is in doubt but is seldom employed because of the potential for anaphylaxis and secondary spread of the infection.

Treatment used to be entirely surgical but currently is a combination of medical therapy with albendazole, surgical removal or PAIR (percutaneous puncture of the cyst, aspiration of fluid, injection of hypertonic saline or ethanol into the cavity, and reaspiration after 15 min). Although comparative studies are limited, PAIR is increasingly used and appears to be very successful in experienced hands.

References

1. McManus DP, Zhang W, Li J, et al. Echinococcosis. Lancet 2003;362:1295–304.
2. Menezes da Silva A. Hydatid cyst of the liver – criteria for the selection of appropriate treatment. Acta Trop 2003;85:237–42.
3. Nasseri Moghaddam S, Abrishami A, Malekzadeh R. Percutaneous needle aspiration, injection, and reaspiration with or without benzimidazole coverage for uncomplicated hepatic hydatid cysts. Cochrane Database Syst Rev 2006;19(2):CD003623.

Case 26

A 30-year-old Caucasian female with congenital tricuspid atresia treated by a Fontan procedure (diversion of venous blood to pulmonary arteries) as an infant presents with increasing abdominal girth and weight over the past 6 months. The CT scan from an outside hospital reports a nodular liver suggestive of cirrhosis and ascites. The patient is transferred to your tertiary hospital for liver transplant evaluation. The patient's social and family histories are unremarkable.

On exam, she has scleral icterus and large abdominal ascites.

Laboratory Parameters Show

WBC 8.6 × 10^3/ul
Hemoglobin 9.8 g/dl
Platelet 68 × 10^3/ul
PT 12 seconds
Tbili 3.0 mg/dl
AST 24 u/l
ALT 33 u/l
Creatinine 1.2 mg/dl
Negative serologies for hepatitis B and C

Questions

1. What would a liver biopsy show?
2. What are the next appropriate tests?
3. Does this patient need transplant? If so, which organ.

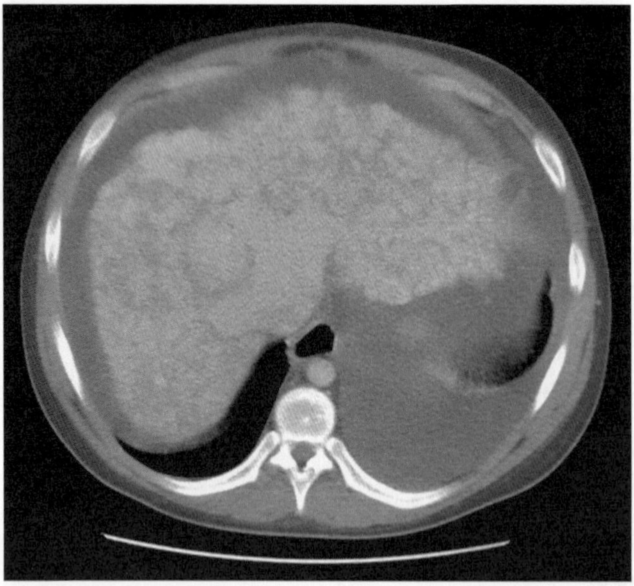

Fig. 26.1 CT scan

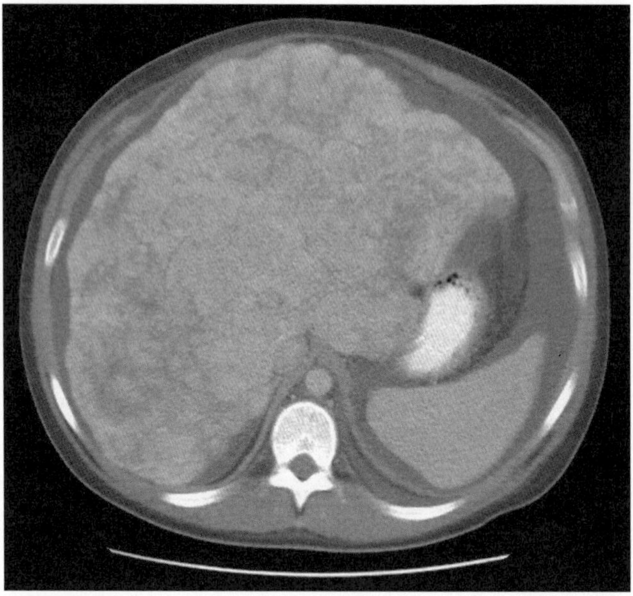

Fig. 26.2 CT scan

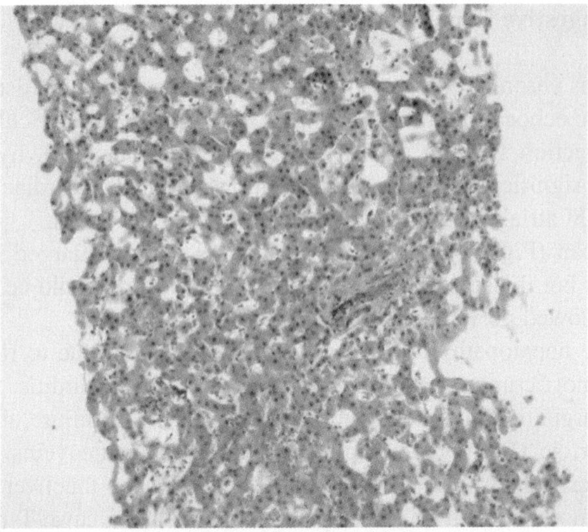

Fig. 26.3 H&E ×100

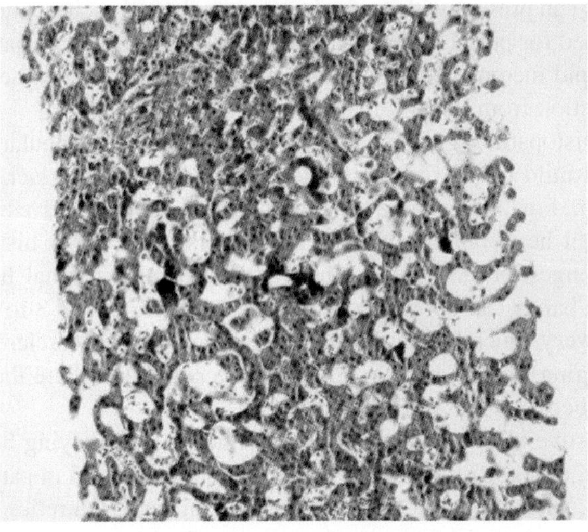

Fig. 26.4 Trichrome ×100

Answer: Congestive Hepatopathy

The patient has chronic right heart failure from congenital heart disease. She needs a transthoracic echocardiogram which showed normal left ventricular size and left ventricular ejection fraction (LVEF) 60%, no tricuspid valve, hypoplastic right ventricle, and significant right to left intracardiac shunt. The cardiac catheterization confirmed right atrial dilation and obstructed Fontan pathways.

The CT scan (Figs. 26.1 and 26.2) shows a nodular enlarged liver consistent with cirrhosis but the spleen is a normal size. Endoscopy could be performed and in this case showed no varices.

Congestive hepatopathy is passive hepatic congestion due to right-sided heart failure. The most common etiologies are constrictive pericarditis, mitral stenosis, tricuspid regurgitation, and cor pulmonale. In right heart failure, the transmission of right ventricle (RV) pressure directly into the hepatic veins causes passive hepatic congestion. In case of congestive hepatopathy, the liver appears to be enlarged and nodular with dilated hepatic veins and vena cava. Typically, patients have few symptoms although severe heart failure can lead to elevated liver enzymes and bilirubin and occasionally overt jaundice. The bilirubin is usually more elevated than would be suggested by the mild if any elevation in alkaline phosphatase. Chronic cases can present with tender hepatomegaly and ascites, and splenomegaly can be confused for portal hypertension from liver disease. A pulsatile liver can be seen in tricuspid incompetence and the hepatojugular reflex can be used to differentiate congestion from Budd–Chiari syndrome.

The liver histopathology (Fig. 26.3) shows marked centrilobular and sinusoidal dilatation and mild portal fibrosis without cirrhosis (note the lack of blue on the trichrome stain, Fig. 26.4). These are classic features of congestive hepatopathy due to chronic right heart failure. Nutmeg liver refers to the gross histology with red areas from congestion and contrasting yellow/brownish normal liver. In chronic cases, fibrous bands can extend from the central vein in zone 3 to the portal tract which looks very much like cirrhosis but is termed cardiac sclerosis and differs from the bridging fibrosis seen in advanced liver disease where the fibrous bands form bridges between portal tracts.

The congestive hepatopathy is reversible once the underlying heart problem is treated as long as significant fibrosis has not developed. Even in patients with "cardiac cirrhosis," decompensated liver disease is unusual. Diuretics can be used to reduce the preload to the heart, and can control ascites and reduce the hepatic congestion.

In this case, the patient was recommended to undergo a heart transplant evaluation instead of liver transplantation as the biopsy showed minimal fibrosis. Very occasionally combined heart liver transplant is required.

References

1. Giallourakis CC, Rosenberg PM, Friedman LS. Liver in heart failure. Clin Liver Dis 2002;6:947–67.
2. Myers RB, Spodick DH. Constrictive pericarditis: clinical and pathophysiologic characteristics. Am Heart J 1999;138:219–32.

Part II
Advanced Liver Disease

Cases 27–65

Case 27

A 73-year-old Caucasian woman presented with hematemesis. She had been diagnosed with cryptogenic cirrhosis several years previously but her disease was well compensated. She was seen at a local hospital and underwent esophagogastroduodenoscopy (EGD) that demonstrated no signs of esophageal varices but a large mass in the fundus and some nodular changes in the stomach. The concern was for a gastric malignancy. She is transfused and sent to you for further investigation.

Her other medical problems included hypertension for which she takes a diuretic. She denies prior surgery and does not drink alcohol or abuse drugs.

Her physical exam reveals a comfortable lady with stable vital signs. She is not icteric and her abdomen is soft and nontender. Her spleen is just palpable.

Laboratory Parameters When She is Seen After Transfer

Hb 11.6 g/dl
Platelets 94,000/μl
INR 1.3
Creatinine 0.8 mg/dl
Tbili 1.0 mg/dl
AST 71 iu/l
ALT 23 iu/l
ALP 48 iu/l
Albumin 2.8 g/dl

During the night she develops further hematemesis. She is moved to intensive care and adequately resuscitated.

Questions

1. What is the differential diagnosis?
2. Which test(s) are indicated?
3. What is the best management scenario?

J. Ahmad, *Hepatology and Transplant Hepatology: A Case Based Approach*,
DOI 10.1007/978-1-4419-7085-5_2,

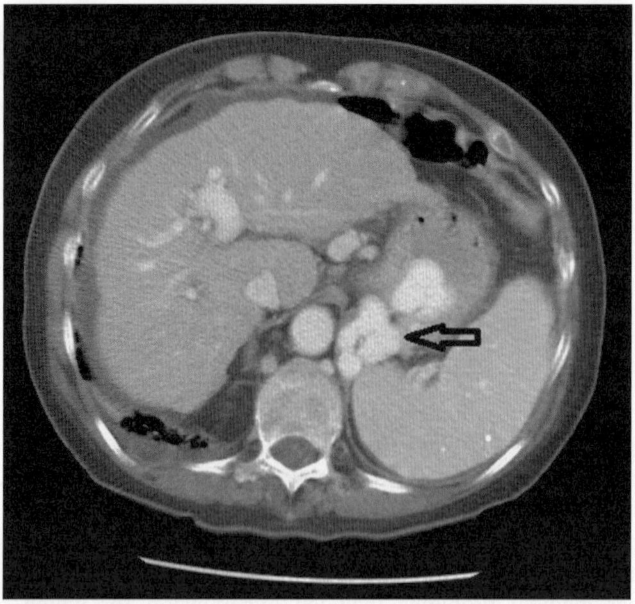

Fig. 27.1 CT scan

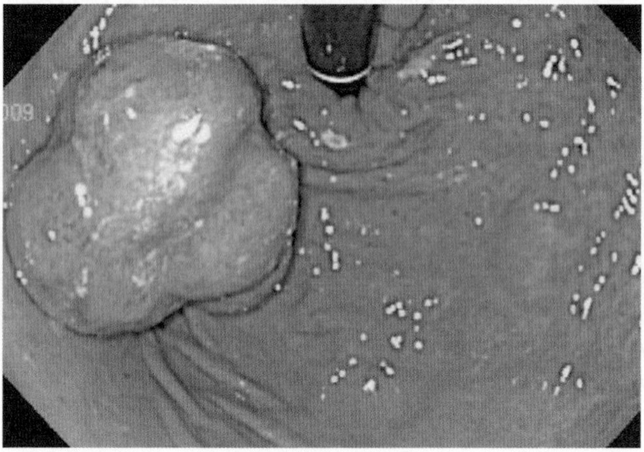

Fig. 27.2 EGD image

Answer: Large Fundal Varices

The CT scan (with i.v. contrast, Fig. 27.1) demonstrates large varices filling in the proximal stomach which are confirmed on the EGD image (Fig. 27.2). The liver has a nodular contour consistent with cirrhosis and there is minimal ascites. The endoscopic image has the scope in a retroflexed position and shows a mass in the fundus which could be confused with a tumor.

The differential diagnosis is essentially all causes of GI bleeding, but these should be separated into portal hypertensive and non-portal hypertensive causes in a patient with known cirrhosis. The latter will include ulcer disease, malignancy, and a Dieulafoy lesion, while the former includes variceal bleeding (esophageal or gastric) and severe portal hypertensive gastropathy.

The laboratory values suggest well-compensated disease but this does not exclude significant portal hypertension.

The initial work up should include an imaging study such as a CT scan or ultrasound scan (USS) (with Doppler). The latter is important to document the patency of the portal vein. However, after adequate resuscitation, repeat EGD is required. Pharmacological therapy with intravenous octreotide should be standard in patients with suspected portal hypertensive bleeding and should be started prior to the EGD, and antibiotics have also been shown to reduce mortality in this situation.

The patient has isolated gastric varices and several red spots are seen on the EGD image which are indicative of recent bleeding. Endoscopic treatment of isolated gastric varices is of limited benefit, although cyanoacrylate has shown some promise (but is not available in the United States). Band ligation of such large varices would be inadvisable but could be tried if the varices were smaller (which is a judgment call).

If the portal vein is open, the patient should undergo transjugular intrahepatic portosystemic shunting (TIPS) which controls bleeding in the majority of cases. Hence, it is important to document portal vein patency prior to EGD if possible since this will influence how aggressive you should be with endoscopic treatment.

References

1. Garcia-Tsao G, Sanyal AJ, Grace ND et al. Prevention and management of gastroesophageal varices and variceal hemorrhage in cirrhosis. Hepatology 2007;46:922–38.
2. Chau TN, Patch D, Chan YW et al. "Salvage" transjugular intrahepatic portosystemic shunts: gastric fundal compared with esophageal variceal bleeding. Gastroenterology 1998;114:981–7.

Case 28

A 54-year-old man presents for liver transplant evaluation. He has a history of cirrhosis secondary to hepatitis C and alcohol. His liver disease has been complicated by ascites and encephalopathy and he has small varices although no history of GI bleeding.

His past medical history is unremarkable without evidence of diabetes, heart or lung disease, or prior surgeries. Medications include diuretics and lactulose.

He has a remote history of drug use and quit drinking over a year ago when he first developed ascites. He is married with grown up children and is still working in a local hardware store. His family history is unremarkable.

His review of symptoms is significant for mild abdominal discomfort and ankle edema. He has some mild shortness of breath and has noticed decreased exercise tolerance over the last year and he has had to take a lighter schedule at work.

On exam he is alert and oriented. His vital signs are normal with BP 120/75, pulse 106 and regular and he is afebrile. His respiratory rate is 22 per min. He has significant palmar erythema and multiple spider nevi on his face, anterior and posterior upper trunk. There is no scleral icterus.

Cardiovascular system reveals normal heart sounds and an added sound immediately after the second heart sound. Chest reveals clear lung fields. He is more comfortable lying flat. He has a liver edge palpable 2–3 cm below the right costal margin but no splenomegaly. There is dullness in the flanks and +ankle edema.

Laboratory Studies

Hb 12.3 g/dl
Platelets 73,000/μl
WBC 6.2 × 10^3/μl
INR 1.3
Creatinine 1.1 mg/dl
Tbili 1.4 mg/dl
AST 37 iu/l
ALT 34 iu/l
GGTP 83 iu/l
ALP 89 iu/l
Albumin 2.6 g/dl
Chest X-ray normal

Questions

1. As well as the standard work up for liver transplant are there any other tests you would consider?
2. What is the significance of his cardiac exam?
3. How is the diagnosis confirmed?
4. What is the prognosis after transplant and what is it based on?

O_2 saturation on room air 91%

pH 7.42
PaO_2 54 mmHg
$PaCO_2$ 28mmHg

Aa gradient (on room air)
$= (150 - 5/4(PaCO_2)) - PaO_2$
= 61 mmHg

Answer: Hepatopulmonary Syndrome

This patient's O_2 saturation on room air in the absence of lung or heart disease is suggestive of hepatopulmonary syndrome (HPS) which is a diagnosis that is frequently undetected. Patients undergoing liver transplant evaluation should have an arterial blood gas.

HPS is defined by an increased alveolar–arterial gradient on room air with evidence of intrapulmonary vascular abnormalities or dilatations (IPVDs) occurring in patients with liver disease and in the absence of intrinsic lung disease. IPVDs are thought to arise due to poor clearance or excess production of pulmonary vasodilators and inhibition of circulating vasoconstrictors by the cirrhotic liver likely mediated through nitric oxide. The resultant dilation of the pulmonary vasculature leads to a large right to left shunt, which is not a true anatomical shunt as it partially responds to increased FiO_2.

The prevalence of HPS varies but it is thought to be 5–50% in cirrhotic patients. HPS can also occur in non-cirrhotic portal hypertension and occasionally acute liver disease. Mild abnormalities are very common. If the PaO_2 is less than 60 mmHg, this is very suggestive of HPS in patients with cirrhosis and no underlying cardiopulmonary disease.

HPS typically presents with dyspnea but often is initially asymptomatic and underdiagnosed. There does not appear to be a correlation between severity of liver disease and degree of hypoxemia although HPS is an independent predictor of death in patients with cirrhosis.

This patient's cardiac exam shows evidence of a hyperdynamic circulation and in HPS there is usually an elevated cardiac output, decreased systemic and pulmonary vascular resistance, and decreased arterial-mixed venous oxygen content difference. As HPS progresses it can lead to decreased oxygenation induced by changes in posture such as platypnea – increase in dyspnea when sitting or standing upright and relieved by lying down or orthodeoxia – desaturation in the upright position relieved in a recumbent position.

The reason it is important to make a diagnosis of HPS is that it negatively impacts outcome after liver transplantation, particularly with a PaO_2 less than 60 mmHg.

The diagnosis can be confirmed in several ways. Contrast-enhanced echocardiography is used to document the presence of IVPDs. This can be performed with dye (indocyanine green) or agitated saline producing bubbles (bubble echo). In the absence of shunts, the dye/bubbles should only be seen in the right heart as the dye/bubbles do not clear the pulmonary capillary circulation. With a right to left shunt, the dye/bubbles will be seen in the left heart, within 3 heartbeats for an intracardiac shunt and 3–6 heartbeats for an intrapulmonary shunt.

Other methods for the detection of shunting include technetium labeled macroaggregated albumin (MAA) scanning. The labeled MAA should not traverse the pulmonary capillary bed but will be seen in the kidneys or brain, if intracardiac or intrapulmonary shunting is present. Pulmonary angiography should be reserved for cases where the diagnosis is still not certain after contrast echocardiography or MAA scan.

Routine chest imaging is typically normal in HPS. Lung function assessments can be abnormal although in a non-specific pattern. The diffusion capacity for carbon monoxide (DLCO) is usually decreased. Arterial blood gases in HPS are abnormal. A PaO_2 of less than 80 mmHg on room air is usual and the Aa gradient is usually greater than 20 mmHg.

The shunt fraction gives an estimate of the degree of shunting and requires measuring the PaO_2 while breathing 100% O_2 for 20 min. The formula is:

$$Qs/Qt = ([PAO_2 - PaO_2] \times 0.003)/[([PAO_2 - PaO_2] \times 0.003)+5]$$

where Qs is the shunt flow and Qt is the total flow and PAO_2 is the alveolar partial pressure of oxygen and PaO_2 is the arterial partial pressure of oxygen.

The normal shunt fraction is 5%. Anything above 20–30% increases the risk of poor outcome after transplantation.

The only effective treatment for HPS is liver transplantation. Case reports detail the use of various agents including somatostatin analogues, methylene blue and indomethacin and are usually unsuccessful. TIPS has also been tried with limited improvement.

Several case series have documented good outcome after liver transplantation in selected patients with HPS. Although survival is not at levels seen in patients without HPS, the survival benefit of transplant is significant. Resolution of HPS after transplant is variable and can be seen after a few days or up to a year.

Most patients will need a model for end stage liver disease (MELD) exception as biological MELD scores are seldom at a level where transplant is likely, particularly in patients with blood type A or O.

References

1. Hoeper MM, Krowka MJ, Strassburg CP. Portopulmonary hypertension and hepatopulmonary syndrome. Lancet 2004;363:1461.
2. Krowka MJ, Mandell MS, Ramsay MA et al. Hepatopulmonary syndrome and portopulmonary hypertension: a report of the multicenter liver transplant database. Liver Transpl 2004;10:174.

Case 29

A 51-year-old man presents to the emergency room complaining of difficulty swallowing for the last few hours. He has a history of alcoholic cirrhosis and continues to drink. His liver disease has been complicated by variceal bleeding in the past and he has undergone band ligation of grade II esophageal varices, the last being 3 months ago but did not follow-up for a repeat session. He also has ascites controlled on diuretics and some mild encephalopathy.

According to his girlfriend who is with him he has been otherwise well without fever, abdominal pain or weight loss. He was out with a group of friends at a local bar drinking heavily when he first noted the symptoms but he is still intoxicated and difficult to comprehend.

His exam demonstrates normal vital signs. He is alert but mildly confused. There are no localizing neurological signs and his abdomen is mildly distended with normal bowel sounds. He has mild ankle edema.

Laboratory Studies

Hb 10.6 g/dl
Platelets 58,000/μl
INR 1.7
Creatinine 1.4 mg/dl
Tbili 3.3 mg/dl
AST 48 iu/l
ALT 17 iu/l
Albumin 2.4 g/dl

Questions

1. Is an endoscopy indicated or should he undergo imaging with oral contrast first?
2. If yes-how should the patient be sedated?

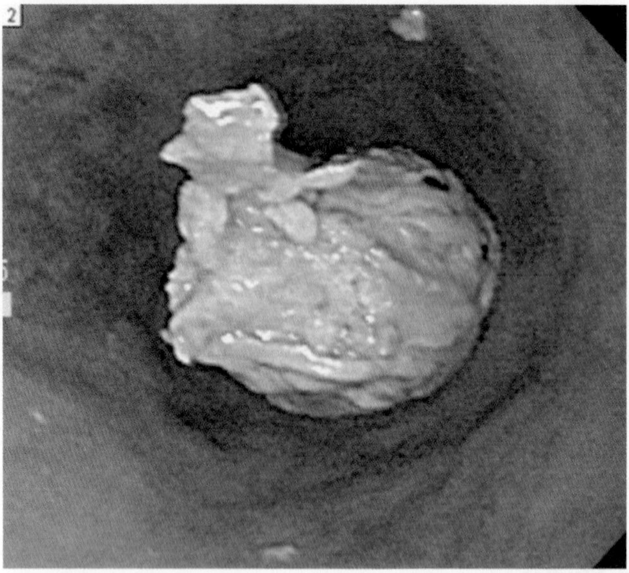

Fig. 29.1 EGD image

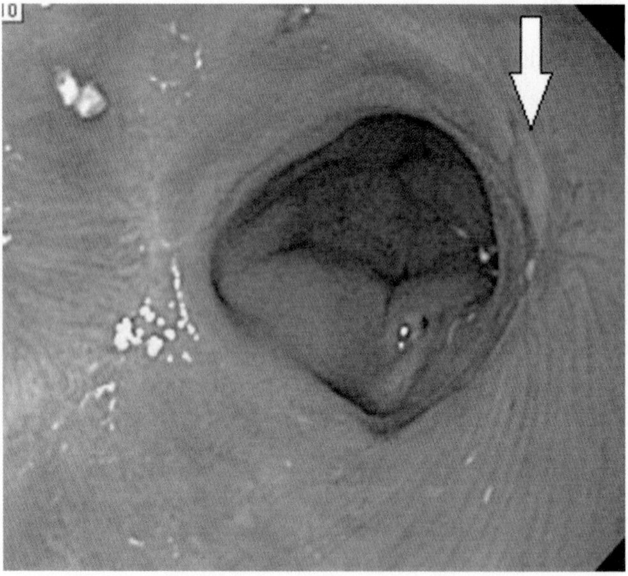

Fig. 29.2 EGD image

Answer: Esophageal Stricture Secondary to Band Ligation

This man is not doing himself any favors. He has decompensated cirrhosis and yet continues to drink. He has developed dysphagia and the sudden onset is suggestive of a food bolus impaction. A contrast study in this situation would be inadvisable due to the risk of aspiration. This will also be an issue in terms of sedating the patient if an EGD is planned.

The patient actually underwent EGD under general anesthesia, since we were concerned about airway protection in the event of a bolus impaction, but also given his inebriated state. In general, anesthesiologists I have worked with would much prefer to intubate a patient like this rather than use moderate sedation. This patient may have proved particularly difficult to sedate using midazolam. Propofol would be an option but the airway would not be protected. There is some literature comparing moderate sedation with general anesthesia in this situation that suggests no real difference in outcome, but I would caution against sedation without airway protection in such a patient.

The images show a food bolus (Fig. 29.1; he was eating chicken wings with the beer) that was easily removed but there was an underlying stricture as seen in Fig. 29.2 with the arrow pointing to a pressure ulcer. The stricture was from repeated banding, which is actually surprisingly uncommon. Reviewing the literature on many studies of banding, strictures are very uncommon, particularly compared to sclerotherapy.

The patient still had varices proximal to the stricture and underwent dilation using a 10 mm pneumatic balloon with some relief. He was instructed to chew thoroughly and drink plenty of fluid with meals (not alcohol!). There is no literature on the best way to dilate such a stricture but we felt it was safer to use a balloon and avoid the proximal varices rather than Savary or Maloney push dilators.

References

1. Schmitz RJ, Sharma P, Badr AS et al. Incidence and management of esophageal stricture formation, ulcer bleeding, perforation, and massive hematoma formation from sclerotherapy versus band ligation. Am J Gastroenterol 2001;96:437–41.
2. Villanueva C, Miñana J, Ortiz J et al. Endoscopic ligation compared with combined treatment with nadolol and isosorbide mononitrate to prevent recurrent variceal bleeding. N Engl J Med 2001;345:647–55.

Case 30

A 52-year-old man presents to your clinic for follow-up. He has a history of cirrhosis secondary to hepatitis C and alcohol but has been abstinent for several years. His hepatitis C was treated in the past with pegylated interferon but he did not respond.

His disease has been well compensated without ascites or encephalopathy, although he has small varices on endoscopy. It has been over a year since his last visit.

He has no past medical history and is only taking some milk thistle. He is not working and continues to smoke. He has a remote history of intravenous drug use.

On exam, his vital signs demonstrate weight 205 pounds, BP 120/70, pulse 65 and he is afebrile. He has mild palmar erythema, no scleral icterus and normal cardiovascular and respiratory systems.

Abdominal exam demonstrates a palpable liver edge and a spleen tip but no ascites and no ankle edema. He has no asterixis.

Laboratory Studies

Hb 12.5 g/dl
Platelets 64,000/μl
INR 1.5
Creatinine 1.2 mg/dl
Tbili 1.9 mg/dl
AST 47 iu/l
ALT 34 iu/l
ALP 112 iu/l
Albumin 2.7 g/dl
AFP 12ng/ml

Questions

1. What options, if any are available to this patient?
2. Is he a candidate for liver transplant?

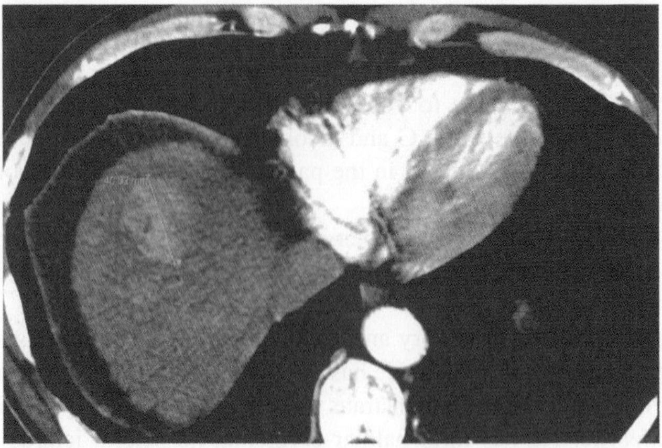

Fig. 30.1 CT scan

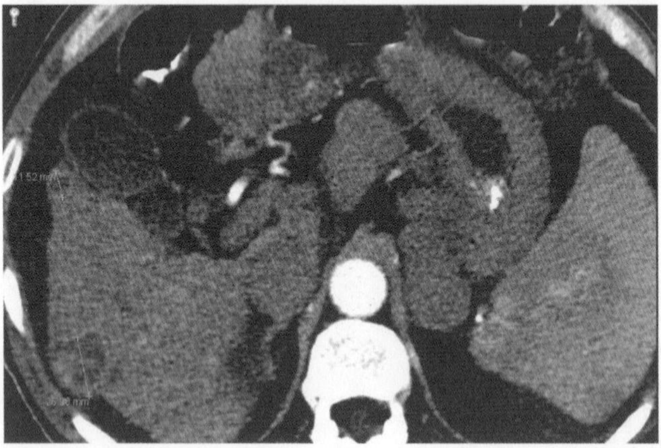

Fig. 30.2 CT scan

Answer: Multifocal Hepatocellular Carcinoma

This gentleman has developed at least three lesions in the liver. The largest is hypervascular and is shown in the first image. It measures 4 cm in diameter. Two smaller lesions are seen in the lower image and appear not to enhance but still are suspicious for hepatocellular carcinoma (HCC). The liver has a nodular contour and the spleen is enlarged consistent with cirrhosis and portal hypertension.

The approach to HCC is well described in American Association for the Study of Liver Diseases (AASLD) guidelines (referenced below). The important points to remember are that biopsy is seldom required to make a diagnosis. Any hypervascular lesion in a cirrhotic liver is considered to be HCC until proven otherwise and biopsy runs the risk of seeding the needle track with HCC cells. I have seen a case of recurrent HCC in the abdominal wall of a patient after liver transplant that had had a liver biopsy a year prior to transplant.

The size and number of lesions are important. A seminal paper published in the 1990s established the Milan criteria that determined that patients with a single lesion less than 5 cm, or three lesions less than 3 cm without vascular invasion or metastases, had good 4-year survival after liver transplant, compared to patients transplanted beyond these criteria. Based on this, the current MELD organ allocation system in the USA allows for an exception of 22 points if the patient's actual MELD score is lower than this (which is invariably the case) in patients who have a T2 tumor (so within Milan criteria but also a single lesion needs to be greater than 2 cm in diameter).

Other studies have suggested that the Milan criteria are too strict and lesions up to 6.5 cm should be considered for transplant (the UCSF criteria) and some regions in the USA would provide a MELD exception for lesions this size.

The options for this patient are limited. He could get chemoembolization or radiofrequency ablation of the larger lesion. Systemic chemotherapy is rarely effective for HCC.

A live donor liver transplant is still an option for this patient since he would not need a MELD exception for a deceased donor organ. However, it should be made clear to the patient and the donor that there is a very significant risk of HCC recurrence.

References

1. Mazzaferro V, Regalia E, Doci R et al. Liver transplantation for the treatment of small hepatocellular carcinomas in patients with cirrhosis. N Engl J Med 1996;334:693–9.
2. Bruix J, Sherman M. Management of hepatocellular carcinoma. Hepatology 2005;42:1208–36.

Case 31

A 46-year-old male presents to the ER with pain and abdominal distension. He has a history of alcoholic cirrhosis that has been complicated by ascites, encephalopathy and the presence of esophageal varices on endoscopy although he denies any bleeding.

For the last 24 h, he has experienced increasing abdominal pain, mainly periumbilical with nausea and vomiting. He has had no fever.

He is currently on a small dose of diuretics, lactulose, and nadolol.

He still smokes but quit drinking about a year ago. His ex-wife is with him but his social situation is poor as he lives alone and has recently lost his job. He has no children.

On exam, he has mild tachycardia but normal blood pressure. He is afebrile. He has mild scleral icterus.

His cardiovascular and respiratory systems are normal. His abdomen is distended with a fluid thrill but is tympanitic with increased bowel sounds. He has a 4–5 cm umbilical hernia that is tender and can be reduced with difficulty.

Laboratory Studies

Hb 12.4 g/dl
Platelets 59,000/μl
INR 1.6
WBC 13.5 × 10^3/μl
Tbili 3.1 mg/dl
AST 48 iu/l
ALT 32 iu/l
ALP 89 iu/l
Albumin 2.8 g/dl
Creatinine 2.4 mg/dl

Plain abdominal films show small bowel with air–fluid levels and a decompressed colon.

Questions

1. Does this patient need any further testing?
2. What is important to calculate?
3. Should this patient undergo surgery?
4. What if the hernia becomes strangulated, does this change the decision?

Calculated MELD score: 24

Answer: Risk Assessment in Cirrhotic Patients Undergoing Surgery

This is a common scenario in a busy hospital. A patient with liver disease who has a condition that likely needs surgery, in this case small bowel obstruction from his umbilical hernia.

He really does not need any other investigation but he needs nasogastric suction, intravenous fluids and analgesia as required and hopefully he will improve with these conservative measures. The problem will arise if he does not improve or if the clinical situation deteriorates such as strangulation of the hernia.

In general, elective surgery should be avoided in patients with decompensated liver disease. Several predictive models exist to determine the risk of morbidity and mortality after surgery in such patients, but the risk depends on the severity of liver disease and also the type and urgency of the surgery. This patient has a Child–Pugh score of 10 or 11 making him a Child's C and his MELD score is given as 24. He is at very high risk of decompensation and surgery should be avoided if at all possible. However, if he worsens and has a potentially fatal disorder (strangulated hernia would count), then he needs to be operated on.

Several studies have quantified the risk depending on the type or surgery and its urgency. In cirrhotic patients undergoing abdominal surgery, Child's class A, B, and C correspond to postoperative mortality of 10, 30, and 80%, respectively. The Child–Pugh score is somewhat subjective and in recent years, the MELD score has been used to assess mortality in liver patients. The MELD score incorporates three biochemical measurements into a complex logarithmic formula – the total bilirubin concentration, serum creatinine, and the international normalized ration (INR). Patient scores range from 6 to 40, with 6 reflecting "early" disease and 40 "severe" disease. The largest study of almost 800 cirrhotic patients undergoing major digestive, orthopedic, or cardiac surgery demonstrated that the MELD score correlated with short-term and long-term mortality extending out to 20 years. For each point increase in the MELD score above 8, there was a 14% increase in 30-day and 90-day mortality. The type of surgery is important but all emergent surgery increases the risk.

Unfortunately, it is all too common to see a patient in the liver clinic who was referred for decompensated liver disease who states that they were completely well until they underwent elective surgery several months ago, or worse still, someone is transferred from another institution as an inpatient and had a recent umbilical hernia repair and now is draining ascites from the wound and has developed hepatorenal syndrome (HRS).

The reasons for worsening of liver disease after surgery are unclear but may reflect circulatory changes brought on by surgery or anesthesia resulting in impaired hepatic vascular flow.

References

1. Malik SM, Ahmad J. Preoperative risk assessment for patients with liver disease. Med Clin North Am 2009;93:917–29.
2. Teh SH, Nagorney DM, Stevens SR et al. Risk factors for mortality after surgery in patients with cirrhosis Gastroenterology 2007;132:1609–1611.

Case 32

A 30-year-old Filipino woman presents with a 4-month history of progressive fatigue, jaundice, severe, generalized pruritus, dark urine, and pale stool. She has no history of abdominal pain, nausea, vomiting, no prior history of jaundice or viral hepatitis. She takes no medications and there is no family history of liver disease. She has had a prior cholecystectomy.

Physical examination reveals excoriations on skin from scratching. She has marked scleral icterus, no hepatosplenomegaly or ascites. No cutaneous stigmata of chronic liver disease.

Lab Results

Total bilirubin 19 mg/dl
Direct bilirubin 13.7 mg/dl
ALP 1833 iu/l
GGTP 1756 iu/l
ALT 194 iu/l
AST 216 iu/l
Albumin 3.2 g/dl
Prothrombin time 21 seconds

Ultrasound shows mild hepatomegaly. There is no biliary ductal dilation, patent hepatic vessels, absent gall bladder, no splenomegaly or ascites.

Questions

1. How would one classify the pattern of this patient's jaundice and abnormal liver enzyme elevation?
2. What is the differential diagnosis?
3. What additional diagnostic procedure should be performed?

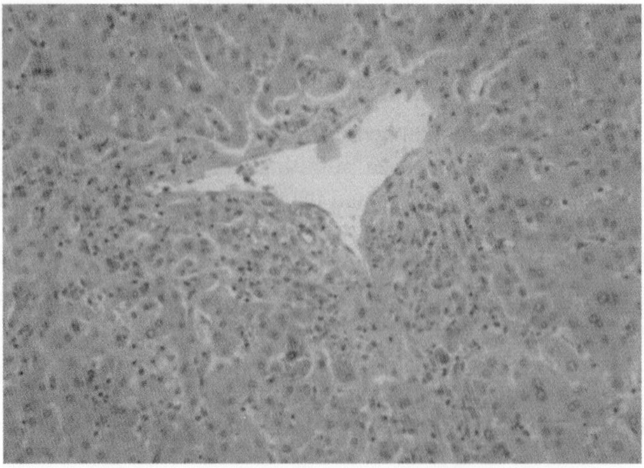

Fig. 32.1 Liver biopsy H&E ×200

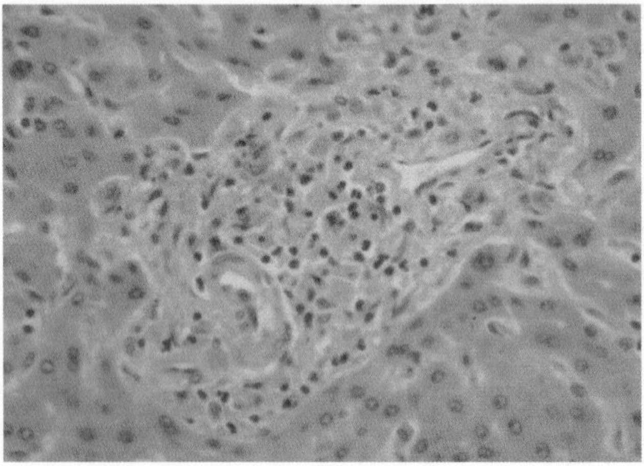

Fig. 32.2 Liver biopsy H&E ×400

Answer: Idiopathic Adulthood Ductopenia

This patient has cholestatic jaundice and more specifically *intrahepatic* cholestasis by virtue of the fact that the ultrasound does not demonstrate biliary ductal dilation.

Additional blood tests showed negative ANA, ASMA, and AMA. Her serum ACE level was normal and quantitative immunoglobulins revealed normal IgG and IgM levels.

Due to concern for a biliary process despite the negative ultrasound, she underwent an ERCP but the cholangiogram was normal without evidence of biliary duct beading or strictures.

The images show her liver biopsy. The first is at low power (Fig. 32.1) demonstrating brownish deposits, consistent with severe chronic cholestasis. There is also an absence of interlobular bile ducts in the portal area.

At higher power (Fig. 32.2), a portal tract is seen and confirms the absence of bile ducts and the presence of a mild chronic inflammatory infiltrate, including lymphocytes, neutrophils, and plasma cells.

The differential diagnosis is lengthy and includes:

Primary biliary cirrhosis (PBC)
Small duct primary sclerosing cholangitis (PSC)
Autoimmune cholangitis
Drug-induced cholestasis
Ischemic bile duct damage
Benign recurrent intrahepatic cholestasis
Cholestasis of pregnancy
Infectious cholangiopathy
Total parenteral nutrition
Sepsis-related cholestasis
Chronic liver allograft rejection
Graft versus host disease
Infiltrative disorders: sarcoidosis, amyloid, cystic fibrosis, lymphoma
Idiopathic adulthood ductopenia

As can be seen, all autoimmune serologies were negative and many of the other possible diagnoses were excluded as they were not clinically applicable.

A liver biopsy confirmed extreme paucity of bile ducts and a diagnosis of *idiopathic adulthood ductopenia* was made. The patient underwent successful orthotopic liver transplantation.

This condition was first described by Jurgen Ludwig in 1988, is similar to the infantile condition, Alagille's syndrome and has an obscure natural history. Orthotopic liver transplantation is the only effective treatment. It is diagnosed in an adult patient with biochemical cholestasis, biopsy evidence of ductopenia (loss of interlobular or septal bile ducts in at least 50% of portal tracts). The diagnosis also requires a negative AMA, normal cholangiogram, no history of infantile cholestasis, no exposure to drugs or toxins that could produce cholangitis and no evidence of sarcoidosis or malignancy.

References

1. Ludwig J, Wiesner RH, La Russo NF. Idiopathic adulthood ductopenia: a cause of chronic cholestatic liver disease and biliary cirrhosis. J Hepatol 1988;7:193–9.
2. Sherlock S. The syndrome of disappearing intrahepatic bile ducts. Lancet 1987;2:493–6.

Case 33

A 47-year-old male presents with several episodes of hematemesis and melena. He has a history of cirrhosis secondary to alcohol and hepatitis C, which has been complicated in the past by multiple admissions for variceal hemorrhage, encephalopathy, and ascites. He continues to drink alcohol and has been very noncompliant in terms of follow-up.

He has previously undergone band ligation of esophageal varices and a TIPS was placed 2 years ago. He has also undergone coil embolization of gastric varices and several revisions of his TIPS, the last being several months ago.

He has not taken any prescribed medication for more than a month after his prescriptions ran out.

Exam demonstrates a disheveled looking man with a BP of 120/80 and pulse 104 beats per minute, regular.

He is alert and oriented and his abdomen is mildly distended. Melena is noted on rectal exam.

Laboratory Parameters

Hb 7.6 g/dl
Platelets 62,000/μl
INR 1.5
Creatinine 0.8 mg/dl
Tbili 2.5 mg/dl
AST 88 iu/l
ALT 48 iu/l
GGTP 495 iu/l

After adequate resuscitation, he undergoes upper GI endoscopy that demonstrates small esophageal varices but large varices in the cardia with red wale signs but no active bleeding. Imaging a month ago had shown a patent TIPS and a significant splenorenal shunt.

Question

1. What treatment options are available for this patient (in the USA)?

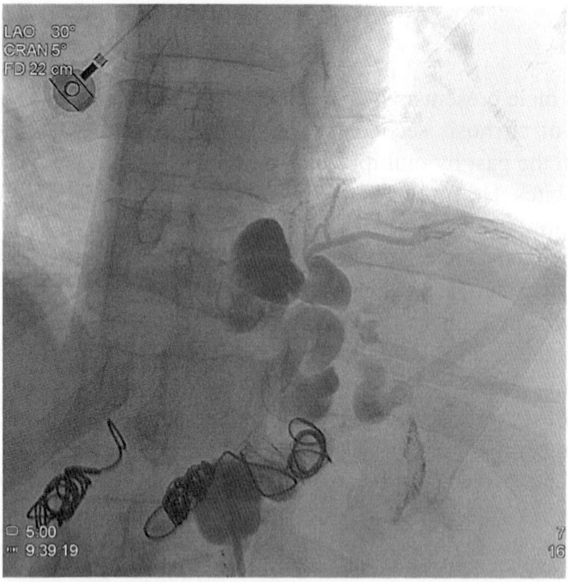

Fig. 33.1 Angiogram pre-treatment

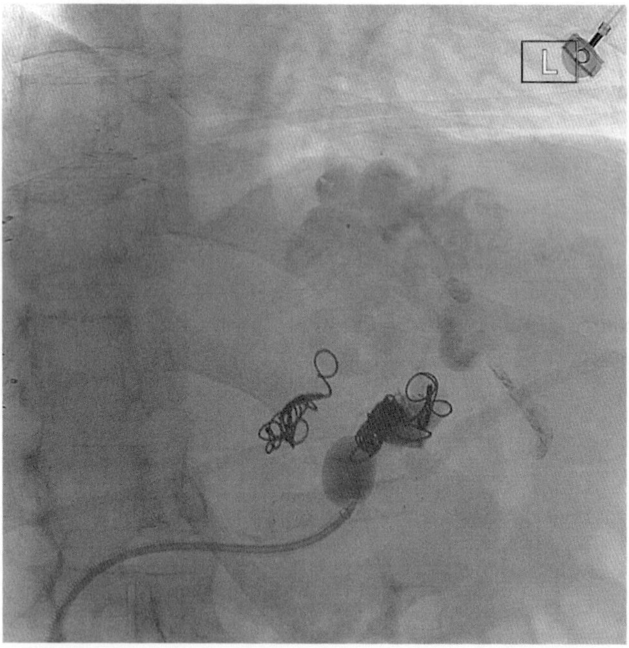

Fig. 33.2 Angiogram post-treatment

Answer: Balloon Occluded Retrograde Transvenous Obliteration of Varices

This gentleman continues to bleed despite aggressive treatment. He has undergone endoscopic therapy and also TIPS and then an attempt at coil embolization of gastric varices with access through the TIPS. His endoscopy shows gastric varices with stigmata of recent bleeding and he has a low hemoglobin. His continued drinking and poor compliance mean that he is not a good transplant candidate.

His options are limited, particularly in the USA, where cyanoacrylate is not available outside of a study setting.

One potential solution that is increasingly used in Asia is balloon occluded retrograde transvenous obliteration (BRTO). This procedure involves passing a catheter into the inferior vena cava through the femoral vein. The catheter is passed into the left renal vein and then the splenic vein through a splenorenal shunt. The gastric varices can be identified coming off the splenic vein and a balloon is inflated and foam or coils can be deployed to prevent retrograde flow.

In Figs. 33.1 and 33.2, previously place coils can be seen. A catheter is visible with a balloon inflated and filling of large gastric varices is readily apparent. Figure 33.2 was taken 20 min after the injection of a foam sclerosant into the varices and markedly reduced flow is seen.

The patient did well for several months after this but expired from other complications of his liver disease.

There is limited data comparing BRTO with other modalities of treatment. One study compared BRTO to cyanoacrylate injection and found similar initial success rates but noted increased rebleeding with injection therapy.

Complications of BRTO include balloon rupture such that sclerosant can leak into the systemic circulation and can cause pulmonary embolism or recurrent gastric variceal bleeding due to the sclerosant not obliterating the varices. In addition, there is some data that the portosystemic pressure gradient can rise following BRTO with concomitant worsening of esophageal varices.

References

1. Hong CH, Kim HJ, Park JH et al. Treatment of patients with gastric variceal hemorrhage: endoscopic N-butyl-2-cyanoacrylate injection versus balloon-occluded retrograde transvenous obliteration. J Gastroenterol Hepatol 2009;24:372–8.
2. Park SJ, Chung JW, Kim HC et al. The prevalence, risk factors, and clinical outcome of balloon rupture in balloon-occluded retrograde transvenous obliteration of gastric varices. J Vasc Interv Radiol 2010;21:503–7.

Case 34

A 28-year-old woman is admitted to the ICU with a 2-week history of abdominal pain, nausea, vomiting, generalized malaise, and fevers to 103°F. There is no history of bleeding or confusion.

There is no relevant prior medical problems and no history of prescription or over the counter/herbal medications, including no acetaminophen. She denies recent travel or sick contacts. There is no history of alcohol, drugs, tattoos, or blood transfusions.

Physical examination reveals a young woman with mild icterus, no oral mucocutaneous lesions, no stigmata of chronic liver disease. Vital signs show she is febrile to 102°F, blood pressure 110/60, HR 95.

Her abdomen has mild diffuse tenderness with no guarding or rebound. No hepatosplenomegaly or ascites is appreciated. She is alert and oriented without asterixis.

Admission Lab Results

Total bilirubin 2.9 mg/dl
AST 20,300 iu/l
ALT 14,050 iu/l
ALP 93 iu/l
GGTP 250 iu/l
Albumin 3.0 g/dl
INR 10.6 (PT 117 s)
WBC 23.2 (25% bands)
Platelets 55 × 10^9
Hgb 13.4 g/dl
Creatinine 0.7 mg/dl

Questions

1. What is this patient's clinical diagnosis?
2. What is the differential diagnosis for her elevated LFT's?
3. How should she be managed?

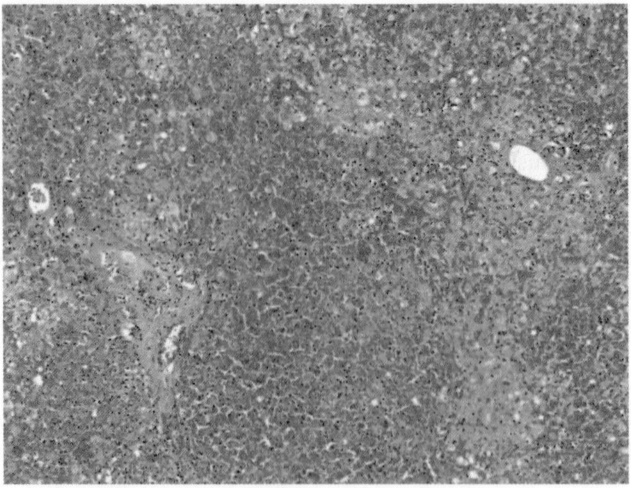

Fig. 34.1 Liver biopsy H&E ×100

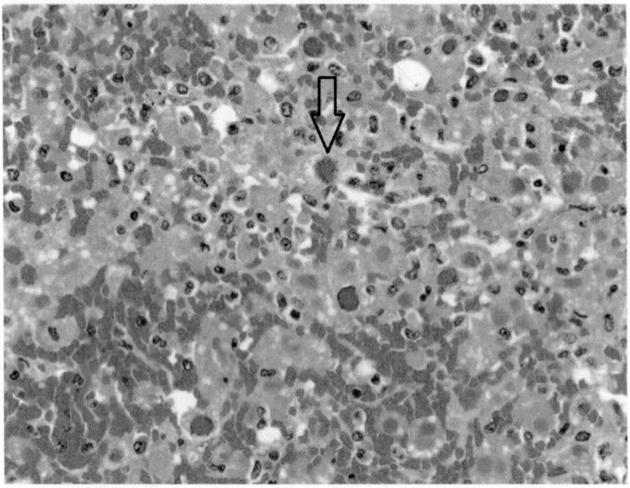

Fig. 34.2 Liver biopsy H&E ×250

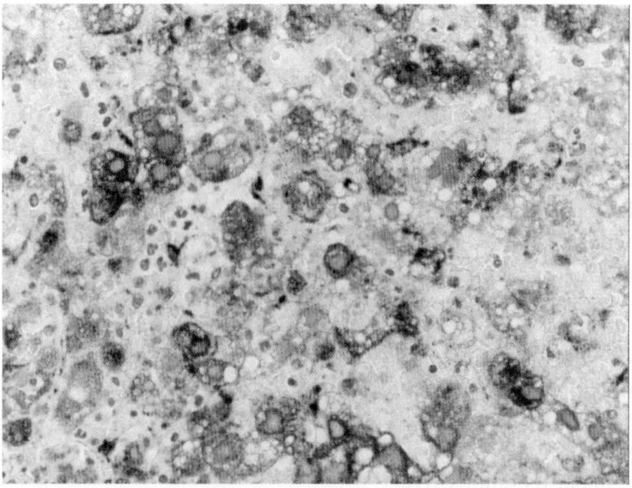

Fig. 34.3 Liver biopsy immunostain

Answer: Acute Herpes Simplex Virus (HSV) Hepatitis

The clinical diagnosis is that of "acute severe hepatitis". The liver enzymes are indicative of a marked hepatocellular or necroinflammatory injury pattern.

By definition, the patient does not yet fulfill criteria for "fulminant hepatic failure" as she has no clinical encephalopathy. The original description of fulminant hepatic failure by Trey and Davidson in 1970 was that of the onset of altered mental status (hepatic encephalopathy) within 8 weeks of initial symptoms in an otherwise healthy individual without preexisting liver disease.
The differential diagnosis for acute, severe hepatitis includes:

- Acetaminophen overdose
- Autoimmune hepatitis
- Viral hepatitis (hepatitis A, B, E, HSV, CMV, EBV)
- Drug-induced
- Ischemic hepatitis (shock liver)
- Wilson's disease

The patient is at high risk of progressing to fulminant hepatic failure and should be managed in a liver transplant center and monitored closely for the development of hepatic encephalopathy, which could indicate the presence of cerebral edema. Frequent neurologic checks are required.

Hospital course: within 18 h of admission, the patient had a rapid deterioration in her clinical condition with the development of grade 4 encephalopathy requiring intubation, ARDS requiring mechanical ventilation, acute renal failure, pancreatitis (amylase 9,600, lipase 8,300), DIC, gastrointestinal bleeding, and severe acidosis. The patient ultimately died despite aggressive medical care.

A postmortem examination revealed massive, hemorrhagic hepatic necrosis involving 99% of the parenchyma as seen in Fig. 34.1. There were intranuclear inclusions (*arrowed* in Fig. 34.2) and an immunostain was positive for *herpes simplex virus* (Fig. 34.3). Serologies yielded a (+) *HSV-1 IgM antibody*.

HSV-1 and HSV-2 produce a wide variety of illnesses including mucocutaneous infections, CNS infections, and occasional infections of visceral organs (which could be life threatening). *HSV hepatitis* is a rare disease in adults, but does have a high mortality, especially if not diagnosed early. The disease can occur in immunocompetent patients, often characterized by the absence of mucocutaneous involvement.

Other clues to the diagnosis:

- High fevers
- Marked liver transaminase elevation
- Relatively low total bilirubin level
- Leukopenia (although not seen in the case presented here)

When suspected, IV acyclovir should be administered immediately. Liver transplant ought to be considered in patients where medical management fails to improve the disease course.

References

1. Trey C, Lipworth L, Chalmers TC et al. Fulminant hepatic failure: presumable contribution to halothane. N Engl J Med 1968;279:798–801.
2. Norvell JP, Blei AT, Jovanovic BD et al. Herpes simplex virus hepatitis: an analysis of the published literature and institutional cases. Liver Transpl 2007;13:1428–34.

Case 35

A 58-year-old woman was admitted with a 2-week history of progressive jaundice, dark urine, acholic stool, and abdominal distension. She had been in her usual state of health until 6 weeks previously. There was no personal or family history of liver disease, no risk factors for viral hepatitis, no history of alcohol use. Medical history was significant for locally invasive infiltrating ductal Ca of the left breast 6 years previously (estrogen receptor (ER) positive, progesterone receptor (PR) negative), for which she underwent mastectomy with axillary node clearance followed by adjuvant chemotherapy and tamoxifen.

Physical examination revealed scleral icterus, mild hepatomegaly with a liver edge three fingers below right costal margin, no splenomegaly and moderate ascites. There were no cutaneous stigmata of chronic liver disease and no asterixis.

Lab Results

Total bilirubin 6.8 mg/dl
Direct bilirubin 4.0 mg/dl
AST 250 iu/l
ALT 100 iu/l
ALP 260 iu/l
GGTP 451 iu/l
Albumin 2.4 g/dl
INR 1.5
Plt 95,000/μl
Hb 13.5 g/dl

Questions

1. How would you evaluate this patient further for the etiology of her liver disease?
2. What is the differential diagnosis for the radiographic appearance shown?

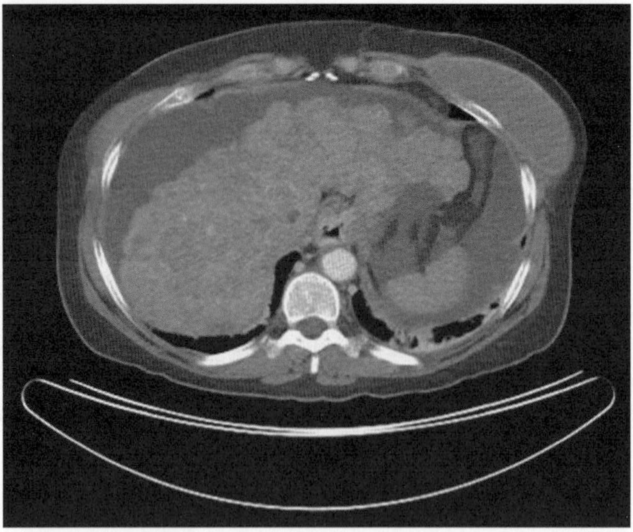

Fig. 35.1 CT scan

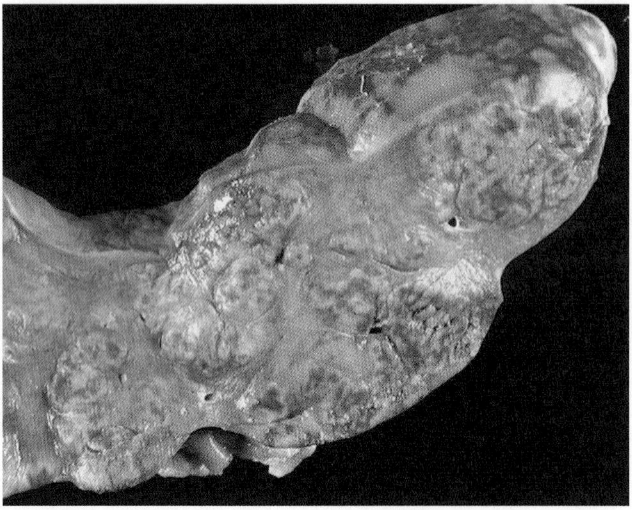

Fig. 35.2 Autopsied liver

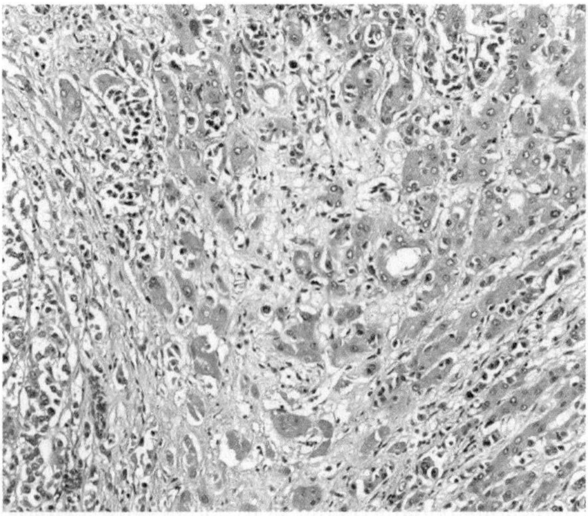

Fig. 35.3 Imunohistochemical stain

Answer: Metastatic Breast Cancer Leading to Pseudocirrhosis

The triphasic CT scan of the abdomen reveals a nodular contour of the liver with heterogeneous attenuation consistent with cirrhosis as well as moderate ascites, but no biliary ductal dilation or splenomegaly.

At first glance, this case appears to be that of decompensated cirrhosis. The patient presents with features of liver failure: jaundice, hypoalbuminemia, prolonged INR, and a cirrhotic appearing liver with evidence of portal hypertension (ascites).

The puzzling issues are that she has no clear risk factors for chronic liver disease, the onset of liver failure has been rather rapid, and she does carry a history of prior malignancy.

Further work-up included:

Serologies for viral, autoimmune, and metabolic etiologies of cirrhosis: all negative.

CEA 250 ng/ml (normal < 5): markedly elevated, raising suspicion of metastatic breast cancer. Ascitic fluid analysis showed a high serum-ascites albumin gradient (SAAG) >1.1 (indicating portal hypertension) and negative cytology.

^{18}F-FDG-labeled PET-CT scan (Fig. 35.1): inhomogeneous uptake consistent with cirrhosis but no focal areas of increased uptake to suggest FDG-avid malignancy.

A liver biopsy was planned; however, the patient had a massive variceal bleed that could not be controlled endoscopically. An emergent TIPS reduced the hepatic portal venous pressure gradient from 30 to 9 mmHg. Despite this, the patient later died and an autopsy revealed the cause of death to be related to the massive variceal hemorrhage and diffuse pulmonary alveolar damage.

The autopsy also revealed grossly evident tumor infiltration of the liver by metastatic tumor (pale, confluent areas in Fig. 35.2). Histopathology (Fig. 35.3) shows diffuse liver infiltration by a poorly differentiated, highly desmoplastic adenocarcinoma. Immunohistochemical stains were positive for CEA and ER, but negative for PR.

The differential diagnosis for a *nodular-appearing liver* on CT imaging includes: cirrhosis, nodular regenerative hyperplasia (NRH), and "*pseudocirrhosis*", where the hepatic histology shows evidence of extensive fibrosis, representing a profound desmoplastic response to the infiltrating tumor. This case is an example of "pseudo-cirrhosis." The only way to differentiate these three entities is via liver biopsy.

It is interesting that the PET-CT did not unequivocally demonstrate metastatic breast cancer in our patient's liver. In one study, this radiologic modality has a 93% sensitivity, 79% specificity, 82% positive predictive value, and 92% negative predictive value.

References

1. Nascimento AB, Mitchell DG, Rubin R et al. Diffuse desmoplastic breast carcinoma metastases to the liver simulating cirrhosis at MR imaging; report of two cases. Radiology 2001;221;117–21.
2. Shirkhoda A, Baird S. Morphologic changes of the liver following chemotherapy for metastatic breast carcinoma: CT findings. Abdom Imaging 1994;19:39–42.
3. Moon DH, Maddahi J, Silverman DH et al. Accuracy of whole-body Fluorine-18-FDG PET for the detection of recurrent or metastatic breast carcinoma. J Nucl Med 1998;39:431–435.

Case 36

A 52-year-old Caucasian male presents to his primary care physician with a 1-week history of fatigue, malaise, and anorexia. Over the last 2 days, he has noticed darkening of his urine and lightening in the color of his stools. He denies any fevers or chills, abdominal pain or pruritus. Remainder of review of symptoms is negative. He has a medical history significant for noninsulin-dependent diabetes. He has been on metformin and pioglitazone for over 3 years and is on no over the counter or herbal medications. He has not been on any recent antibiotics. He is married with three healthy children and works full time as an automotive mechanic. He drinks 6–8 beers on weekends and has no history of illicit drug use. His father died at the age of 59 from a sudden heart attack.

Physical exam is notable for a middle aged male in no apparent distress. He is afebrile with a heart rate of 98 beats per minute. His BMI is 29.5 kg/m^2. He is jaundiced with scleral icterus. Abdominal exam is soft and nontender without hepatosplenomegaly. He has no lymphadenopathy. He is mentating well and has no asterixis. There are no stigmata to suggest chronic liver disease.

Laboratory Parameters

Tbili 8.5 mg/dl
Direct 6 mg/dl
AST 1696 iu/l
ALT 3310 iu/l
ALP 155 iu/l
GGTP 229 iu/l

Normal renal function and hemogram
INR 1.4

Questions

1. What is the differential diagnosis?
2. What test(s) should you order?
3. What are potential treatment options?

HBs Ag: +
anti HBs: negative
anti HBc Total: +
anti HBc IgM: +
HBe Ag +
HBe Ab –
HBV DNA: 3,511,928 iu/ml

Answer: De Novo Acute Hepatitis B Infection

The liver enzyme abnormalities in this case are primarily hepatocellular in nature. The extreme elevations in transaminases with marked elevation in bilirubin narrow the differential diagnosis to a handful of disease entities, including: acute viral, autoimmune hepatitis, and drug-induced liver injury. Although the degree of injury would be categorized as "severe" based on the elevation in liver function tests and bilirubin, the patient does not fulfill criteria for acute liver failure as there is no evidence of encephalopathy or coagulopathy. In addition to supportive care and careful monitoring for evidence of impending liver failure, laboratory testing should be sent for hepatitis A, B, C and an autoimmune panel. A right upper quadrant ultrasound would be reasonable to ensure no evidence of underlying chronic liver disease.

The patient's serologies indicate acute hepatitis B infection. The first detectable viral marker is HBsAg followed by hepatitis B e antigen (HBeAg) and HBV DNA. Titers may be high during the incubation period, but HBV DNA and HBeAg levels begin to fall at the onset of illness and may be undetectable at the time of peak clinical illness. Core antigen does not appear in blood, but antibody to this antigen (anti-HBc) is detectable with the onset of clinical symptoms. The positive IgM antibody is the hallmark of an acute hepatitis B infection.

The Center for Diseases Control estimate between 140 and 320,000 cases of acute hepatitis B yearly in the USA. About 30% of patients develop symptoms with nearly 15,000 requiring hospitalization. Symptoms usually develop 2–4 months following exposure to the virus. Transmission of the virus is predominantly via sexual contact, percutaneous exposure (IVDU), or vertical transmission (mother to child). As is the case in the patient above, a significant number of times the etiology of transmission is never determined. The highest concentration of the virus is found in blood, semen, vaginal discharge, breast milk, and saliva. The time period between exposure and onset of symptoms is referred to the "incubation period." The most common symptoms are fatigue, anorexia, abdominal pain, and jaundice. As opposed to hepatitis A infection, fever is uncommon in HBV.

AST and ALT levels increase to between 500 and 5,000 iu/l and fall after the acute phase. Serum bilirubin seldom increases above 10 mg/dl. Alkaline phosphatase and prothrombin time are usually normal or mildly elevated.

The virus is spontaneously cleared in 95% of adults with acute infection, with the remainder of individuals developing chronic infection. This is in contrast to neonates and children infected with hepatitis B where a *majority* will develop chronic infection. Because of the natural history and spontaneous clearance, treatment is almost never needed in adults with acute hepatitis B infection. Although some small studies suggest that antivirals such as lamivudine may prevent the progression of severe infection to fulminant status and because of their excellent safety profile may be considered in rare, severe cases. Acute liver failure develops in 0.5–2% and is associated with fatality in up to 93% of cases without liver transplantation.

From 1990 to 2002, the incidence of reported cases of acute hepatitis B declined by 67% secondary to routine vaccination in children and adolescents. The incidence, however, has increased by 5% in men above the age of 19, 20% in men above the age of 40, and 30% in women above the age of 40. The highest incidence is seen in African Americans and Hispanics.

The gentleman in this case was discharged on hospital day 4 when his enzymes began a downward trend. Recommendations were given to the patient and his family to avoid sharing of razor blades and toothbrushes. His spouse was vaccinated against HBV.

The patient was seen in follow-up and at 4 months he developed complete normalization of his enzymes and seroconversion with the appearance of surface antibody:

HBsAg –, anti HBs 290 miu/ml, anti HBcore total +, anti HBcore IgM –, HBeAg –, HBeAb +, HBV DNA undetectable.

References

1. Kao JH. Diagnosis of hepatitis B virus infection through serological and virological markers. Expert Rev Gastroenterol Hepatol 2008;2:553–62.
2. Schmilovitz-Weiss H, Ben-Ari A, Sikuler E et al. Lamivudine treatment for acute severe hepatitis B: a pilot study. Liver Int 2004;24:547–51.

Case 37

A 53-year-old man presents to the emergency room with hematemesis. He has a history of cryptogenic cirrhosis and has been evaluated for liver transplant in the past but was felt to be early based on a low MELD score.

His wife is with him and states that he was feeling fine up until a few hours ago when he started complaining of some abdominal discomfort. There has been no fever or chills and as far as she is aware, his bowels have been moving normally without blood or change in stool color. His appetite has been good and there has been no weight loss.

His liver disease has been well compensated in the past and his only medication includes a small dose of beta-blocker.

He does not smoke or drink and works fulltime.

In the ER, he looks comfortable but anxious. His vital signs are BP 110–75, pulse 64 and he is afebrile.

He has a few spider nevi but no scleral icterus. His heart and lungs are normal. Abdominal examination demonstrates an enlarged liver and spleen but no ascites or ankle edema. While being examined, he has another episode of hematemesis with what appears to be a very large amount of fresh blood and clots.

Initial Laboratory Studies

Hb 7.4 g/dl
Platelets 56,000/μl
INR 1.5
Tbili 1.9 mg/dl
AST 38 iu/l
ALT 32 iu/l
ALP 101 iu/l
GGT 49 iu/l
Albumin 2.9 g/dl
Creatinine 0.8 mg/dl

He is emergently intubated, resuscitated and transferred to the intensive care unit and started on a somatostatin analogue, and antibiotics. Endoscopy shows actively bleeding large esophageal varices and a large amount of fresh blood and clot in the stomach obscuring the fundus. Despite several attempts at endoscopic treatment, the bleeding cannot be controlled.

Questions

1. What is/are the next option(s)?
2. What imaging is required in the ICU?

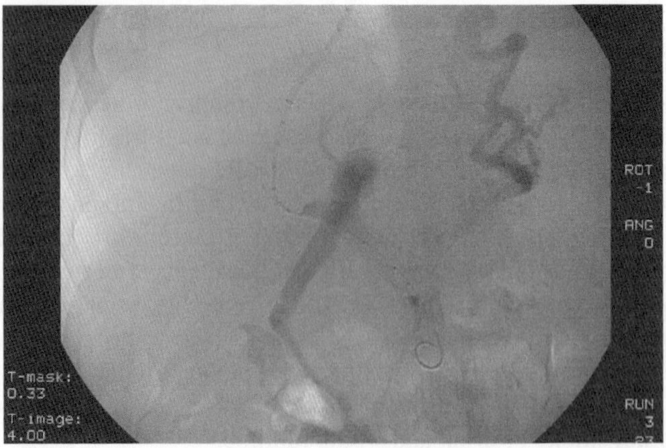

Fig. 37.1 Angiogram

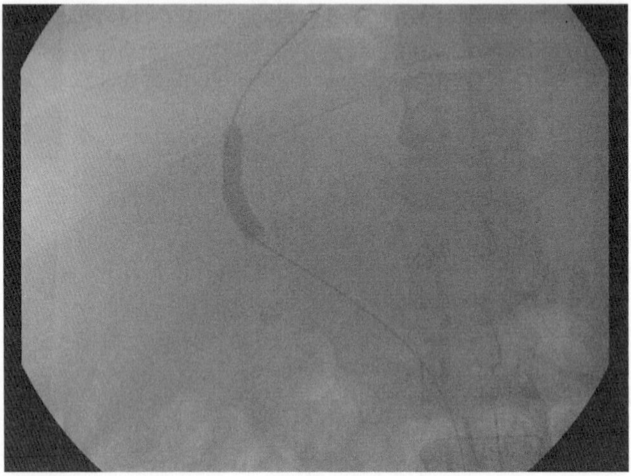

Fig. 37.2 Angiogram

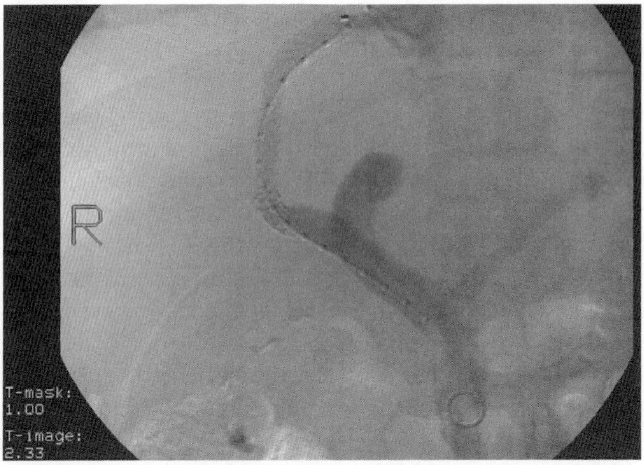

Fig. 37.3 Angiogram

Answer: Transjugular Intrahepatic Portosystemic Shunt (TIPS) as Salvage Therapy for Variceal Bleeding

This gentleman has a life-threatening problem. He has actively bleeding esophageal varices that cannot be controlled despite pharmacological therapy with a somatostatin analogue (in the USA this would typically be octreotide) and endoscopic therapy. In addition, he may have bleeding gastric varices but the fundus is obscured. Endoscopic treatment of bleeding esophageal varices is successful 80–90% of the time, but this figure is not nearly as high with gastric variceal bleeding.

The definition of failure of endoscopic therapy is controversial but most authorities would agree that inability to stop bleeding with two endoscopies within 14 days is reasonable. This patient has failed endoscopic therapy since he continues to bleed even after the first procedure. An appropriate intervention for short-term cessation of bleeding at this time would be balloon tamponade. Several balloons are available including the Sengstaken-Blakemore tube (which has gastric and esophageal balloons and a single gastric suction port), the Minnesota tube (a Sengstaken-Blakemore tube with an esophageal suction port as well), and the Linton-Nachlas tube (which has a single gastric balloon). These can be used for 12–24 h to control ongoing bleeding. At some point, the patient should get a bedside ultrasound to ensure that the portal vein is patent.

Figures 37.1–37.3 show insertion of a TIPS which involves the creation of a low-resistance connection between the hepatic vein and the intrahepatic portion of the portal vein by an interventional radiologist. The connection is kept patent by the deployment of an expandable metal stent across it, so that some of the portal venous blood flow is shunted to the systemic circulation, thereby decreasing portal pressure and decreasing variceal bleeding. Several studies have shown that TIPS is very effective for refractory variceal hemorrhage. The TIPS is formed by passing a needle catheter via the transjugular route into the hepatic vein and wedging it there. The needle is then extruded into the liver parenchyma and attempts are made to find a branch of the intrahepatic portion of the portal vein. Figure 37.1 shows the catheter in place in the portal vein. A series of balloon catheters are then used to dilate the tract from the hepatic vein to the portal vein (Fig. 37.2) and the stent, which is typically a 10-mm diameter covered wire mesh device, is inserted (Fig. 37.3).

To assess the response, pressures are measured. In this patient, the pre-TIPS angiogram demonstrated hepatofugal flow from the portal system into a prominent paraumbilical vein and left coronary vein (top right of first image). The wedged pressure in the hepatic vein was 40 mmHg (a measure of portal pressure) and the free hepatic vein pressure was 16 mmHg giving a portosystemic gradient of 24 mmHg pre-TIPS consistent with portal hypertension. After the TIPS, the gradient dropped to 9 mmHg and the post-TIPS angiogram demonstrated flow through the TIPS shunt with decreased filling of the paraumbilical vein and left coronary vein.

The main complication of TIPS is the development of portosystemic encephalopathy (PSE), which occurs 30% of the time and can be debilitating. We typically will start the patient on lactulose prior to TIPS. Very occasionally, a TIPS needs to be deliberately occluded due to severe PSE (usually in elderly patients). Regular imaging is suggested after TIPS with Doppler sonography to ensure patency, although newer covered stents have lower stenosis rates.

References

1. Rossle M, Haag K, Ochs A et al. The transjugular intrahepatic portosystemic stent-shunt procedure for variceal bleeding. N Engl J Med 1994;330:165–71.
2. Boyer TD, Haskal ZJ. The role of transjugular intrahepatic portosystemic shunt in the management of portal hypertension. Hepatology 2005;41:386.
3. Sanyal AJ, Freedman AM, Luketic VA et al. Transjugular intrahepatic portosystemic shunts for patients with active variceal hemorrhage unresponsive to sclerotherapy. Gastroenterology 1996;111:138–46.
4. Chau TN, Patch D, Chan YW et al. "Salvage" transjugular intrahepatic portosystemic shunts: gastric fundal compared with esophageal variceal bleeding. Gastroenterology 1998;114:981–7.

Case 38

A 31-year-old Caucasian female nurse of Spanish/Portuguese descent was evaluated by her primary care physician for complaints of fatigue and lower extremity paresthesiae. A thyroid mass was palpated on exam that prompted a biopsy revealing papillary thyroid cancer. Her only other medical history is heterozygosity for factor V Leiden deficiency without prior thrombus, for which she is maintained on 81 mg of aspirin daily. The patient was employed full time as a nurse; however, she was no longer able to work due to her current symptoms. She is separated and has one healthy 7-year-old son. She previously smoked 1/2 pack of cigarettes per day, drinks seldomly, and has no history of illicit drug use. She has two tattoos, the first obtained 12 years ago. Her mother died at the age of 37 from sudden cardiac death, which was thought to be related to heart failure. Several other family members on her mother's side have had early death from a variety of diseases and all had the same fatigue and paresthesiae, and were thin (with some suggestion of a bulimia type eating disorder due to constant vomiting). Review of systems is positive for constipation, light headedness, and blurred vision from her right eye. The patient undergoes thryoidectomy and removal of 2.2 cm papillary thyroid cancer with no evidence of vascular invasion or lymph node metastases. She is treated successfully with postoperative radiation.

She is referred to the liver clinic by her oncologist because of abnormal liver tests in a mixed pattern.

Physical exam is notable for a healthy young female with a BMI of 25.8 kg/m^2. Her supine blood pressure is 118/62 with a heart rate of 62, upon standing she does complain of light headedness and her repeat blood pressure is 88/42 with a heart rate of 96. She has no stigmata to suggest chronic liver disease. Her abdominal exam is normal.

She has normal renal function and hemogram.

Questions

1. What is the diagnosis?
2. Is liver transplantation a viable option?
3. How would the diagnosis of thyroid cancer affect her status as a candidate?

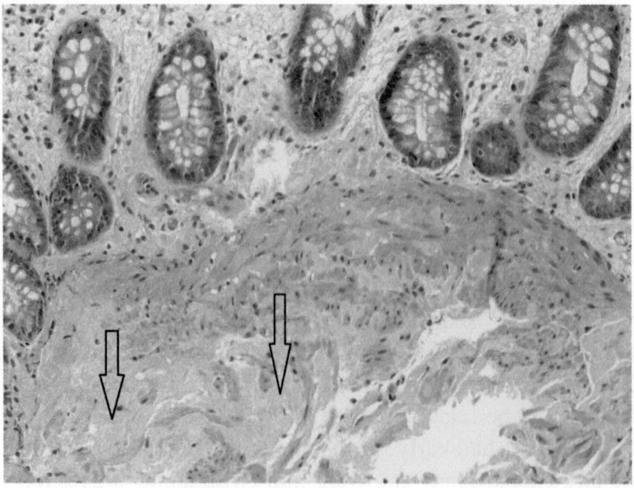

Fig. 38.1 Rectal biopsy H&E ×100

Answer: Familal Amyloidosis and Liver Transplantation

This patient has familial amyloid polyneuropathy (FAP). FAP is an autosomal dominant multisystemic fatal disorder, characterized by a progressive peripheral neuropathy and autonomic neuropathy with neural and systemic amyloid deposits. The disease is caused by a mutant gene on chromosome 18. The amyloid protein in type 1 FAP (the most common form) is the variant transthyretin in which methionine is a substitute for valine at position 30 (TTR Met 30). More than 90% of TTR Met 30 is produced by the liver.

Amyloidosis is a generic term that refers to the extracellular tissue deposition of fibrils composed of low molecular weight subunits of a variety of proteins, many of which circulate as a constituent of plasma. There are at least 25 different human protein precursors of amyloid fibrils known.

As in this particular case, a majority of patients with FAP present with peripheral polyneuropathy: pain, sensory loss, and motor disability. Gastrointestinal dysfunction may also develop, including constipation, diarrhea, and sometimes fecal incontinence. A rectal biopsy can show amyloid, particularly on a congo red stain, but can also be seen on a standard H&E stain as shown in Fig. 38.1 with the amorphous pink material between the smooth muscle fibers in the muscularis mucosa. Difficulty in gastric emptying with nausea and vomiting are also frequent. Cardiovascular symptoms range from orthostatic hypotension to different arrhythmias and first and second degree atrioventricular block. Kidney involvement typically manifests as proteinuria with the reduction of the glomerular filtration rate and decreased creatinine clearance.

Although cases of FAP type 1 may be found all over the world, the most important clusters are in Portugal and Sweden. Frequently, the disease is present in either the father or the mother and there are also other family members affected.

Since more than 90% of TTR Met 30 is produced within the liver, it is expected that liver transplantation will stop disease progression and that TTR Met 30 will clear from the serum. The first orthotopic liver transplantation for FAP patients was performed in 1990. Since 1995, over 1,500 liver transplantations for FAP have been performed, on average 110 patients with FAP are transplanted per year (http://www.fapwtr.org/ram1.htm).

It is now established that liver transplantation for symptomatic patients with FAP is an acceptable treatment for the disease and at the current time the only way to halt disease progression. Key points which have been gained from the experience with transplantation in these patients include:

1. The earlier the transplant after the onset of symptoms the better the outcome.
2. Caution should be warranted before listing patients with longstanding disease (greater than 6 years) as many of these patients will not have regression of their signs and symptoms.
3. Consideration should be given to combined heart–liver transplantation in those patients with orthostatic hypotension and cardiac arrhythmias
4. A complete screening of renal function should be performed and combined liver–kidney transplantation should be considered in patients with moderate-to-severe kidney involvement.

5. Domino transplant seems to be a safe way to increase donor offers and so far there is no evidence of FAP de novo in the recipient.

At the present time, there is no consensus on the optimum window of time between presumed cure of various extrahepatic malignancies and liver transplantation, and each case needs to taken individually. As recommended in the current AASLD guidelines on liver transplantation, close consultation was obtained with oncology before listing this patient for liver transplantation.

The patient in this case received a living donor liver transplant from her 27-year-old sister who tested negative for FAP. The patient's liver upon explant showed intact architecture with predominantly portal-based amyloid deposits and was used in a domino fashion to transplant a 67-year-old woman with HCV cirrhosis and HCC.

References

1. Okamoto S, Wixner J, Obayashi K et al. Liver transplantation for familial amyloidotic polyneuropathy: impact on Swedish patient's survival. Liver Transpl 2009;15:1229–35.
2. Yamamoto S, Wilczek HE, Nowak G et al. Liver transplantation for familial amyloidotic polyneuropathy (FAP): a single-center experience over 16 years. Am J Transplant 2007;7:2597–604.

Case 39

A 25-year-old Caucasian female is admitted to the hospital with a 2-week history of right upper quadrant pain, bloating, nausea, vomiting, and malaise. She endorses chills, but no fevers and has noticed that her urine has become "cola colored." The patient is single and is sexually active in a monogamous relationship. She has three tattoos and a prior stint with IV heroin; however, she has been clean for several years. She has been drinking a moderate amount of alcohol for the last 7 years, and very heavy amounts for the last 1 year, consuming 5–7 mixed drinks including vodka daily. Her last drink was 2 days prior to admission. She also smokes one-half pack of cigarettes per day. She has been told in the past that she has hepatitis C, although she has never been treated. She has no other significant medical history. She takes a daily oral contraceptive pill. Her parents and younger brother are in good health.

Physical exam reveals a young female who is profoundly jaundiced with deep scleral icterus. Temperature is 100.2°F with a heart rate of 106 beats per minute; her BMI is 26.2 kg/m^2. She is in no distress and answers questions appropriately although she is lethargic and drifts to sleep several times during your exam. Her abdomen is distended and she has pain to palpation in the right upper quadrant. Her liver is palpable 5 cm below her right costal margin. A hepatic bruit is auscultated in the right upper quadrant. She has no splenomegaly, but shifting dullness is positive. She has 1+ pitting edema bilaterally, palmar erythema but no asterixis.

Laboratory Data Are Notable for

WBC 18,000 with 91% Neutrophils
Hg 12 g /dl; MCV 109 fL
Platelets 155,000/μl
PT 20 seconds (normal 8–10); INR 2.2
Tbili 14.5 mg/dl (conjugated 11)
AST 202 iu/l
ALT 81 iu/l
AP 120 iu/l
GGTP 685 iu/l
Albumin 3.3 g/dl
Normal electrolytes and renal function
HCV Ab +
PCR undetectable

Questions

1. What is the differential diagnosis?
2. How would you characterize the severity and prognosis of the patient's illness?
3. What treatment if any would you recommend?

Hounsfield units:
Liver 16
Spleen 42

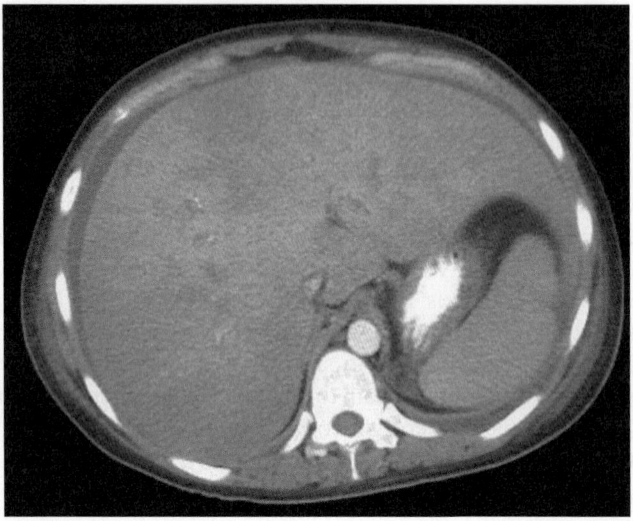

Fig. 39.1 CT scan

Answer: Severe Acute Alcoholic Hepatitis

This young patient has the hallmark clinical features of severe acute alcoholic hepatitis: low-grade fever, jaundice, tender hepatomegaly, leuckocytosis, and moderate elevation of AST compared to ALT. Other physical exam findings may include a hepatic bruit, which is reported in >50% of cases and if heard is pathognomonic for the disease. Approximately 25–30% of patients with alcoholic hepatitis present with manifestations of portal hypertension (ascites, varices, encephalopathy), which may be a consequence of advanced fibrosis and cirrhosis or the result of transient portal venous obstruction from hepatic swelling. Up to 50% of patients presenting with acute alcoholic hepatitis will have underlying cirrhosis.

The spectrum of alcoholic liver disease ranges from asymptomatic fatty liver to alcoholic hepatitis to decompensated cirrhosis. Fatty liver or hepatic steatosis is the most common form of alcoholic liver disease and is reversible with abstinence from alcohol intake. Its first clinical manifestation is typically asymptomatic hepatomegaly. As a consequence of preferential alcohol oxidation, the liver develops fatty deposition. Alcoholic fatty liver is rarely diagnosed clinically because most patients are asymptomatic and do not seek medical attention. However, up to 90% of alcoholics have steatosis. Fatty liver can occur within hours after a large alcohol binge. It represents a direct effect of ethanol and can occur despite an adequate nutritional state. The CT scan image (Fig. 39.1), in this case, reveals an enlarged fatty liver (Hounsfield units of the liver are much lower when compared with the spleen; i.e., the liver is less dense, correlating with severe fatty infiltration).

The diagnosis of acute alcoholic hepatitis can almost always be made on clinical grounds and rarely is a liver biopsy needed. In the rare case, where the diagnosis is uncertain a liver biopsy may be obtained revealing hepatoceullular disarray; polymorphonuclear cell infiltration in the parenchyma; Mallory's hyaline bodies (seen in approximately one-third of cases), which are clumps of intermediary cytokeratin filaments due to tubulin–acetaldehyde adducts; and some degree of steatosis, cholestasis, fibrosis, and necrosis. The presence of neutrophils is a hallmark of alcoholic hepatitis and is unusual in chronic viral hepatitis.

Alcohol is metabolized primarily through the liver. Once alcohol is ingested and absorbed through the gut, it is metabolized by both gastric and hepatic alcohol dehydrogenase to acetaldehyde. Acetaldehyde is in turn oxidized by the liver using aldehyde dehydrogenase and the microsomal ethanol-oxidizing system, cytochrome P450 2E1 (CYP2E1).

Heavy alcohol consumption is considered >20 g/day in women and >80 g/day in men. The incidence of cirrhosis is significantly increased in men who consume >40–60 g/day. Approximately 20% of men drinking >12 beers/day will go on to develop cirrhosis in 10 years.

It is estimated that 30% of patients with alcoholic hepatitis are infected with HCV.

A high prevalence (25–65%) of hepatitis C virus infection has been recognized in alcoholics. Such patients tend to have more severe disease, decreased survival, and an increased risk of HCC.

There are several characteristic laboratory abnormalities in patients with alcoholic liver disease, but no lab test in particular is diagnostic. The most common pattern of LFT abnormality is a disproportionate elevation of serum AST to ALT. This ratio is usually greater than 2, a value that is rarely seen in other forms of liver disease. The absolute value of serum AST and ALT are usually less than 500 iu/l (and typically less than 300). The unusual variant "alcoholic foamy degeneration" which is characterized by jaundice and hyperlipidemia can elevate AST as high as 700.

Other lab abnormalities include: marked elevation in GGTP, macrocytosis as a result of poor nutritional status and B12 and folate deficiencies; thrombocytopenia as a result of primary bone marrow hypoplasia or splenic sequestration due to splenomegaly from portal hypertension. Leuckocytosis is a hallmark lab finding and correlates closely with the severity of the hepatic injury.

The presentation of alcoholic hepatitis can be dramatic and many times carries a grave prognosis. The prognosis of alcoholic liver disease depends upon its severity. Several predictive models have been proposed, which can also help to guide therapy. The Maddrey's discriminant function is perhaps the most widely used. It takes into account the elevation in prothrombin time and Bilirubin: 4.6 × (patient's PT – control PT) + total bilirubin. Scores ≥32 are considered severe and warrant consideration for treatment. More recently, the MELD score has been used to prognosticate outcome, with a score of >11 considered severe disease.

Therapy is generally supportive and many times futile. Survival in patients admitted to an intensive care unit is approximately 5%, This is especially true when there is concomitant renal failure. In addition to strict abstinence, aggressive nutrition and supplementation, treatment of withdrawal, several studies have shown a role for steroids (prednisolone) or pentoxyfylline. Appropriate patients who have been abstinent for at least 6 months should be considered for liver transplantation.

The patient in the case presented was started on pentoxyfylline 400 mg po TID. Despite treatment, however, over the next several months, the patient deteriorated with the onset of ascites, renal failure, and eventually variceal bleeding requiring endoscopic band ligation. After 6 months of abstinence and formal alcohol rehab, the patient underwent successful liver transplantation. She was seen in the clinic 1 year after her transplant and is doing well and has remained abstinent from all drugs and alcohol.

References

1. Maddrey WC, Boitnott JK, Bedine MS et al. Corticosteroid therapy of alcoholic hepatitis. Gastroenterology 1978;75:193–9.
2. Akriviadis E, Botla R, Briggs W et al. Pentoxifylline improves short-term survival in severe acute alcoholic hepatitis: a double-blind, placebo-controlled trial. Gastroenterology 2000;119:1637–48.
3. Rambaldi A, Saconato HH, Christensen E et al. Systematic review: glucocorticosteroids for alcoholic hepatitis – a Cochrane Hepato-Biliary Group systematic review with meta-analyses and trial sequential analyses of randomized clinical trials. Aliment Pharmacol Ther 2008;27:1167–78.

Case 40

A 33-year-old Caucasian male with a past medical history significant only for psoriasis, presents to a local emergency room with progressively worsening right flank pain over the last 1 month. He also reports some mild nausea and early satiety. He has unintentionally lost 7 pounds during this period. The remainder of his review of systems is negative. Specifically he denies any dysuria, fevers, or chills. The patient takes a proton pump inhibitor as required for reflux. He has undergone an appendectomy and left inguinal hernia repair over 20 years ago. He is married with one 8-year-old daughter. The patient works in a shipping yard. He smokes 1/2 pack of cigarettes for 15 years. He drinks socially. There is no history of blood transfusions or tattoos. He admits to experimenting with nasal cocaine in high school.

Physical exam is notable for a young gentleman who is slightly anxious, but otherwise appears well. His BMI is 26.7 kg/m^2. He has no stigmata to suggest chronic liver disease. The patient is tender in his right upper and lower quadrant. Liver edge is palpable 4 cm below the right costal margin. There is no splenomegaly. The remainder of the physical exam is normal.

Laboratory Data

Tbili 1.5 mg/dl
AST 22 iu/l
ALT 28 iu/l
AP 66 iu/l
GGTP 88 iu/l

Albumin 4.2 g/dl
INR 1

AFP 2 ng/ml
CEA 1.2 ng/ml
CA 19-9 0.8 iu/ml

UA: negative

Renal function, hemogram and electrolytes are all normal
Workup for chronic liver disease including HCV is negative

Questions

1. What is the differential diagnosis?
2. What additional testing if any would you recommend?
3. What treatment if any would you recommend?

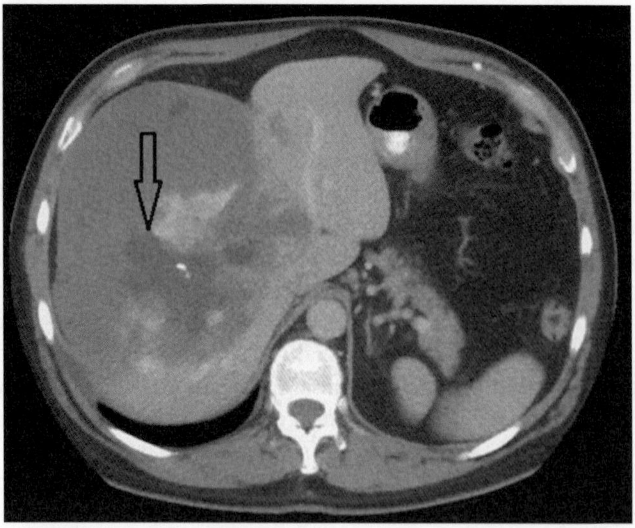

Fig. 40.1 CT scan

Answer: Fibrolamellar Hepatocellular Carcinoma

This patient presented in this case is relatively young with no evidence to suggest chronic liver disease. Tumor markers are normal and CT scan shows a large heterogenous mass with central scar in what otherwise appears to be normal liver parenchyma (Fig. 40.1). Although the differential would include typical HCC, focal nodular hyperplasia, metastatic tumor, hepatic abscess, and giant cavernous hemangioma, the most likely diagnosis given the clues would be fibrolamellar hepatocellular carcinoma (FLHCC).

FLHCC was first described in 1965 as a distinctive form of primary HCC. Controversy exists as to whether FLHCC is a distinct entity or a morphological variant of HCC. The two differ in many ways including patient demographics, risk factors, tumor markers, and prognosis.

The reported incidence of FLHCC seems to vary by geographical region. The incidence of FLHCC in the USA was reported to be 1–2% of the total HCC cases versus 5.8% of all liver cancers in a Mexican cohort.

More than 85% of all FLHCC cases occur in individuals aged <35 years with the average age being 25. This is in contrast to primary HCC where the mean age at diagnosis is between 50 and 65 years of age. Also in apposition to HCC where males are affected nearly 2:1 compared to females, FLHCC shows an equal frequency among gender.

The etiology of FLHCC is still unknown, although some reports have linked occult HBV and focal nodular hyperplasia and long-term oral contraceptive and estrogen use to the formation of FLHCC there is no solid evidence to suggest causality. In contrast to typical HCC, FLHCC generally occurs in patients without chronic liver disease and cirrhosis.

The diagnosis of FLHCC is made on the combination of clinical presentation, imaging studies, and negative tumor marker, however, pathological diagnosis remains the gold standard. Macroscopically, about 75% of cases have a prominent central scar. Microscopically, FLHCC usually consists of malignant hepatocytes that are well differentiated in a background of noncirrhotic liver. The pathological diagnosis of FLHCC is based upon the following: large tumor cells with deeply eosinophilic cytoplasm, the presence of macronucleoli and abundant fibrous stroma arranged in thin parallel lamellae around tumor cells and is cleary distinguishable from conventional HCC in the hands of an experienced pathologist.

At presentation, 70% of FLHCC patients have metastatic lymphadenopathy. Nearly half of patients develop distant metastasis.

Liver function tests are typically normal or only mildly elevated. Commonly used markers for HCC such as alpha fetoprotein are of little help in diagnosing FLHCC, as only a small proportion of patients show minor elevations.

On CT scan, tumors are typically sharply demarcated with a central scar, sometimes with calcification, usually occurring in an otherwise noncirrhotic, normal appearing liver. The lesion seen on CT scan is usually hypodense, which may show marked enhancement after contrast injection.

Overall, the key to successful management of FLHCC is early diagnosis. As is being considered for the patient in the current case, the cornerstone for treatment is surgical resection and lymph node dissection. The outcome of patients with FLHCC after surgical resection is usually good. A 50–75% cure rate has been reported after complete surgical resection. In cases in which partial hepatectomy is not technically feasible because of size or extension, liver transplantation should be considered. However, recurrence occurs in about half of patients within 3.5 years of transplant. If resection and liver transplantation are not options, chemotherapy or hepatic artery chemoembolization can be used as an alternative treatment approach.

References

1. Liu S, Chan KW, Wang B et al. Fibrolamellar hepatocellular carcinoma. Am J Gastroenterol 2009;104:2617–24.
2. Ichikawa T, Federle MP, Grazioli L et al. Fibrolamellar hepatocellular carcinoma: imaging and pathologic findings in 31 recent cases. Radiology 1999;213:352–61.

Case 41

A 43-year-old Caucasian female with no significant past medical history was in her usual state of health until 1 week prior to presentation when she developed what she described as "flu-like symptoms," including fever up to 102°F, anorexia, diarrhea, epigastric fullness and discomfort (mostly in her right quadrant), malaiase, and myalgias. At the onset of her symptoms, the patient did take approximately 2 g of acetaminophen daily for three days. Her fevers subsided, but the remainder of her symptoms persisted which prompted a visit to her local emergency room. After admission into the hospital and administration of intravenous fluids, the patient states that she feels much better. She denies any cough, her urine appears darker than normal, but she denies any dysuria. The patient and her family returned from visiting her in-laws over the Christmas holiday in Monterrey, Mexico 2 weeks prior to the onset of her symptoms. None of her family members are ill. Her only surgical history is the removal of a benign ovarian cyst over 4 years ago. She takes a daily multivitamin, oral contraceptive (which she has been on since the age of 32) and as needed ibuprofen and acetaminophen. She denies any herbal medications or recent antibiotics. The patient works as an accountant at a pediatric hospital. She has been married for over 20 years now and has three young children all in good health. The patient works part-time as a babysitter/nanny. The patient's husband owns a local seafood restaurant, and occasionally, the patient helps in the preparation of food products. The patient occasionally drinks wine. There are no other habits or high risk behavior. The patient's father died of colon cancer at the age of 81.

Physical examination is notable for a generally well-appearing, middle-aged female in no distress accompanied by her entire family. Temperature is 100.8°F and vital signs are stable. She has mild scleral icterus. She has no stigmata of chronic liver disease. Her lungs and heart are normal. Her abdomen is soft, although she is mildly tender in her right upper quadrant. Her liver edge is smooth and is palpable three fingerbreadths below her right costo vertebral angle. She has no shifting dullness, and extremities are without edema. She is mentating well and has no asterixis.

Laboratory Data

Tbili 3.0 mg/dl (direct 2.2); bilirubin peaked at 6.5 mg/dl
AST 2540 iu/l
ALT 3380 iu/l
ALP 125 iu/l
Amylase and Lipase normal
WBC 4,700 with 38% lymphocytes (3% atypical)
INR 1.2

Questions

1. What is the differential diagnosis?
2. What additional testing if any would you recommend?
3. What treatment if any would you recommend?
4. When can the patient safely return to work?

ANA, Smooth muscle Antibody, Immunoglobulins WNL
HBsAg –

Anti-HB core Total negative
HCV Ab –
Anti HAV Total Ab +
Anti HAV IgM Ab +
EBV IgG Ab +
EBV IgM Ab –

Right Upper Quadrant Ultrasound with Dopplers reveals:
Increased perioportal echogenicity throughout the liver; no focal hepatic masses and no intrahepatic biliary dilation. Marked circumfrential gallbladder wall thickening which almost completely obliterates the lumen of the gallbladder. No discrete shadowing stone is identified. Patent and appropriately directed flow within the hepatic vasculature.

Answer: Acute Hepatitis A Infection

This patient has an acute severe hepatitis but no evidence of coagulopathy or encephalopathy to categorize it as acute liver failure. The degree of hepatocellular injury and the onset of fever and diarrhea, in addition to the multiple risk factors (travel, work exposure) would place acute hepatitis A virus (HAV) at the top of the differential diagnosis. The presence of HAV IgM confirms the diagnosis.

HAV is a nonenveloped RNA virus in the hepatovirus genus of the picornavirus family. Hepatitis A has an incubation period of approximately 4 weeks. Its replication is limited to the liver, but the virus is also present in bile, stool, and blood during the late incubation period and acute preicteric phase of illness. Despite persistence of virus in the liver, viral shedding in feces, viremia, and infectivity diminish rapidly once jaundice is apparent.

HAV is transmitted almost exclusively by the fecal-oral route. Person-to-person spread of HAV is enhanced by poor personal hygiene and overcrowding: large ouTbilieaks as well as sporadic cases have been traced to contaminated food, water, milk, frozen fruit, and shellfish.

In developing countries, exposure, infection, and subsequent immunity are almost universal in childhood. With improvements in personal hygiene and sanitation, the frequency of subclinical childhood HAV infection will continue to decline (Fig. 41.1). In turn, a susceptible cohort of adults emerges and the likelihood of clinically apparent and severe HAV infection may increase. Hepatitis A infection tends to be more symptomatic in adults. Travel to endemic areas is a common source of infection for adults of nonendemic areas.

Antibodies to HAV (anti-HAV) can be detected during acute illness when serum aminotransferase activity is elevated and fecal HAV shedding is still occurring. This early antibody response is predominantly of the IgM subclass and persists for several months. The detection of acute hepatitis A is made by demonstrating anti-HAV IgM. During convalescence, however, anti-HAV of the IgG subclass becomes the predominant antibody. IgG antibodies will remain detectable indefinitely and are thought by most experts to provide lifelong immunity to the host.

The incubation period for HAV ranges from 15 to 45 days (mean 4 weeks). The prodromal symptoms of acute viral hepatitis are generally systemic and quite variable. Constitutional symptoms of anorexia, nausea and vomiting, fatigue, malaise, arthralgias, myalgias, and headache may precede the onset of jaundice by 1–2 weeks. A low-grade fever (100–102°F) is often present in hepatitis A. With the onset of clinical jaundice, the constitutional symptoms usually diminish. A substantial proportion of patients with acute hepatitis A never become icteric. Patients may complain of abdominal discomfort as the result of tender hepatomegaly. Complete clinical and biochemical recovery is expected within 1–2 months in nearly all cases of hepatitis A.

The serum aminotransferases show variable increase during the prodromal phase and precede the rise in bilirubin level. The level of elevation in these enzymes does not correlate well with the severity of illness or degree of liver cell damage. Peak levels vary from 400 to 4,000 iu or more. These levels are usually reached at the time the patient is clinically jaundiced. The serum bilirubin may continue to rise despite falling aminotransferase levels. In most instances, the total bilirubin is equally divided between the conjugated and unconjugated fractions.

As in this case, virtually all previously healthy patients with hepatitis A recover completely from their illness with no clinical sequelae. The case fatality in hepatitis A is very low (approximately 0.1%) and almost always occurs in the setting of advanced age or underlying debilitating disease. A small proportion of patients with hepatitis A experience relapsing hepatitis weeks to months after apparent recovery from acute infection. Relapses are characterized by recurrence of symptoms, aminotransferase elevations, occasionally jaundice, and fecal excretion of HAV. Another unusual variant of acute hepatitis A is cholestatic hepatitis, characterized by protracted cholestatic jaundice and pruritus. Rarely, liver test abnormalities may persist for months or even up to a year. Even when these complications of hepatitis A occur, it remains a self-limiting disease and does not progress to chronic liver disease.

Physical isolation of patients with hepatitis A is rarely necessary except in the case of fecal incontinence. Because most patients hospitalized with hepatitis A excrete little if any HAV, the likelihood of transmission from these patients during their hospitalizations is low. Hospitalized patients may be discharged when there is substantial symptomatic improvement, a significant downward trend in the ezymes levels, and normalization of PT. Mild aminotransferease elevation should not be considered a contraindication to the gradual resumption of normal activity.

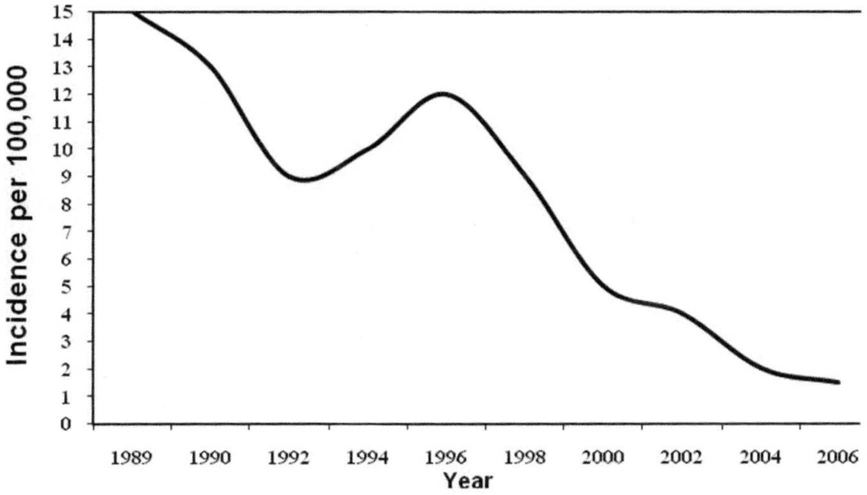

Fig. 41.1 Incidence of acute hepatitis A virus infection, by year – United States, 1989–2006

References

1. Brundage SC, Fitzpatrick AN. Hepatitis A. Am Fam Physician 2006;73:2162–8.
2. Jeong SH, Lee HS. Hepatitis A: clinical manifestations and management. Intervirology 2010;53:15–9.

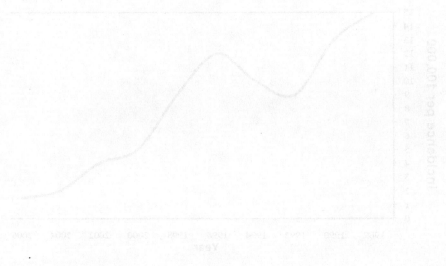

Case 42

A 19-year-old white male with a past medical history significant for attention deficit-hyperactivity disorder (ADHD) presents to his local emergency room with a one day history of severe nausea and nonbloody emesis. The patient reported some abdominal discomfort and fatigue. Remainder of review of systems was negative, although the patient did report feeling depressed after a "big-time fight" with his girlfriend. The patient denied any suicidal or homicidal ideation. He had his tonsils and adenoids removed 3 years ago. His prescription medications include amphetamine and dextroamphetamine for ADHD and venlafaxine which he has recently started on for anxiety. He denied any recent antibiotics, herbal, or over-the-counter medications. The patient lives with his mother and is coping with the recent separation of his parents. He has a 9-year-old healthy sister. He denies alcohol, but he does smoke one pack of cigarettes per day and smokes marijuana on weekends. He denies any intravenous drug use. He has a tattoo of his girlfriend's name which he obtained 1 year ago. His relationship with his girlfriend is monogamous, and he says he always uses protection. He has a family history significant for alcohol abuse and depression.

Physical examination is notable for a thin (BMI 19.1 kg/m^2) somewhat ill-appearing Caucasian male. He is afebrile, heart rate is 101 per minute, and blood pressure is 142/66. He answers questions appropriately, and there is no asterixis. He has no stigmata of chronic liver disease. He is nonicteric. Cardiac and pulmonary exam are normal. His abdomen is soft; bowel sounds are normal, but he is mildly tender in right quadrant. There is no appreciable hepatosplenomegaly.

Table 42.1 Laboratory data

Hospital day	Tbili (mg/dl)	AST (iu/l)	ALT (iu/l)	ALP (iu/l)	INR	BUN (mg/dl)	Cr (mg/dl)
1	1.8	32850	24750	95	3.3	13	0.8
3	2.4	1290	4400	101	1.9	48	5.7
7	0.9	56	330	88	1.0	15	1.8

pH 7.27; lactate 2.9
WBC 9,400/μl
Amylase 350 iu/l, Lipase 780 iu/l
Acetaminophen level 12 (44 h after ingestion)
Right Upper Quadrant US with Dopplers
Normal liver, normal hepatic flow

Questions

1. What is the differential diagnosis?
2. How would you assess the degree of liver injury and what models can be used to help predict prognosis?
3. What treatment if any would you recommend?

Table 42.2 King's college criteria for liver transplantaiton in acute liver failure secondary to acetaminophen

Arterial pH <7.3 (irrespective of the grade of encephalopathy), or
Grade III or IV encephalopathy, and
Prothrombin time > 100 s, and
Serum creatinine > 3.4 mg/dl

Answer: Acute Hepatitis Secondary to Intentional Acetaminophen Ingestion

Initially, this patient adamantly denied taking any excessive medications. When his liver tests returned and he was further questioned, he eventually admitted to ingesting a "fistful" of Tylenol®, estimated to be just over 16 g (50 × 325 mg tablets).

The massive elevations (nearly 1,000× upper limits of normal) and exclusively hepatocellular injury, elevated INR, and development of acute tubular necrosis all point towards acetaminophen toxicity as the cause of liver injury.

Acetaminophen (*N*-acetyl-p-aminophenol; APAP; paracetamol) is the most widely used analgesic-antipyretic in the United States. Although safe when taken at prescribed doses, overdose can cause severe and sometimes life-threatening hepatic injury. Acetaminophen has become the most common etiology of acute liver failure in the United States and accounts for more intentional and unintentional overdoses and overdose deaths each year in the US than any other pharmaceutical agent.

The maximum recommended dose in a 24 h period in adults is 4 g. Toxicity is likely to occur with a single ingestion >12 g over a 24 h period. Virtually all patients who ingest doses >350 mg/kg develop severe liver toxicity unless appropriately treated.

Acetaminophen is rapidly and completely absorbed from the intestinal tract. Serum concentrations peak between one-half and 2 h after an oral dose. At therapeutic doses, 90% of acetaminophen is metabolized in the liver to sulfate and glucuronide conjugates, which are then excreted in the urine. Approximately 2% is excreted in the urine unchanged. The remaining acetaminophen is metabolized via the hepatic cytochrome P450 mixed function oxidase pathway to a toxic, highly reactive intermediate *N*-acetyl-p-benzoquinoneimine (NAPQ1). Appropriate acetaminophen doses produce a small amount of NAPQ1 which is rapidly conjugated with hepatic glutathione, forming nontoxic cysteine and mercaptate compounds that are excreted in the urine. However, with toxic doses of acetaminophen, the sulfation and glucuronidation pathways become saturated, and more acetaminophen is metabolized to NAPQ1 via cytochrome P450. When hepatic glutathione stores are depleted by approximately 75%, NAPQ1 begins to react with hepatocytes and leads to injury and necrosis. There is evidence that conditions that deplete stores of glutathione, such as malnutrition and a period of fasting may predispose patients to acetaminophen toxicity.

Clinical manifestations of acetaminophen poisoning are divided into four stages:

1. (0.5–24 h): nausea, vomiting, diaphoresis, pallor, lethargy, and malaise, though some patients may remain asymptomatic. Lab studies are typically normal.
2. (24–72 h): laboratory evidence of hepatotoxicity is seen in nearly all patients within 36 h; and occasionally nephrotoxicity; stage one symptoms may resolve and patient may appear to improve clnically; as stage two progresses patient may develop RUQ tenderness and liver enlargement and PT may elevate.
3. (72–96 h): LFTs peak from 72 to 96 h after ingestion. The systemic symptoms of stage 1 reappear in conjunction with jaundice and encephalopathy.

4. (4 days to 2 weeks): patients who survive stage III enter a recovery phase that is usually completed 1 week after ingestion.

Histological changes in the liver vary from cytolysis to centrilobular necrosis. The centrilobular region (zone III) is preferentially involved because it is the greatest area of concentration of CYP2E1 and therefore the site of maximal production of NAPQ1. Histological recovery lags behind clinical recovery and may take up to 3 months.

Acute renal failure due primarily to acute tubular necrosis occurs in 25% of patients with significant hepatotoxicity and in more than 50% of those with frank hepatic failure.

All patients with a clear history of acetaminophen or suspected of overdose should undergo measurement of serum acetaminophen concentration. If any doubt exists about the time of ingestion, a serum concentration should be obtained immediately at the time of presentation. A serum concentration should also be obtained 4 h following the time of acute ingestion or presentation.

Management consists of supportive care, prevention of drug absorption, and, when appropriate, the administration of antidotes, namely, *N*-acetylcysteine (NAC).

Treatment with NAC is recommended for all patients with liver tenderness, elevations of aminotransferases, supratherapeutic serum acetaminophen concentrations (greater than 20 mcg/ml), and those with history of excessive ingestion, risk factors for toxicity, and acetaminophen concentrations >10 mcg/ml. If a patient has a detectable acetaminophen concentration but is without signs, symptoms, or risk factors for toxicity and without elevations of aminotransferases, then treatment is likely not necessary.

The outcome of acetaminophen intoxication is nearly always good if NAC is given in a timely fashion. No deaths have been reported in any of the large studies of acetaminophen overdose provided NAC was given within 10 h of ingestion, regardless of the initial serum acetaminophen concentration.

Several statistical models have been developed for predicting the outcome in patients with acute liver failure, including the MELD. Perhaps the most widely recognized of these models, however, is the King's College Criteria (see table above). This model was developed in a cohort of over 500 patients who were managed between 1973 and 1985. Recommendations for liver transplantation were based upon the results. The predictors of outcome were stratified according to whether the ALF was caused by acetaminophen or "other" causes. The positive and negative predictive values of the Kings College Criteria for mortality in patients with acetaminophen-induced ALF (not including patients who were transplanted) are 88 and 65%, respectively

The patient in this case was administered NAC as soon as his enzyme elevation was noted. His transaminases dramatically normalized, and although he developed oliguric renal failure secondary to ATN, he never required renal replacement therapy. He was eventually discharged to an inpatient psychiatric ward on hospital day 6.

References

1. Larson AM. Acetaminophen hepatotoxicity. Clin Liver Dis 2007;11:525–48.
2. Smilkstein AU, Knapp GL, Kulig KW et al. Efficacy of oral *N*-acetylcysteine in the treatment of acetaminophen overdose. Analysis of the national multicenter study (1976 to 1985). N Engl J Med 1988;319:1557–62.
3. O'Grady JG, Alexander GJ, Hayllar KM et al. Early indicators of prognosis in fulminant hepatic failure. Gastroenterology 1989;97:439–45.

Case 43

A 43-year-old male presents to the emergency room with confusion and jaundice. He is a heavy drinker and has been drinking even more heavily recently following separation from his wife. He complains of abdominal discomfort and nausea. He has no other medical history. He has been laid off work recently due to his alcoholism.

He smokes and admits to drinking 20–30 beers on a daily basis and has been drinking vodka in addition over the last 2 weeks.

He is cirrhotic based on imaging from 2 years ago when he presented to the outpatient clinic with abnormal liver tests.

He is on no prescribed medication.

On examination, vital signs are stable. He is obviously confused with asterixis. He has palmar erythema, scleral icterus, and an enlarged liver and spleen. Skin reveals jaundice and multiple 5–10 mm lesions as shown in the photographs.

Laboratory Studies

Total bilirubin 25.6 mg/dl
Direct bilirubin 19.7 mg/dl
AST 154 iu/l
ALT 47 iu/l
ALP 135 iu/l
GGTP 657 iu/l
Albumin 2.2 g/dl
INR 1.9

Questions

1. What is the relevance of the skin lesions – are they always pathological?
2. How many lesions are considered significant?
3. Is there a recognized distribution in patients with liver disease?
4. Is the etiology of his liver disease relevant?

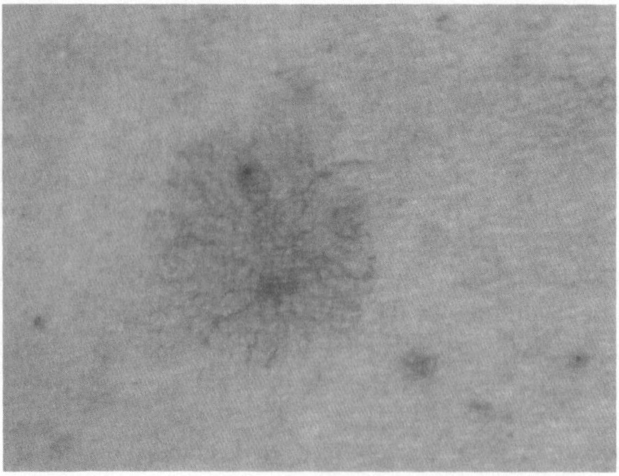

Fig. 43.1

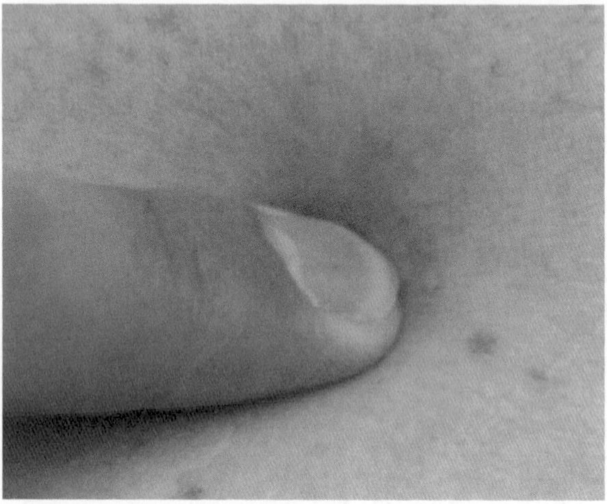

Fig. 43.2

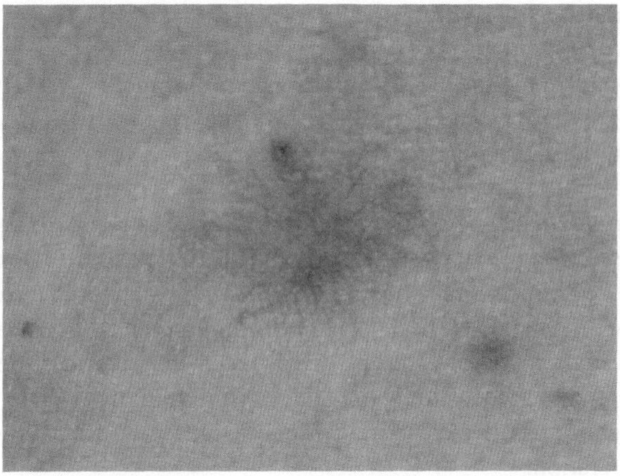

Fig. 43.3

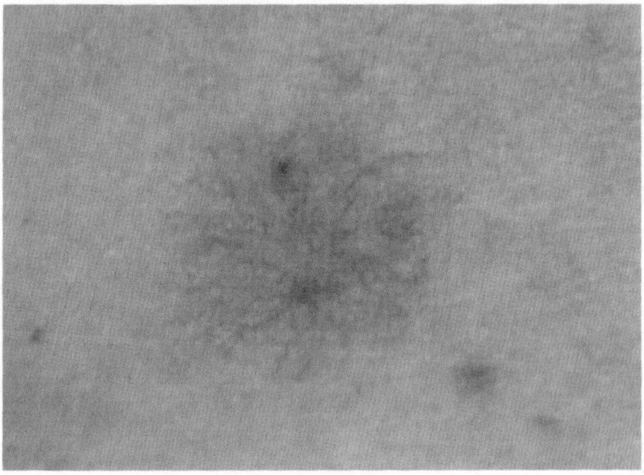

Fig. 43.4

Answer: Spider Nevi (Angioma)

Figures 43.1–43.4 show the classic appearance of a spider nevus. There is a central arteriole and capillaries extending outwards. They blanch with pressure and then refill from centrally when the pressure is released.

They are seen in 10–15% of healthy children and young adults. They are commonly seen in pregnancy, and in women where there appears to be a relationship with the menstrual cycle, and in high output states such as thyrotoxicosis. In liver disease, they are common in cirrhosis, particularly if alcohol is the etiology.

The number is thought to be relevant with more than 5–7 indicative of pathology. The distribution follows that of the superior vena cava, so lesions are seen above the nipple line, face, shoulders, and upper extremities.

The pathogenesis is unclear but is related to dilation of existing vessels rather than neoproliferation.

Some studies have suggested that their presence together with other markers of liver disease is indicative of increased hepatic fibrosis in patients with chronic hepatitis C.

References

1. Khasnis A, Gokula RM. Spider nevus. J Postgrad Med 2002;48:307–9.
2. Li CP, Lee FY, Hwang SJ et al. Spider angiomas in patients with liver cirrhosis: role of alcoholism and impaired liver function. Scand J Gastroenterol 1999;34:520–3.
3. Romagnuolo J, Jhangri GS, Jewell LD et al. Predicting the liver histology in chronic hepatitis C: how good is the clinician? Am J Gastroenterol 2001; 96:3165–74.

Case 44

A 64-year-old woman presents to your outpatient office because of worsening ankle edema. She has a history of cirrhosis likely from significant alcohol use but quit drinking several years ago. Her liver disease has been complicated by encephalopathy, and she has mild portal hypertension based on imaging and endoscopy.

Her past medical history is significant for hypertension and a hysterectomy many years ago for a nonmalignant condition.

Her current medications include a thiazide diuretic and lactulose.

She is an ex-smoker but denies drug use. Her alcohol history is significant for daily drinking including spirits and beer up until 4 years ago.

She is widowed and comes to the appointment with an adult daughter.

Her family history is notable for several family members with alcoholic liver disease.

Her review of symptoms is significant for the ankle edema and some shortness of breath on exertion but no chest pain, weight loss, or abdominal distension. She does feel very fatigued.

On exam, she is alert and oriented. Her vital signs show BP 140/85, pulse 82 and regular, and she is afebrile. She has mild palmar erythema and a few spider nevi. There is no scleral icterus.

Cardiovascular system reveals normal heart sounds with a pansystolic murmur heard best at the left sternal edge, and chest reveals a few bibasilar crackles. Her abdomen is soft and nontender. The liver is palpable several cms below the right costal margin and she has a spleen tip in the left upper quadrant. There is some dullness in the flanks, and she has 2+ ankle edema.

Laboratory Studies

Hb 11.2 g/dl
Platelets 57,000/μl
INR 1.4
Creatinine 1.4 mg/dl
Tbili 1.9 mg/dl
AST 52 iu/l
ALT 39 iu/l
GGTP 120 iu/l
ALP 188 iu/l
Albumin 2.7 g/dl

Questions

1. What test(s) would you order?
2. How is the diagnosis confirmed?
3. What is/are the treatment option(s)?
4. Does this condition recur after transplant?

Dobutamine stress test

Right ventricular pressure 40 mmHg

Answer: Portopulmonary Hypertension

This lady has symptoms and signs suggestive of portopulmonary hypertension (PPHTN). This condition is defined by pulmonary arterial hypertension in the setting of portal hypertension in the absence of other causes of pulmonary hypertension.

The pulmonary symptoms typically include dyspnea on exertion, chest pain, fatigue, orthopnea, and syncope. Exam can demonstrate right ventricular overload with tricuspid incompetence (as in this case), worsening ascites, and dependent edema. Her laboratory studies also suggest some hepatic congestion.

The diagnosis cannot be made clinically but is suspected on echocardiography and confirmed by right heart catheterization. This lady should undergo a stress echocardiogram, which is a good screening test for pulmonary hypertension. The right ventricular pressure is elevated and should prompt referral to a cardiopulmonary specialist and right heart catheterization to make a diagnosis. Pulmonary artery hypertension is defined by a mean pulmonary artery pressure (MPAP) >25 mmHg at rest and a pulmonary capillary wedge pressure (PCWP) <15 mmHg.

The pathogenesis of PPHTN is unclear but may occur on the background of genetic susceptibility as there are cases of familial pulmonary hypertension related to dysfunction of the bone morphogenetic protein receptor type II. Some studies suggest that the underlying portal hypertension leads to porto-systemic collaterals and substances that normally would be metabolized in the liver mediate the pulmonary hypertension. Multiple cytokines and hormones have been implicated including serotonin, IL-1, vasoactive intestinal peptide, glucagon, endothelin-1, and thromboxane B2.

The hyperdynamic circulation seen in cirrhosis and chronic thromboembolism may also play a role. Pulmonary histology in PPHTN demonstrates in situ thrombosis, pulmonary arteriopathy, and vasoconstriction.

It is important to make a diagnosis of PPHTN as it negatively impacts outcome after liver transplantation, particularly with a MPAP >35 mmHg.

Treatment can be by liver transplantation, which has a good outcome in patients with a MPAP below 35 mmHg. Higher MPAP and increased peripheral vascular resisitance (PVR) (>250 dynes s cm^{-5}) are associated with significant mortality after transplantation, and MPAP >50 mmHg is an absolute contraindication to transplant.

The medical therapy of PPHTN has increased over the last few years and involves vasodilatory agents including epoprostenol (Flolan), sildenafil (Revatio), iloprost, and bosentan, best administered in the setting of a pulmonary hypertension clinic. The data is based on case series rather than randomized controlled trials, but the goal is to reduce MPAP and decrease PVR to acceptable levels for transplant. There is very limited data to demonstrate improved outcome after transplant in patients treated with these agents.

Several case series have documented good outcome after liver transplantation in selected patients with PPHTN. Although survival is not at levels seen in patients without PPHTN, the survival benefit of transplant is significant. Resolution of PPHTN after transplant is usual, and there is no evidence that it recurs.

References

1. Hoeper MM, Krowka MJ, Strassburg CP. Portopulmonary hypertension and hepatopulmonary syndrome. Lancet 2004;363:1461.
2. Colle IO, Moreau R, Godinho E et al. Diagnosis of portopulmonary hypertension in candidates for liver transplantation: a prospective study. Hepatology 2003;37:401.
3. Krowka MJ, Mandell MS, Ramsay MA et al. Hepatopulmonary syndrome and portopulmonary hypertension: a report of the multicenter liver transplant database. Liver Transpl 2004;10:174.

Case 45

A 57-year-old Asian male presents to the emergency room with hematemesis. The patient has been recently diagnosed with non-small cell lung cancer. The cancer has not yet been treated. He is not known to have liver disease.

His current medications include aspirin and atenolol for hypertension.

The patient also reports a history of intermittent dysphagia to solid food for the last several weeks.

He is a heavy smoker with a 42 pack-year smoking history. He denies use of alcohol or drugs.

The patient is admitted to the intensive care unit and intubated for airway protection. He undergoes an emergent upper endoscopy which shows large masses starting right below the upper esophageal sphincter. The masses progressively became thinner distally.

Laboratory Parameters Show

WBC 9×10^3/uL
Hb 9.0 g/dl
Tbili 0.9 mg/dl
AST 34 U/l
ALT 45 U/l
Creatinine 1.2 mg/dl

Questions

1. What is the pathogenesis of these lesions?
2. What is the long-term prognosis?

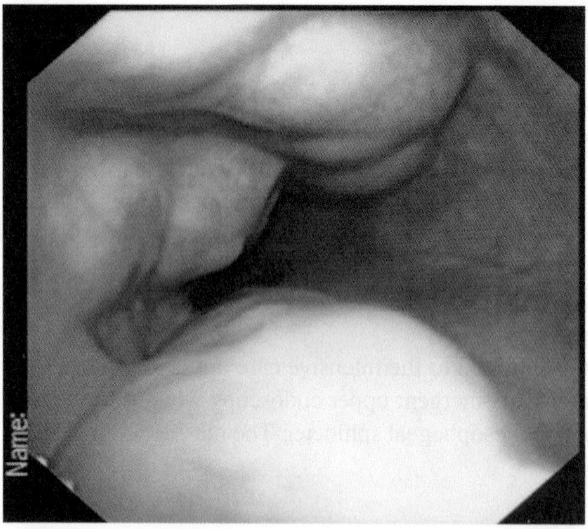

Fig. 45.1 Upper esophagus at 20 cm from the incisors

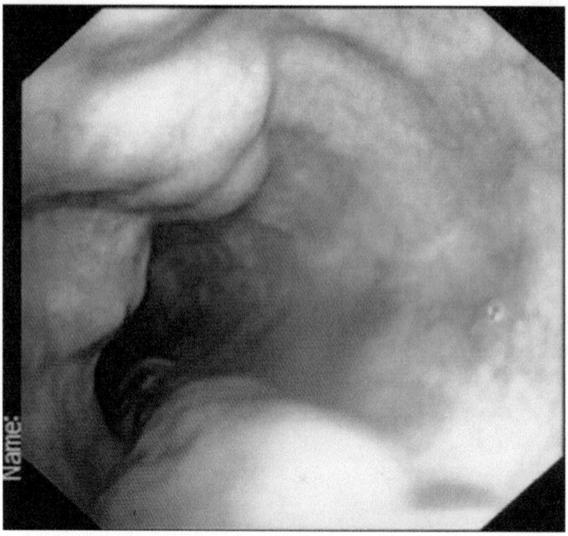

Fig. 45.2 Mid esophagus distally

Answer: Downhill Varices

The EGD pictures (Figs. 45.1 and 45.2) demonstrate large esophageal varices extending from the upper esophagus to the mid esophagus. The varices become thinner and disappear in the mid to distal esophagus. Downhill varices are a result of obstruction of the superior vena cava (SVC). When the SVC is obstructed superior to the azygous vein, venous blood is redirected downhill as it flows through the esophageal veins into the azygous vein. This results in development of downhill varices in the upper to mid esophagus. The most common etiologies of downhill varices are malignancies such as lung cancers and mediastinal tumors. Other potential etiologies include mediastinal fibrosis, substernal goiter, and trauma from central intravenous line placement. The patient may also have other signs of SVC obstruction such as dyspnea, dysphagia, facial and arm swelling, plethora, and headache. Because malignancy is the most common etiology, the prognosis from bleeding is often poor.

Band ligation and sclerotherapy can be attempted, but data on their efficacy is limited and would be expected to cause significant discomfort this high in the esophagus.

References

1. Cotran RS, Kumar V, Collins T (eds). Robbins Pathologic Basis of Disease, 6th ed. Philadelphia, PA: WB Saunders; 1999, pp 845–901.
2. Sherlock S, Dooley J. Diseases of the Liver and Biliary System, 10th ed. Oxford, United Kingdom: Blackwell Science; 1997, pp 135–80.
3. Felson B, Lessure AP. "Downhill" varices of the esophagus. Dis Chest 1964;46:740–6.

Case 46

A 47-year-old man presents to your outpatient clinic for follow-up. He has a history of cirrhosis secondary to hepatitis C. He attempted treatment in the past but could not tolerate the side effects and developed worsening depression.

His disease has been well compensated with minimal ascites controlled on diuretics and no encephalopathy. He has grade 1 esophageal varices on endoscopy.

His past medical history is significant for hypertension and some mild depression. He works as a schoolteacher. He denies current tobacco or alcohol but has a remote history of intranasal cocaine use.

His current medications include paroxetine, furosemide 40 mg daily, spironolactone 100 mg daily, and metoprolol 25 mg daily.

On exam, his vital signs demonstrate weight 165 pounds, BP 135/75, and pulse 62, and he is afebrile. He has no scleral icterus and normal cardiovascular and respiratory systems.

Abdominal exam demonstrates a soft nontender abdomen without organomegaly and no ascites and no ankle edema. He has no asterixis.

Laboratory Studies

Hb 12.5 g/dl
Platelets 64,000/μl
INR 1.5
Creatinine 1.2 mg/dl
Tbili 1.9 mg/dl
AST 47 iu/l
ALT 34 iu/l
ALP 112 iu/l
Albumin 2.7 g/dl
AFP 257 mcg/l

Questions

1. What options if any are available to this patient?
2. What is the treatment that is illustrated, and has it worked?
3. Is he a candidate for liver transplant?

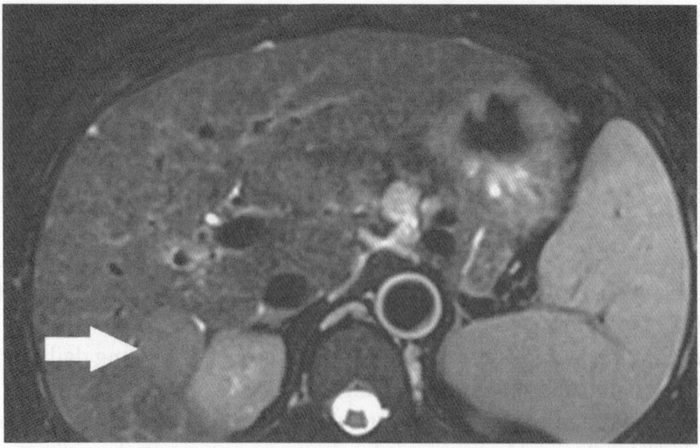

Fig. 46.1 CT scan

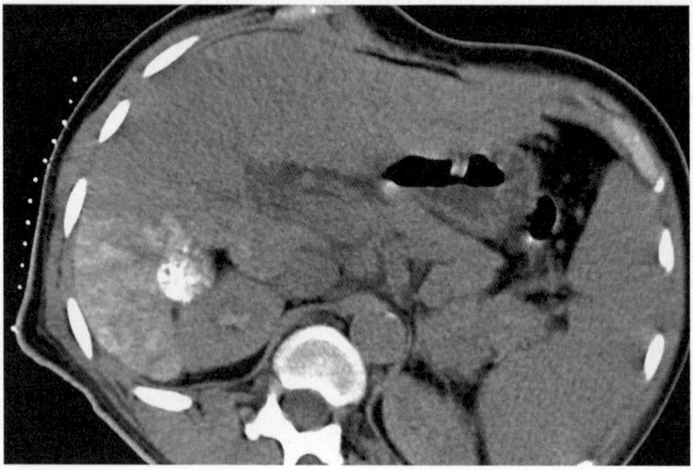

Fig. 46.2 CT scan

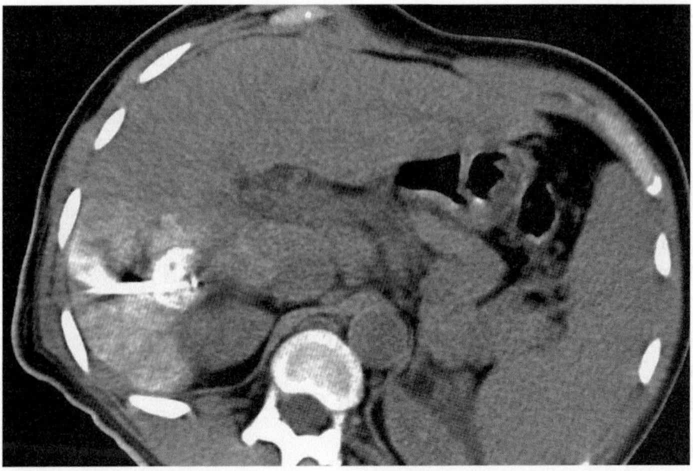

Fig. 46.3 CT scan

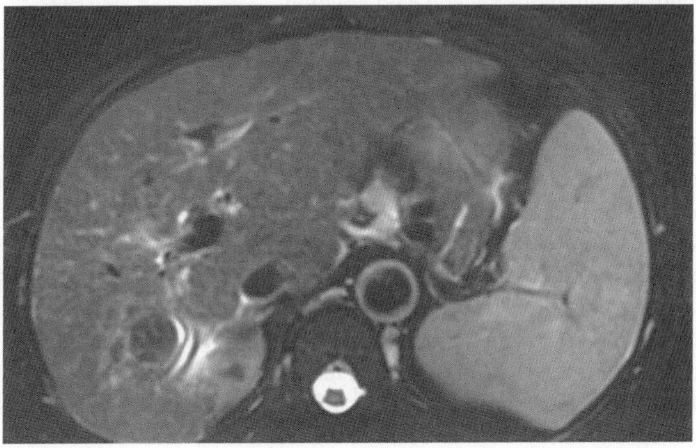

Fig. 46.4 Follow up CT, after 2 months

Answer: Treatment of Solitary Hepatocellular Carcinoma (HCC)

This man has developed HCC, which is increasingly common in the United States in people with cirrhosis secondary to hepatitis C. Some studies suggest that the yearly incidence of HCC may be anywhere from 3 to 8% in patients with hepatitis C cirrhosis.

The MRI images (Figs. 46.1–46.3) show a 3 cm lesion in the posterior right lobe (arrowed in Fig. 46.1). Figure 46.2 shows the lesion after transarterial chemoembolization has been administered, and the third image (Fig. 46.3, CT) shows a radiofrequency ablation probe being placed into the lesion. The follow-up MRI 2 months later (Fig. 46.4) shows the treated lesion which did not enhance, suggesting successful treatment.

Multiple treatment modalities exist for HCC including:

- Surgical resection
- Liver transplantation
- Transarterial chemoembolization (TACE)
- Radiofrequency ablation (RFA)
- Percutaneous ethanol or acetic acid ablation
- Cryoablation
- Radiation therapy
- Systemic chemotherapy

The basic algorithm for management of HCC is shown in the first reference below, but essentially, the decision to use which treatment modality is based on center preference and also severity of underlying liver disease.

Resection is a good treatment option for HCC as it can be potentially curative. A single HCC confined to the liver without evidence of vascular invasion in a patient without portal hypertension, and well-preserved hepatic function would be an ideal candidate. Very good 5-year survival rates have been reported.

Liver transplant for HCC is discussed in another case.

TACE uses the fact that the majority of the blood supply to HCCs is derived from the hepatic artery so that eliminating hepatic arterial supply to the tumor should cause ischemia. In addition, chemotherapy can be given directly to the tumor. The chemotherapy is often given with lipiodol, which promotes intratumoral retention of chemotherapy drugs. After the chemotherapy has been delivered, the hepatic artery branch can be occluded in a variety of ways.

TACE is usually not curative but is used as a bridge to transplant for larger tumors, but there is limited data on its efficacy compared to other modalities.

RFA involves the application of radiofrequency thermal energy directly to the lesion. This causes the temperature of the tissue to rise, and when it reaches beyond 60°C, cells begin to die, resulting in a necrosis of tumor cells.

RFA is a reasonable option for patients who are not candidates for resection but typically only works well for lesions less than 4 cm. Again, it is often used as a bridge to transplant, but there is limited data for outcome after RFA compared to other treatments.

Reference

1. Bruix J, Sherman M. Management of hepatocellular carcinoma. Hepatology 2005;42:1208–36.

Case 47

A 52-year-old man presents with bright red blood per rectum. He has a history of cirrhosis secondary to alcohol and is still drinking. His liver disease has been complicated by ascites, but he denies encephalopathy or spontaneous bacterial peritonitis (SBP). He has undergone endoscopy and colonoscopy in the last year at his local hospital and states that they were "OK".

His bowels have been moving normally with a normal stool color up until yesterday when he noticed blood in the toilet bowl. He denies abdominal pain or fever.

Upon presentation to the emergency room he is witnessed to have further bleeding per rectum with bright red blood but also several large clots.

He has been taking diuretics but no other medications.

He is divorced, lives alone and is not working.

On exam, he looks comfortable and is alert and oriented.

Pulse is 110 beats per minute, regular, blood pressure 95/60

His abdomen is soft, and the flanks are dull. Extremities reveal mild ankle edema.

Rectal exam demonstrates dark red clots.

Laboratory Studies

Hb 9.3 g/dl
Platelets 35,000/μl
INR 1.8
BUN 21 mg/dl
Creatinine 1.7 mg/dl
Tbili 2.5 mg/dl
AST 89 iu/l
ALT 45 iu/l
Albumin 2.6 g/dl

Questions

1. What should you do next?
2. What are the treatment options for this condition?

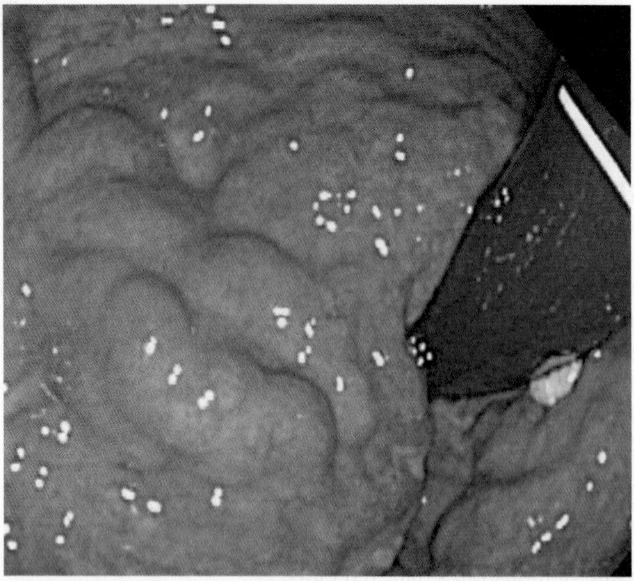

Fig. 47.1 Endoscopic image

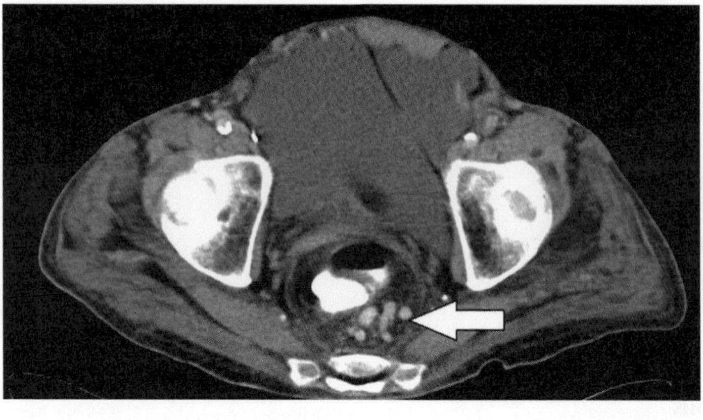

Fig. 47.2 CT scan of the pelvis

Answer: Rectal Varices

The endoscopic image (Fig. 47.1) demonstrates significant rectal varices seen on retroflexion (the black tube on the right is the scope). The CT image of the pelvis (Fig. 47.2) shows the varices around the distal rectum (arrowed). Scrolling up through the images showed a single vessel running all the way from the perirectal varices up to the splenic vein.

The differential diagnosis here is essentially all the causes of bright red blood per rectum including hemorrhoids, diverticular bleeding, arteriovenous malformations and tumor.

In a patient with portal hypertension, ectopic varices also have to be considered. An upper source of GI bleeding could be a possibility but is unlikely given the relatively well-maintained hemodynamics and hemoglobin.

The usual algorithm for lower GI bleeding includes resuscitation and then colonoscopy. The timing of the colonoscopy will depend on the degree of bleeding.

In this patient, there was significant bleeding, and we elected to proceed with colonoscopy after a rapid purgative preparation.

The rectal varices were immediately evident, and there was no evidence of any blood proximal to the rectum.

Treatment of rectal varices is based on very limited data. Banding or sclerotherapy does not appear to be effective. I have on one occasion used the gastric balloon of a Blakemore tube inserted into the rectum to control torrential bleeding from huge rectal varices. Unfortunately, the patient died after a prolonged intensive-care course.

There is anecdotal data that in bleeding ectopic varices – treatment with TIPS and/or embolisation by a radiologist can control bleeding. In this case, the bleeding stopped spontaneously, and we elected not to try a TIPS due to his elevated MELD score although the patient may have had some decompression based on the CT images showing a single vessel supplying the rectal varices from the splenic vein.

Reference

1. Vangeli M, Patch D, Terreni N et al. Bleeding ectopic varices – treatment with transjugular intrahepatic porto-systemic shunt (TIPS) and embolisation. J Hepatol 2004;41:560–6.

Case 48

A 25-year-old man presents with jaundice. He is otherwise asymptomatic but does admit to dark urine and pale stool. The jaundice has gradually worsened over the last few weeks and he is now complaining of itching. No one else has been sick, and he denies any foreign travel.

He denies fever or abdominal pain, and his appetite is good with a stable weight.

He has no other past medical history that he is aware of but knows he has had an abdominal surgery as an infant. He takes no medications.

He does not smoke or drink.

He is married with a young child. He works as a carpenter.

His family history is not available as he was adopted as a toddler. He is not aware of his birth parents and is not in contact with his foster parents.

On exam, he looks comfortable and is alert and oriented. He is obviously jaundiced.

Pulse is 70 beats per minute, regular, blood pressure 115/60, and he is afebrile.

His abdomen is soft and nontender. There is a midline scar in the epigastric area extending into the right upper quadrant. Extremities reveal no edema.

Laboratory Studies

Hb 14.2 g/dl
Platelets 74,000/μl
INR 1.5
Creatinine 1.1 mg/dl
Tbili 22.5 mg/dl (direct 19.1 mg/dl)
AST 109 iu/l
ALT 75 iu/l
ALP 457 iu/l
GGT 987 iu/l
Albumin 3.2 g/dl

Questions

1. What should you do next?
2. What are the treatment options for this condition?

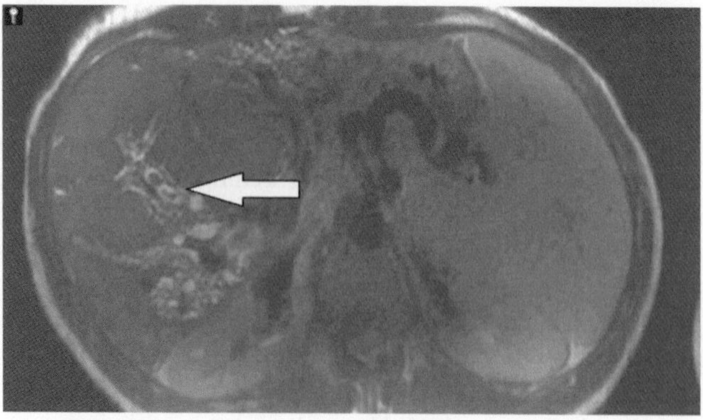

Fig. 48.1 MRI abdomen

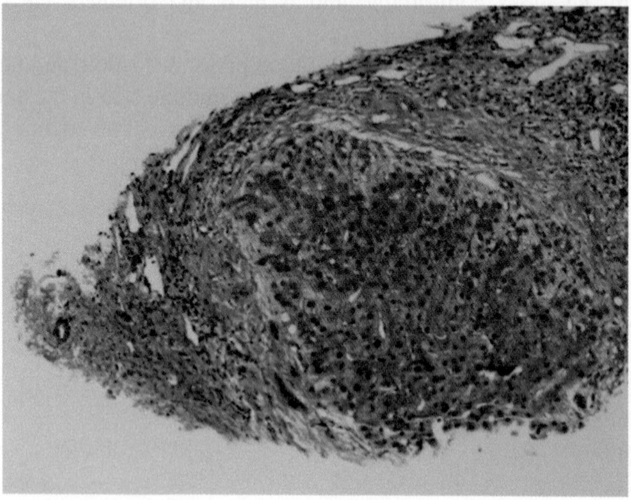

Fig. 48.2 Liver biopsy H&E ×100

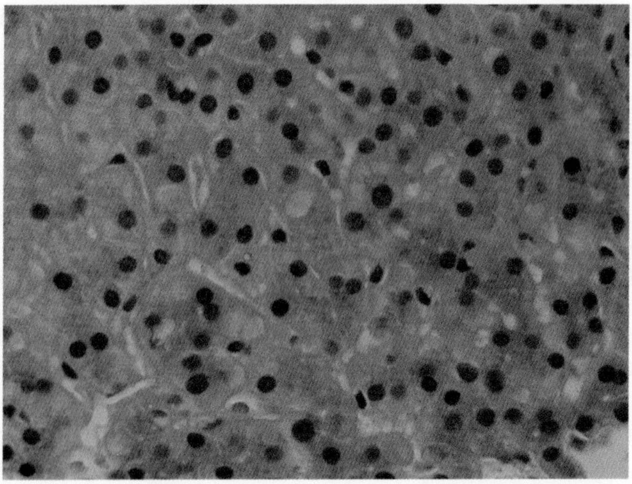

Fig. 48.3 Liver biopsy H&E ×250

Answer: Biliary Cirrhosis After Kasai Procedure for Extra-Hepatic Biliary Atresia as a Child

This young man has an obstructive picture with jaundice and pale stool and dark urine. The differential diagnosis includes posthepatic causes of jaundice such as biliary obstruction from stones or tumor, on intrahepatic causes such as cholestatic liver disease. In this case, he states he had surgery as an infant. A cholecystectomy would be unusual at that age, but inadvertent damage to the biliary tree during such a procedure could lead to secondary biliary cirrhosis. Typically, this would occur after only a few years and not 20–25 years as in this case.

He does have some evidence of portal hypertension given the low platelet count but looks to be relatively well compensated.

The next best test would be imaging. The MRI (Fig. 48.1) shows evidence of biliary ductal dilation, and there are stones and sludge within the biliary tree (arrowed). On other cuts, it was evident that there was a biliary-enteric anastomosis, and the spleen is big consistent with portal hypertension.

This was actually a patient who had undergone a Kasai procedure (hepatoporto-enterostomy) for extra-hepatic biliary atresia (EHBA) at the age of 1 month. He has developed secondary biliary cirrhosis which is seen in the majority of cases.

This patient was being worked up for liver transplant, and we decided to obtain a tranjugular liver biopsy to assess the degree of liver damage since he had so much biliary obstruction. The low power image (Fig. 48.2) shows a cirrhotic nodule and at higher power (Fig. 48.3) the cholestasis is readily apparent.

EHBA has an incidence of approximately 1 in 10,000–20,000 births and is characterized by inflammation of the bile ducts leading to progressive obliteration of the extrahepatic biliary tract. The diagnosis of BA should ideally be made within the first month of life as multiple studies have demonstrated that the success of biliary drainage using the Kasai procedure is poor after 3 months of age.

The Kasai procedure attempts to restore bile flow from the liver to the proximal small bowel by using a roux-en-Y loop of bowel and a direct anastomosis to the capsule of the liver following excision of the biliary remnant and portal fibrous plate.

If the procedure is successful, the small patent bile ducts drain into the small bowel and relieve the biliary obstruction and prevent nutritional issues from cholestasis.

Biliary cirrhosis usually occurs within 5–10 years, and liver transplantation is required. The outcome after transplant is good with overall survival of approximately 70–80% long term survival. More recent case series have suggested better long-term outcome with early Kasai procedures and perhaps explains this patient's later presentation.

References

1. Chardot C, Carton M, Spire-Bendelac N et al. Prognosis of biliary atresia in the era of liver transplantation: French national study from 1986 to 1996. Hepatology 1999;30:606–11.
2. Shinkai M, Ohhama Y, Take H et al. Long-term outcome of children with biliary atresia who were not transplanted after the Kasai operation: >20-year experience at a children's hospital. J Pediatr Gastroenterol Nutr 2009;48:443–50.

Case 49

A 45-year-old male presents to the emergency room brought in by his family. He has become increasingly jaundiced over the last several days and is mildly confused. His wife states that he "drinks like a fish." His last alcohol was yesterday.

He complains of some mild abdominal pain but otherwise denies fever or chills. His bowels move normally without blood, and he denies dysuria.

His past medical history is significant for diabetes and hypertension, but he has been off medication for several months after he lost his job and his medical insurance. He denies any over-the-counter medications.

His family history is notable for alcohol-related liver disease in his father and several male siblings.

Exam demonstrates an obese male, looking older than stated, with vital signs weight 257 pounds, BP 120/80, pulse 104 regular, and temperature 100°F.

He is not in distress but has mild asterixis. He is obviously icteric and has multiple spider nevi. He has temporal wasting. His heart and lungs are normal but his abdomen is distended with dilated abdominal veins. His liver is markedly enlarged and tender, but his spleen is impalpable. Extremities show ++ ankle edema, and his skin demonstrates jaundice.

Laboratory Studies

Hb 12.6 g/dl
Platelets 246,000/μl
WBC 15.3 × 10^3/μl
INR 2.3
Creatinine 4.3 mg/dl
Tbili 37.5 mg/dl
Direct bili 24.3 mg/dl
AST 210 iu/l
ALT 109 iu/l
GGTP 236 iu/l
ALP 128 iu/l
Albumin 2.5 g/dl

Ultrasound of abdomen

Hetergeneous liver, no ductal dilation, normal-looking kidneys, minimal ascites.

Questions

1. What else is required to make a definitive diagnosis?
2. What is the prognosis?
3. Are there any treatment options other than abstinence from alcohol?

Laboratory Studies 2 Weeks Ago

Hb 13.1 g/dl
Platelets 232,000/μl
WBC 6.7 × 10^3/μl
INR 1.6
Creatinine 1.4 mg/dl
Tbili 3.1 mg/dl

Current urine studies
Urine sodium <5 mEq
Urine protein <200 mg
Urinalysis – no red cells, no casts, no bacteria

Answer: Type I Hepatorenal Syndrome (HRS)

This man presents with classic alcoholic hepatitis, but it has been complicated by type 1 HRS. This is a diagnosis that is actually quite difficult to make (according to the international ascites club) since several other disorders need to be excluded.

There are two types of HRS which by definition occur in patients with cirrhosis, severe alcoholic hepatitis, or fulminant hepatic failure. Type I is defined as at least a 50% lowering of the creatinine clearance to a value below 20 ml/min in less than a 2 week period or at least a twofold increase in serum creatinine to a level >2.5 mg/dl (221 μmol/l). Hence, the lab values shown from 2 weeks ago would fulfill this criterion. Patients do not need to be oliguric although most are. Type II is defined as any renal insufficiency in a patient that has the above liver diseases but does not meet criteria for type I. In general, this is essentially similar to diuretic-resistant ascites.

The absolute definition of HRS is:

- Patient with liver disease/failure and portal hypertension.
- Plasma creatinine >1.5 mg/dl (133 μmol/l) that progresses over days to weeks.
- Absence of any other apparent cause for renal disease, including shock, ongoing bacterial infection, current or recent treatment with nephrotoxic drugs, and the absence of ultrasonographic evidence of obstruction or parenchymal renal disease.
- Urine red cell excretion <50 cells per high power field.
- Urine protein excretion <500 mg/day.
- Lack of improvement in renal function after volume expansion with intravenous albumin (1 g/kg of body weight per day up to 100 g/day) for at least two days and withdrawal of diuretics.

The pathogenesis is related to splanchnic arterial vasodilation in the setting of portal hypertension. This is thought to be mediated by increased production or activity of vasodilators such as nitric oxide, mainly in the splanchnic circulation. In patients with significant liver disease, the cardiac output increases and the systemic vascular resistance decreases despite activation of the renin-angiotensin and sympathetic nervous systems.

The glomerular filtration rate and sodium excretion (usually <10 mEq/day in advanced cirrhosis) decline in this setting along with a fall in mean arterial pressure, despite the intense renal vasoconstriction.

HRS is best considered a reversible form of renal dysfunction in patients with liver failure (cirrhosis or acute liver failure), and treatment aims at improving the vasodilation by using vasoconstrictors. However, the underlying liver disease needs to be taken care of, and this usually means patients with type I HRS need urgent liver transplant evaluation as long as there are no other contraindications.

In the United States, we would typically use a combination of octreotide and midodrine (with intravenous albumin) or norepinephrine as vasoconstrictors. In countries where it is unavailable, the potent vasoconstrictor terlipression is used as it demonstrates a survival benefit in HRS.

In this patient, the prognosis is poor since his discriminant function is greater than 32. In addition, several studies have shown that the MELD score is also a good predictor of mortality in such patients, and his score is >40.

The cause of death in patients with alcoholic hepatitis is usually renal failure, and studies have shown that pentoxifylline is beneficial in this situation.

In this patient, after a trial of fluid, we would typically start him on pentoxifylline along with intravenous albumin.

References

1. Gines P, Schrier RW. Renal failure in cirrhosis. N Engl J Med 2009;361:1279.
2. Salerno F, Gerbes A, Gines P et al. Diagnosis, prevention and treatment of hepatorenal syndrome in cirrhosis. Gut 2007;56:1310.

Case 50

A 49-year-old female is admitted with a chief complaint of "*I wasn't feeling well*". The patient states she was in her usual state of health until 5 days prior to admission when she began to develop severe fatigue. The next day she began to develop nausea, bilious emesis, and darkening of her urine. The patient thought she had the flu and continued to work. Over the next two days, she began to develop right upper quadrant pain, anorexia, chills, and light headedness and finally presented to her local emergency room. She has a past medical history significant only for endometriosis. Over the last several days, she did take a few tablets of acetaminophen and ibuprofen, but otherwise takes no prescription medications, herbals nor has she had any recent antibiotic exposure. The patient lives with her husband of 25 years and their 15-year-old son. She works full-time as a bank teller. She has one tattoo which she obtained over 25 years ago. She has no habits, and there has been no recent travel. The patient's father died at the age of 69 of a pulmonary embolism following an open cholecystectomy.

The patient's husband is being followed in the liver clinic for chronic hepatitis B which was diagnosed over 15 years ago. He underwent a liver biopsy 3 years ago which revealed 1/6 fibrosis and minimal disease activity. The patient was seen in the liver clinic 1 year ago and was a symptomatic; however, his AST and ALT were 64 and 140 respectively. He was HBsAg +, sAb –, core total +, eAg negative, and eAb +. His viral load was 350,000 iu/ml and was being maintained on 10 mg of adefovir. Within the last 2 months, because of a lack of finances, the patient stopped taking his medication. He was last seen about 6 weeks ago complaining of fatigue. His lab work showed ALT 156 and ALT 320, and his DNA was 11,360,000 iu/ml. A resistance panel was performed, revealing the presence of a precore tag mutation. The patient was restarted on adefovir 10 mg in addition to 100 mg of lamivudine.

On physical exam, the patient was febrile at 100.5°F with a heart rate of 90 and blood pressure of 100/50. She was lethargic and confused with asterixis. She was jaundiced with scleral icterus. Cardiac and lung exam were normal. Abdomen was flat with hypoactive bowel sounds. She was very tender in her right upper quadrant. There was no evidence of hepatosplenomegaly. Extremities were without clubbing cyanosis or edema. There were no stigmata to suggest chronic liver disease.

Laboratory Data Revealed

Tbili 7.9 mg/dl (conjugated 4.8 mg/dl)
AST 6380 iu/l
ALT 7319 iu/l
ALP 218 iu/l

INR 4.9
pH 7.50, lactate 3.9
Hemogram, electrolytes, and renal function were all WNL

12 h after admission, repeat labs reveal:

Tbili 12 mg/dl
AST declined to 777 iu/l
ALT 2500 iu/l
INR to 11.5
HBsAg: Non-reactive
HBsAb: 233 miu/ml
HBcAb +
HBcAb IgM +
HBeAb +
HBeAg –
HDV IgM –
HBV DNA: 134,222 iu/ml (58,824 copies/ml)

Questions

1. Does this patient fulfill criteria for acute liver failure?
2. What is the patient's prognosis?
3. What treatment if any would you recommend?

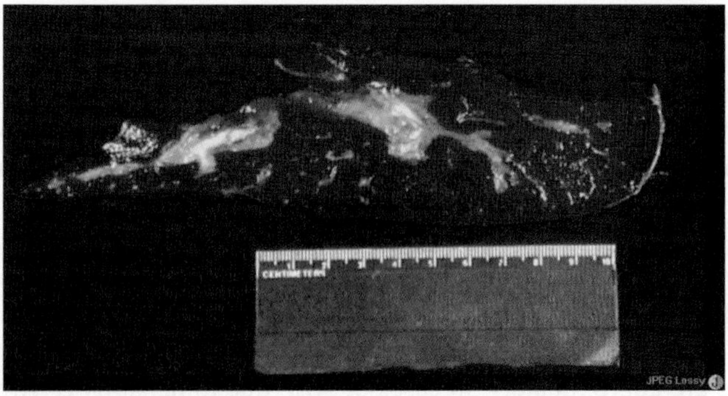

Fig. 50.1 Gross liver specimen

Fig. 50.2 Liver biopsy, H&E low power

Answer: Acute Liver Failure Secondary to Acute De Novo Hepatitis B Virus

The patient fulfills criteria for acute liver failure (ALF): the onset of coagulopathy and encephalopathy in a previous healthy individual. An important point for clinicians to realize is that although many patients with ALF will have elevated bilirubin levels, jaundice is not included in the formal definition. ALF is a rare condition with only approximately 2,000 cases per year in the United States. The most common cause of ALF in the US is acetaminophen toxicity. ALF secondary to HBV develops in less than one percent of patients infected with the virus.

Without liver transplantation, the fatality rate in patients with ALF from HBV is 93%. There are approximately 50 cases of ALF due to hepatitis B Virus (HBV) in the US each year. If detected in time, transplantation can be live-saving, with a 1 year survival of approximately 85%.

The injury in patients with severe hepatitis B infection is a consequence of the patient's violent immune response. The patient's viral serologies in this case provide a unique but telling tale into this immune response. It was during the process of fighting the infection and producing antibodies to the HBV that the patient became acutely ill. Unfortunately, the reaction and liver injury in this case was too far advanced for the patient to recover from. Antivirals would not reverse and would likely not stabilize the acute injury in this case. An argument could be made to administer antivirals to decrease the patient's viral load pre LT in the hopes of decreasing the incidence of recurrent HBV post transplant.

Although the decision tree in patients with ALF secondary to HBV is somewhat easier given the high mortality, knowing when to "pull the plug" on a patient with ALF and send them for LT can be a difficult decision. The clinician must weigh the chances of the patient's spontaneous recovery with the chances of progressive deterioration and multisystem organ failure. Many prognostic models have been proposed to help in this decision-making process.

To the untrained eye, the precipitous fall in the patient's enzyme in the case above may be viewed as an improvement; however, in conjunction with the worsening coagulopathy, this is actually a sign of impending doom and is a consequence submassive hepatocellular necrosis. The gross pathology (Fig. 50.1) of the patients explant reveals a "shriveled" liver weighing only 525 g (normal weight of a female adult liver 1,200–1,400 g). Histology (Fig. 50.2) reveals lobular necrosis with hemorrhage involving over 90% of the liver. Almost no hepatocytes are recognized.

The patient's husband in this case had an acute "flare" in his disease off of antiviral medications. The patient and her husband did have relations during this period. Transmission of HBV among adults is predominantly through sexual contact. HBV is a preventable disease, and all adults with potential exposure risk should be offered vaccination.

References

1. Lee HC. Acute liver failure related to hepatitis B virus. Hepatol Res 2008;38:S9–13.
2. Kim WR. Epidemiology of hepatitis B in the United States. Hepatology 2009;49:S28–34.
3. Wai CT, Fontana RJ, Polson J et al. Clinical outcome and virological characteristics of hepatitis B-related acute liver failure in the United States. J Viral Hepat 2005;12:192–8.

Case 51

A 55-year-old lady presents for elective outpatient endoscopy. She has a history of alcoholic cirrhosis that has been complicated by variceal bleeding 2 months ago when she was first diagnosed with liver disease. She underwent band ligation. She quit drinking at this time but previously had been drinking a bottle of vodka every few days. She developed encephalopathy while she was hospitalized with the bleeding but this is well controlled on lactulose. She has required a small dose of diuretics for ankle edema but has noticed some improvement in her overall condition with abstinence from alcohol.

She has no other medical problems.

Medications include nadolol, lactulose, furosemide, and aldactone. She is also taking a multivitamin and folate.

She is divorced and has no children. She has not worked for several years.

She is still smoking a packet of cigarettes daily but has no history of drug use.

She has a strong family history of alcoholism.

Her review of systems is significant for fatigue but is otherwise negative.

On exam she looks well and is alert and oriented.

Vital signs show BP 105/65, pulse 58, and she is afebrile.

There is mild scleral icterus and multiple spider nevi.

Heart reveals normal S1 and S2 without added sounds. Chest reveals lung fields.

His abdomen is soft and nontender with a spleen easily palpable. There is +ankle edema.

Laboratory Studies

Hb 9.6 g/dl
Platelets 42,000/μl
WBC 3.1 × 10^3/μl
INR 1.8
Creatinine 1.4 mg/dl
Tbili 4.9 mg/dl
AST 89 iu/l
ALT 67 iu/l
GGTP 189 iu/l
ALP 139 iu/l
Albumin 2.4 g/dl

She undergoes endoscopy and representative images (Figs. 51.1 and 51.2) are shown.

Questions

1. Is there an advantage in treating her with band ligation in combination with a beta-blocker or is banding alone sufficient?
2. If she has to undergo TIPS, will this improve her survival?
3. Is she a candidate for shunt surgery?

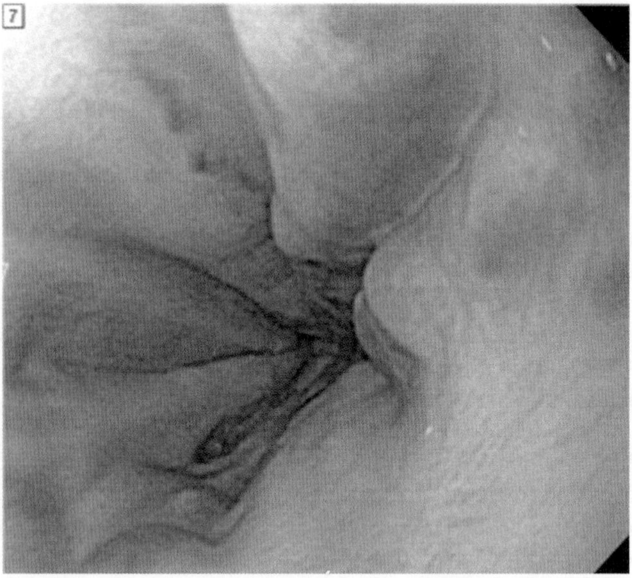

Fig. 51.1 Endoscopic images

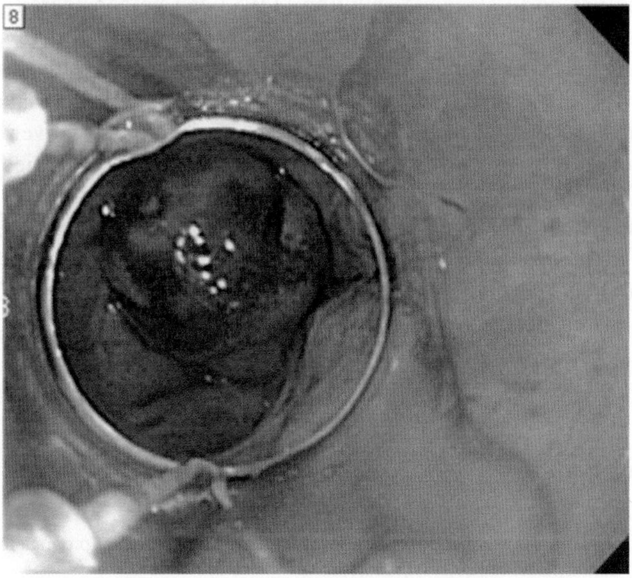

Fig. 51.2 Endoscopic images

Answer: Secondary Prophylaxis of Variceal Hemorrhage

This lady still has grade II esophageal varices with red wale signs at endoscopy (first image). She undergoes repeat band ligation as seen in the second image and likely will need further sessions to try and eradicate her varices.

There is a vast amount of literature on preventing rebleeding after an initial esophageal variceal bleed, and the American Association for the Study of Liver Diseases has published guidelines dealing with this topic.

The patient appears to be on an adequate dose of nadolol as evidenced by her pulse and blood pressure. Nonselective beta-blockers reduce the risk of a primary bleed, and several studies have shown that they reduce the risk of recurrent bleeding by about 40%. Ideally, the efficacy of beta-blockers should be measured by the reduction in hepatic venous pressure gradient, but this requires invasive testing, and most studies use a reduction of 25% in resting hear rate as a surrogate marker.

A combination of beta-blocker and endoscopic therapy with band ligation is better than either treatment alone in preventing rebleeding but does not reduce mortality compared to either treatment. Hence, patients who have experienced variceal bleeding should undergo band ligation until eradication of varices (we typically repeat an endoscopy every 6–8 weeks until varices are no longer present or too small to band) as well as beta-blocker treatment. If patients are intolerant to beta-blockers, band ligation alone is sufficient.

Transjugular porto-systemic shunting (TIPS) can be considered, particularly in patients with continued bleeding despite these measures. Studies comparing TIPS with endoscopic therapy for the prevention of variceal rebleeding found an advantage for TIPS, but this did not extend to a survival benefit and TIPS was associated with more complications such as encephalopathy, liver failure, and repeat intervention for TIPS dysfunction (although these studies were with uncoated TIPS stents).

As illustrated in another case, shunt surgery such as a distal splenorenal shunt is an option to prevent rebleeding but should be reserved for patients with well-maintained liver synthetic function which is not the case here. The ultimate treatment would be liver transplant, but this is contraindicated in patient with such short sobriety.

References

1. Hayes PC, Davis JM, Lewis JA, Bouchier IAD. Meta-analysis of value of propranolol in prevention of variceal hemorrhage. Lancet 1990;336:153.
2. Gonzalez R, Zamora J, Gomez-Camarero J et al. Meta-analysis: combination endoscopic and drug therapy to prevent variceal rebleeding in cirrhosis. Ann Intern Med 2008;149:109.
3. Jalan R, Forrest EH, Stanley AH et al. A randomized trial comparing transjugular intrahepatic portosystemic stent-shunt with variceal band ligation in the prevention of rebleeding from esophageal varices. Hepatology 1997;26:1115.

Case 52

A 25-year-old white female comes to the liver clinic to reestablish care. She initially presented to the children's hospital at the age of 9 with hematemesis. She underwent urgent EGD revealing bleeding esophageal varices and was treated with endoscopic sclerotherapy. She never had recurrent bleeding and never followed-up afterwards. She has been recently diagnosed with a spontaneous left lower extremity blood clot and is found to have protein C deficiency. Before starting her on chronic anticoagulation, given her history of GIB, hematology recommends consultation with you.

The patient states she feels well. She has a history of anxiety and takes as needed benzodiazepines. Two years ago the patient underwent an uneventful laparoscopic cholecystectomy for symptomatic gallstones, an intraoperative liver biopsy revealed mild fibrosis and bile ductular proliferation. Although the patient doesn't know details, she knows her mother is on lifelong warfarin for a history of blood clots. The patient lives with her fiancé and works as a cashier at a convenience store. She smokes one-half pack of cigarettes per day and drinks only on special occasions. There is no history of high-risk behavior.

On exam, she appears well and is not in distress. Her heart rate is 80 beats per minute, blood pressure 110/50; BMI is 27.7 kg/m^2. She has no evidence of scleral icterus or stigmata to suggest chronic liver disease. Her lungs and cardiac exam are normal. Abdominal exam reveals some dilated umbilical veins, no hepatomegaly, but a palpable spleen tip. No appreciable ascites. Her left leg has some mild erythema and trace edema.

An EGD was performed revealing mild-to-moderate portal hypertensive gastropathy (most notable in the fundus) and grade 1 esophageal varices but no evidence of gastric varices.

Laboratory Data Revealed

Tbili 1.8 mg/dl (conjugated 0.2)
AST 32 iu/l
ALT 17 iu/l
AP 94 iu/l
INR 1.1
Alb 3.7 g/dl

Electrolytes and renal function normal
Platelet count of 120,000, remainder of hemogram normal

Questions

1. How would you work up this patient?
2. What are your recommendations regarding anticoagulation?

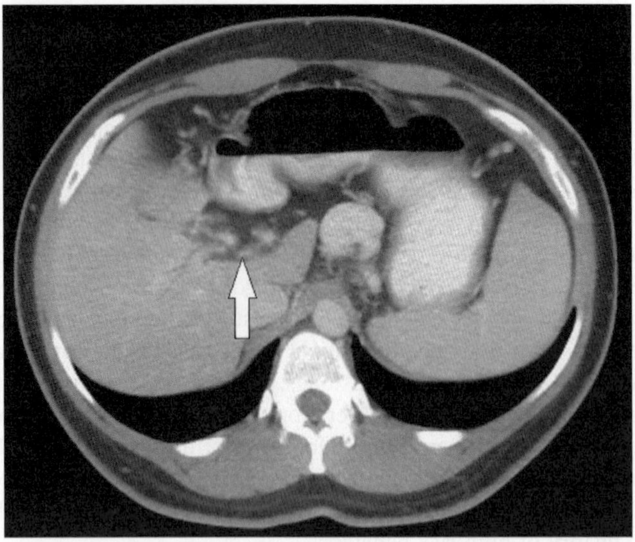

Fig. 52.1 CT scan done (prior to surgery 2 years ago)

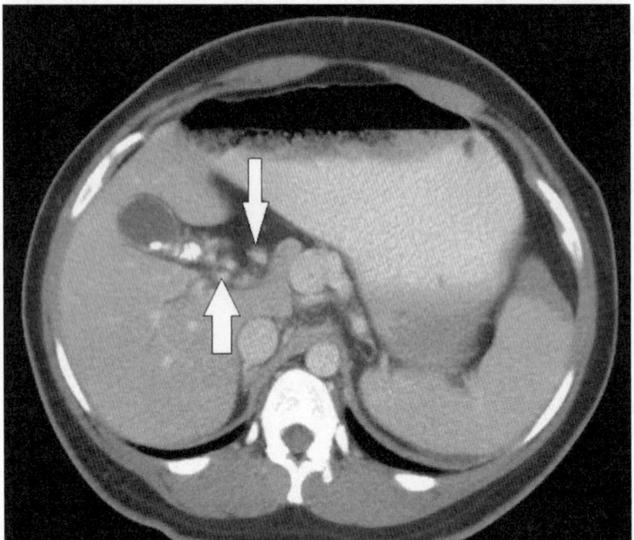

Fig. 52.2 CT scan done (prior to surgery 2 years ago)

Answer: Hypercoaguable State Leading to Portal Vein Thrombosis, Cavernous Transformation and Portal Hypertension

This young lady has portal hypertension, but interestingly, this was first noted as a child, and hence, congenital causes have to be high on the differential diagnosis. The main possibilities include portal vein atresia or portal vein thrombosis. Cirrhosis is uncommon in young children and would be expected to worsen with time and yet this lady did well for many years. The first test to obtain would be an imaging study to look at the liver and hepatic vasculature. CT scan, MRI, or ultrasound all have a potential role.

Portal hypertension is defined by a hepatic venous pressure gradient (HVPG) greater than 5 mmHg. A variety of disorders can cause portal hypertension in the absence of cirrhosis, a condition referred to as "noncirrhotic portal hypertension."

Portal hypertension has been categorized as prehepatic, intrahepatic, or posthepatic based upon the site of obstruction to flow. The clinical consequences of portal hypertension (ascites, varices, and encephalopathy) are similar regardless of the cause or site of obstruction.

Presinusoidal portal hypertension is caused by obstruction to flow through the portal venous system in the extrahepatic portion of the portal vein (extrahepatic presinusoidal portal hypertension; see image one above) or at the level of portal vein branches within the liver (intrahepatic presinusoidal portal hypertension).

The causes of portal vein thrombosis (PVT) vary with age. In adults, approximately 25% of patients with PVT have underlying cirrhosis, with the prevalence correlating with the severity of underlying liver disease. In children, the most common etiology of PVT is thrombophlebitis of the umbilical vein (omphalitis) and ultimately the portal vein. Omphalitis is a rare event in industrialized countries but is estimated to be as high as 6% in the developing world.

No apparent cause for portal vein thrombosis is evident in more than one-third of patients Many of these patients probably have an underlying hypercoagulable state. The following hypercoagulable states have been identified in different studies comparing patients with portal vein thrombosis compared to various controls and should be tested for:

Factor V Leiden
Prothrombin gene mutation
Protein C deficiency
Protein S deficiency
Antithrombin deficiency
MTFR gene mutation that raises homocysteine
Myeloproliferative disorders, in some cases diagnosed only by the presence of a JAK2 617F mutation
Increased factor VIII levels

Chronic portal vein thrombosis develops in patients whose thrombosis does not spontaneously resolve. This may either produce a chronic noncavernous thrombosed portal vein or cavernous transformation of the portal vein. Cavernous transformation refers to the development of collateral blood vessels that bring blood in a hepatopedal manner from the region of obstruction. When seen in a transverse section, as on a CT scan, cavernous transformation gives the appearance of multiple caveolar orifices (white arrows in image two above). Image one above reveals abrupt "cut off" of the portal vein (arrow) at the confluence secondary to extensive thrombus.

More than 85–90% of patients with chronic portal vein thrombosis have esophageal varices, while 30–40% have concomitant gastric varices with bleeding occurring in 50–70% of patients. In contrast to variceal bleeding in patients with cirrhosis, the risks of developing liver failure, encephalopathy, and death are much lower in patients with portal vein thrombosis or other causes of extrahepatic portal vein obstruction without underlying cirrhosis.

Since the liver parenchyma is not directly involved in patients with portal vein thrombosis, a majority of patients have histologically normal livers.

There are few controlled data on which to base clinical decisions in patients with portal vein thrombosis. Thus, treatment should be determined by an individual patient's clinical circumstances, the pathophysiology involved, and the available expertise. A surgical approach can be considered for patients with correctable anatomic abnormalities causing extrahepatic portal vein obstruction, provided there is no cirrhosis.

A 2009 guideline from the American Association for the Study of Liver Diseases recommends consideration of long-term anticoagulation in patients with chronic portal vein thrombosis without cirrhosis who have a permanent risk factor for venous thrombosis that cannot be corrected. In patients with gastroesophageal varices, anticoagulation should not be initiated until adequate prophylaxis for variceal bleeding has been instituted.

The young lady in this case was "cleared" to remain on anticoagulation. She was started on a nonselective beta blocker with titration to a heart rate of 55 beats per minute. Close follow-up was arranged in both the hematology and hepatology clinics given her prior history of noncompliance.

References

1. Sarin SK, Agarwal SR. Extrahepatic portal vein obstruction. Semin Liver Dis 2002;22:43–58.
2. Condat B, Pessione F, Hillaire S et al. Current outcome of portal vein thrombosis in adults: risk and benefit of anticoagulant therapy. Gastroenterology 2001;120:490–7.
3. DeLeve LD, Valla DC, Garcia-Tsao G. Vascular disorders of the liver. Hepatology 2009;49:1729–64.

Case 53

A 53-year-old white female with a past medical history significant for hypertension and hypercholesterolemia is brought to the emergency room with chest pain and syncope. The patient was "found down" in her kitchen by her 14-year-old son. She was diaphoretic, grasping for air, holding her chest, complaining of severe, crushing pain. Upon arrival, emergency medical service (EMS) documented her temperature as 99.1°F, heart rate 116, systolic blood pressure 82, and respiratory rate 22. Her oxygen saturation was 83% on room air. The patient's only other medical history includes long standing hypothyroidism. She underwent a carpal tunnel release on her right hand 4 years ago. Her prescription medications include hydrochlorothiazide and synthroid. She stopped taking her cholesterol medication (rosuvastatin) months ago as she thought it was the cause of her "aching muscles." She does suffer from chronic low back pain and takes as needed ibuprofen and acetaminophen. She took 3 g of acetaminophen two days prior to admission. Her husband notes that she has been complaining of intermittent chest discomfort for the last month. She was scheduled for an evaluation with her primary care physician next week. The patient lives with her husband of 28 years and their three healthy children. She works full-time as a school bus driver. She has a 20 pack year smoking history and currently smokes ten cigarettes per day. She averages between 6 and 8 beers per week. She has two tattoos, the first of which she obtained 25 years ago. Her father passed from pneumonia at the age of 59. He suffered from a debilitating stroke 1 year prior. Her mother died at the age of 66 from postoperative complications following an abdominal aortic aneurysm (AAA) repair. The patient's 57-year-old brother has diabetes.

Physical exam is notable for an obese, middle-aged white female with a BMI of 33.7 kg/m^2. She is awake, but confused. She is diaphoretic and very anxious. Sclerae are nonicteric. JVP is measured at 13 cm. She has rales bilaterally, and an S3 is auscultated on cardiac exam. Her abdomen is soft and nontender. Bowel sounds are normal. Liver edge is smooth and palpable 2 cm below the right costo-vertebral angle. There is no appreciable splenomegaly. She has trace lower extremitiy edema. There are no stigmata suggestive of chronic liver disease.

An EKG reveals ST elevations in the anterior leads. Troponin I is 125.6 ng/ml. The remainder of initial laboratory data are shown below.

The patient is taken emergently for cardiac catheterization. Coronary angiography reveals high grade, three vessel disease. Right heart catheterization reveals pressures consistent with severe biventricular congestive heart failure. An intraaortic balloon pump is inserted, and the patient is taken emergently to the operating room for coronary artery bypass (CABG).

You are consulted on postoperative day 3 for a rising bilirubin. The primary team also asks you "when would it be safe to restart her statin?"

Laboratory Data

On admission

Na 141 mEq/l
BUN 39 mg/dl
Cr 2.6 mg/dl
WBC 15,400/μl
Hb 14 g/dl
Platelets 390,000/μl

Troponin I: 125.6 ng/ml
Tbili 0.8 mg/dl
AST 8690 iu/l
ALT 6888 iu/l
ALP 226 iu/l
INR 1.4
LDH 2480 iu/l

Post CABG day 3

BUN 8 mg/dl
Cr 1.4 mg/dl
Tbili 3.3 mg/dl (conjugated 1.9)
AST 874 iu/l
ALT 290 iu/l
ALP 118 iu/l

Questions

1. What is the differential for the abnormalities noted in liver function tests and the increasing bilirubin level?
2. What further testing would you recommend?
3. What treatment if any would you recommend?
4. When would it be safe to start a statin?

Answer: Ischemic/Hypoxic Liver Injury

There are only a handful of liver injuries which will cause transaminase levels to be in the tens of thousands initially and then drop in half the next day. Perhaps the most commonly encountered of these in the United States is ischemic liver injury. One study quoted a prevalence of 0.9% of all ICU admissions to suffer from ischemic liver injury.

The case presentation here is quite classic. The transaminase levels are remarkably high in the setting of shock (in this case cardiogenic); there is concomitant kidney injury (likely the result of acute tubular necrosis). The elevated LDH is also a clue and makes a viral etiology less likely. As the underlying insult resolves, the transaminase levels improve precipitously.

It is not uncommon for the consult in these cases to be called in several days after admission. The primary team is comforted by the rapid improvement in transaminase levels, but is concerned given the rising total bilirubin.

The term "ischemic hepatitis" was first coined in 1979 to refer to liver injury characterized histologically by centrilobular liver cell necrosis with a sharp increase in serum aminotransferase levels in the setting of cardiac failure.

The etiology of ischemic liver injury is a result of a reduction in hepatic perfusion leading to hepatic anoxia and necrosis. The degree of liver injury is proportional to the amount of liver rendered ischemic. The outcome is dependent upon restoration in hepatic blood flow and oxygen delivery. Global hypotension (as seen in shock/hypotension) typically leads to rapid recovery with no long-term effects, granted there is no significant underlying liver disease. Ischemia resulting from vascular occlusion or injury to the contrary can cause permanent injury and lead to fibrosis and ischemic cholangiopathy.

In one of the larger studies to evaluate this entity, over a 10-year period, 142 episodes of ischemic hepatitis were identified. Four main groups were identified: decompensated congestive heart failure, acute cardiac failure, exacerbated chronic respiratory failure, and toxic/septic shock. The hemodynamic mechanisms responsible for liver injury were different in the four groups. In congestive heart failure and acute heart failure, the hypoxia of the liver resulted from decreased hepatic blood flow due to left-sided heart failure and from venous congestion secondary to right-sided heart failure. In chronic respiratory failure, liver hypoxia was mainly due to profound hypoxemia. In toxic/septic shock, oxygen delivery to the liver was not decreased, but oxygen demands were increased. A "shock" state was present in only 55% of cases. We agree with the authors of this study that the commonly used term "shock liver" should be disregarded, and replaced with "hypoxic liver injury."

The workup in cases like this should be determined on a case-by-case basis but in most instances should be limited and cost-efficient. A right upper quadrant ultrasound with Dopplers to rule out underlying liver disease and vascular occlusion should be performed. Viral serologies are not unreasonable. The bilirubin will typically "lag" behind the transaminase levels and will peak on days 3–5. Avoiding additional hepatic insults is important. Generally supportive care and improving the underlying cause of hypoxia will improve the liver injury. Liver failure is rare in these settings; when it does occur, it almost always occurs in the setting of severe cardiac disease or cirrhosis.

The use of statins in patients with liver disease is a commonly asked question of primary care physicians. Statins have become one of the most widely prescribed medications in the western world. Their beneficial effects in patients with cardiovascular disease are well established. They have an excellent safety profile. The most common clinical hepatic manifestation of statins is asymptomatic elevations in liver enzymes with an incidence of about 3%. In general, however, the incidence of liver enzymes elevations in statin-treated patients has not been consistently different than placebo. The risk of "significant" liver injury is extremely rare, and the risk of acute liver failure has been limited to a handful of case reports.

Understanding the beneficial effects a statin would have for the patient in this particular case, we recommend starting the medication after liver enzymes were closer to normal values. The patient's enzymes returned to near normal after 2 weeks from her initial presentation. She was restarted on her statin medication and repeat enzymes 1 month later were completely normal. We recommend monitoring every 3–4 months for the first year. The patient has had no sequelae from her acute liver injury.

References

1. Henrion J, Schapira M, Luwaert R et al. Hypoxic hepatitis: clinical and hemodynamic study in 142 consecutive cases. Medicine 2003;82:392–406.
2. de Denus S, Spinler SA, Miller K et al. Statins and liver toxicity: a meta-analysis. Pharmacotherapy 2004;24:584–91.

Case 54

A 41-year-old lady presents with several weeks of right upper quadrant pain, abdominal distension, and shortness of breath. She denies any jaundice or change in urine or stool color.

She is otherwise well and has no other medical problems.

She takes no medications and denies over-the-counter or herbal supplements.

She is married and works as a secretary. She has two children who are alive and well.

She denies tobacco or alcohol and does not use illicit drugs.

There is no family history.

Exam shows a lady who is uncomfortable. Vital signs show BP 125/80, pulse 104, respiratory rate 26 per minute, and she is afebrile.

There is mild scleral icterus but no spider nevi or palmar erythema. She is alert and oriented. Heart reveals normal S1 and S2 without added sounds. Chest reveals decreased air entry at the right base with a stony dull percussion note and decreased fremitus.

Her abdomen is distended with a liver that is felt 6 cm below the right costal margin and is tender but not pulsatile. There is a fluid thrill but no dilated abdominal veins. She has 2+ankle edema to the knees bilaterally.

Laboratory Studies

Hb 15.3 g/dl
Platelets 587,000/μl
WBC 16.6 × 10^3/μl
INR 1.5
Creatinine 1.2 mg/dl
Tbili 3.4 mg/dl
AST 238 iu/l
ALT 206 iu/l
GGTP 349 iu/l
ALP 287 iu/l
Albumin 2.9 g/dl

Ultrasound shows ascites and chest x-ray shows a right pleural effusion

Questions

1. What are the other tests required to make a diagnosis?
2. What are the treatment options?
3. What is the long-term prognosis?

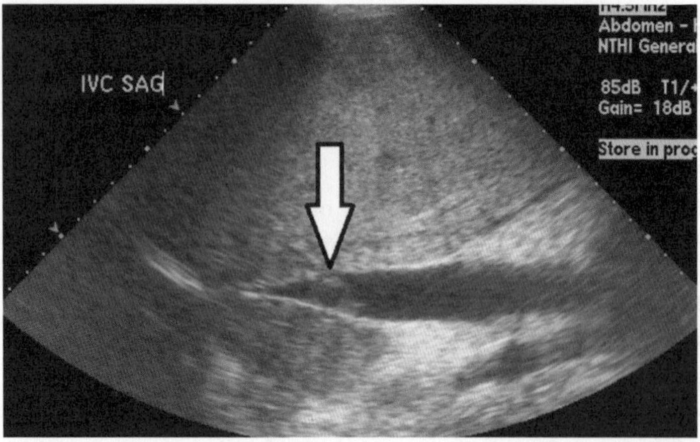

Fig. 54.1 Ultrasound

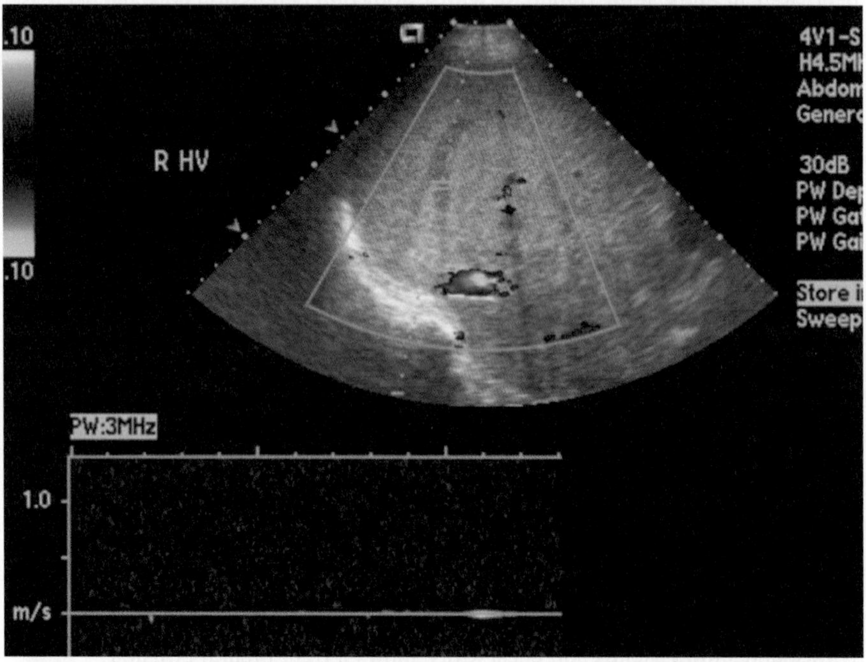

Fig. 54.2 Ultrasound

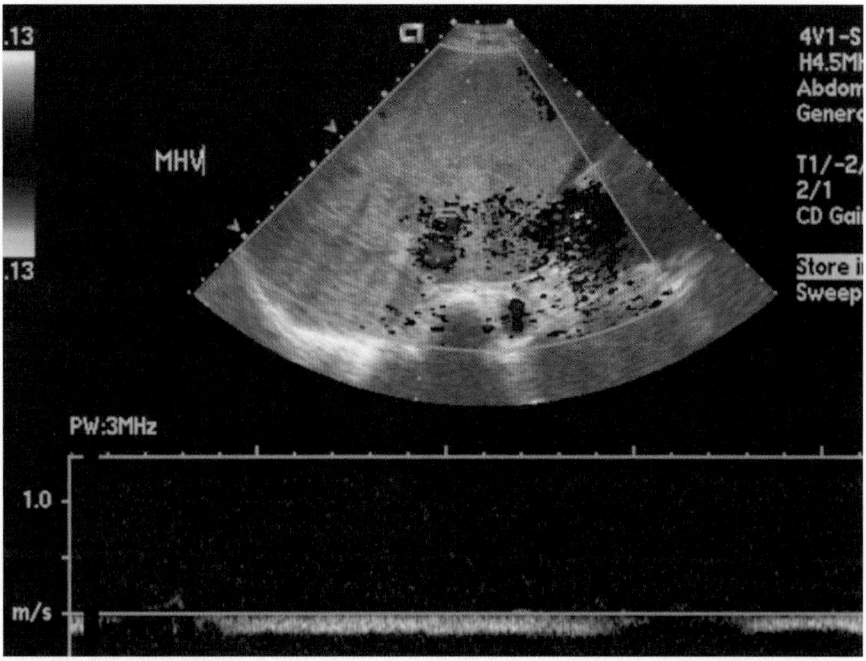

Fig. 54.3 Ultrasound

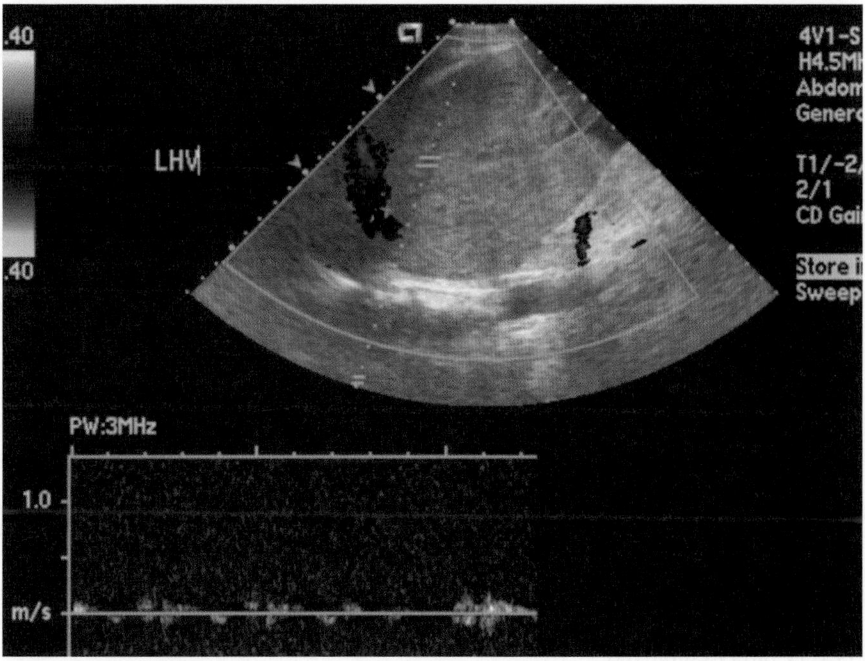

Fig. 54.4 Ultrasound

Answer: Budd–Chiari Syndrome

The ultrasound with Doppler(Figs. 54.1–54.4) shows echogenic material in the inferior vena cava (IVC) that is arrowed (Fig. 54.1), and all of the hepatic veins show no flow and are barely visible indicating complete thrombosis.

Budd–Chiari syndrome (BCS) is defined by obstruction of venous outflow from the liver. This is typically due to hepatic venous or inferior vena caval thrombosis.

This lady has a classic presentation with a relatively acute onset of tender hepatomegaly, ascites and lower extremity edema. In several large case series, most patients will present in this fashion or with chronic disease characterized by portal hypertension and cirrhosis. A few will have fulminant hepatic failure. BCS is more common in women and a quarter of patients will have an overt myeloproliferative disorder (typically polycythemia vera). This lady's elevated hemoglobin and platelet count are very suggestive and subsequent work-up confirmed this was indeed the case.

Laboratory studies typically show a mixed picture of enzyme elevation and mild hyperbilirubinemia. If the disease is not treated encephalopathy and liver failure can ensue.

The diagnosis is typically made as in this case with Doppler imaging showing either thrombosis or lack of flow in the hepatic venous outflow tract. Ct scan or MRI can also be employed and the gold standard is venography. The differential diagnosis includes right heart failure and constrictive pericarditis so echocardiogram is a useful test, particularly as analysis of ascitic fluid can demonstrate a total protein >3.0 g/l, and the serum-ascites albumin concentration gradient can be >1.1 g/dl, as seen in patients with cardiac and pericardial disease.

Liver biopsy is not necessary to make a diagnosis but can be helpful for determining prognosis and for guiding therapy, since patients with advanced fibrosis or cirrhosis are unlikely to improve with revascularization.

Treatment can be medical, radiologic, or surgical depending on the acuity of presentation and severity of the obstruction but is also guided by local expertise. The goal is restore venous outflow and decompress the liver to prevent portal hypertension and its sequelae. It is important to complete a hypercoaguable work up and involve a hematologist in the care of these patients so as not to delay use of anticoagulation or anti-platelet agents. In patients with an acute presentation, direct thrombolytic therapy into the thrombosed vessels has had some success.

This patient was treated with diuretics with a good response and was started on heparin and aspirin while waiting for a diagnosis.

She later underwent a TIPS placement. Recent data would suggest that long-term survival after TIPS is 80%, equivalent to that seen with transplant. There are small case series illustrating the benefit of dilation or stent therapy without TIPS, but this runs the risk of restenosis or reocclusion. Because of the improvement in interventional radiology over the last 10–15 years, nontransplant surgery for BCS is very rarely employed.

Liver transplant is an excellent option for patients with evidence of cirrhosis and decompensation who are not candidates for TIPS. It also has the advantage of correcting potential hematologic etiologies including protein C, protein S, or antithrombin III deficiencies. Several large case series have demonstrated 70–80% 5–10 year survival.

The American Association for the Study of Liver Diseases guidelines for BCS recommend:

- Correcting any underlying risk factor(s) for venous thrombosis.
- Start anticoagulation therapy immediately using low molecular weight heparin and switching to warfarin.
- Maintain permanent anticoagulation therapy unless contraindications/ complications.
- Treat complications of portal hypertension.
- Treat venous obstruction amenable to percutaneous angioplasty/stenting in all symptomatic patients.
- Consider TIPS in patients without ongoing improvement on anticoagulation therapy (with or without angioplasty).
- Consider liver transplantation if TIPS insertion fails or does not improve the patient's condition and in those with fulminant hepatic failure.
- Refer/confer care with a transplant center.

References

1. Menon KV, Shah V, Kamath PS. The Budd–Chiari syndrome. N Engl J Med 2004;350:578.
2. Murad SD, Plessier A, Hernandez-Guerra M et al. Etiology, management, and outcome of the Budd-Chiari syndrome. Ann Intern Med 2009;151:167.
3. De Leve LD, Valla D-C, Garcia-Tsao G. Vascular disorders of the liver. Hepatology 2009;49:1729–64.

Case 55

A 41-year-old man presents to the emergency room with ascites and lower extremity edema. He is not known to have liver disease and in fact was very healthy up until a motor vehicle accident 4 months ago where he was in the passenger seat and his car had a head-on collision with a minivan. Fortunately, he was wearing a seatbelt then and suffered only a fractured tibia that has healed well.

He has noticed increasing abdominal distension over the last few days and now cannot get his shoes on without difficulty. He denies GI bleeding or encephalopathy.

There has been no fever or chills, but he has noticed some shortness of breath.

He denies any prescribed or over the counter medication.

He does not smoke or drink and is married. He has no obvious risk factors for viral hepatitis and no family history of liver disease.

On exam, he looks well with vital signs showing BP 120/75, pulse 92, and he is afebrile. His BMI is 23 kg/m^2. There is no scleral icterus, but he has several spider nevi.

His heart exam is normal, and lungs reveal some decreased air entry at the right base. His abdomen is distended with dullness in the flanks. His liver is palpable just below the right costal margin, and the spleen is easily felt. He has ++ankle edema to the thighs.

Laboratory Studies

Hb 11.2 g/dl
Platelets 64,000/μl
INR 1.3
Tbili 2.1 mg/dl
AST 102 iu/l
ALT 95 iu/l
ALP 149 iu/l
Albumin 2.5 g/dl
Creatinine 1.3 mg/dl

Questions

1. Which is the likely diagnosis?
2. How is the diagnosis made?
3. What treatment options are available?

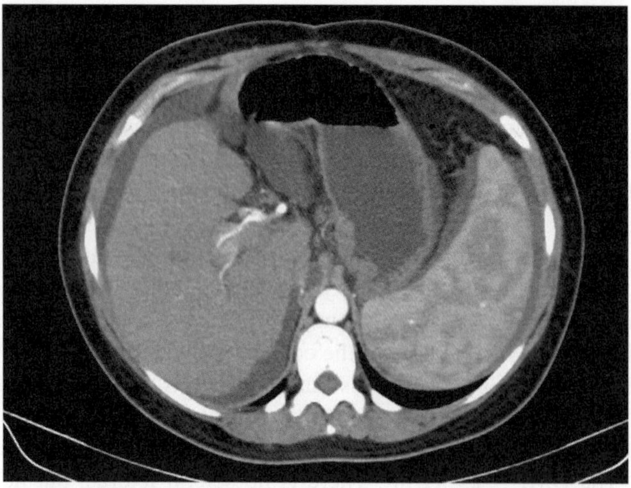

Fig. 55.1 CT image

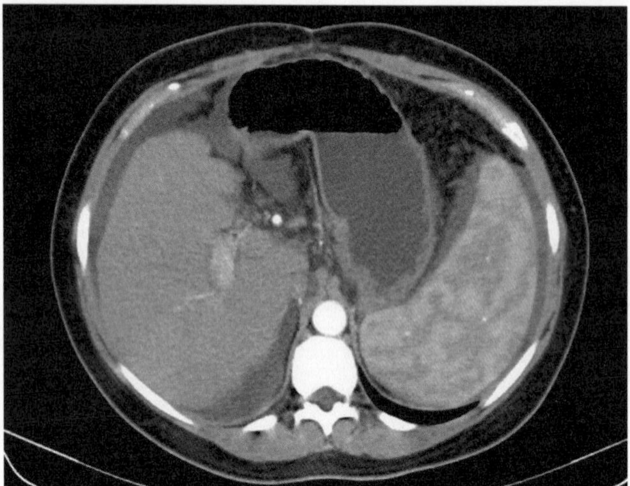

Fig. 55.2 CT image

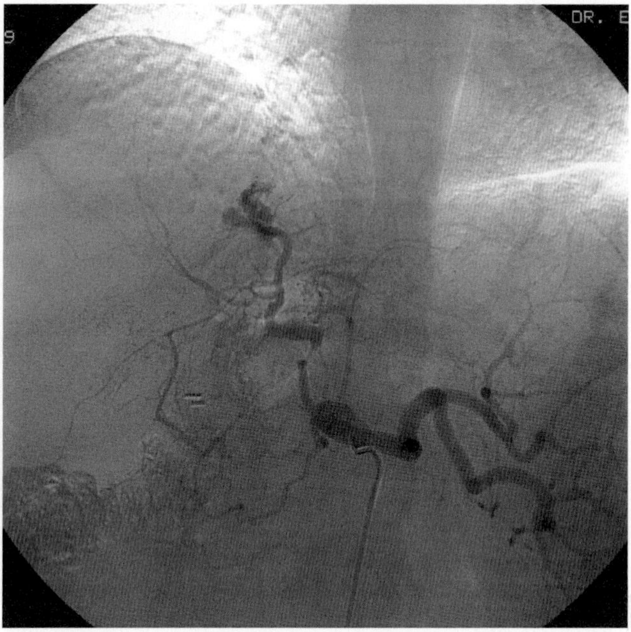

Fig. 55.3 Angiogram

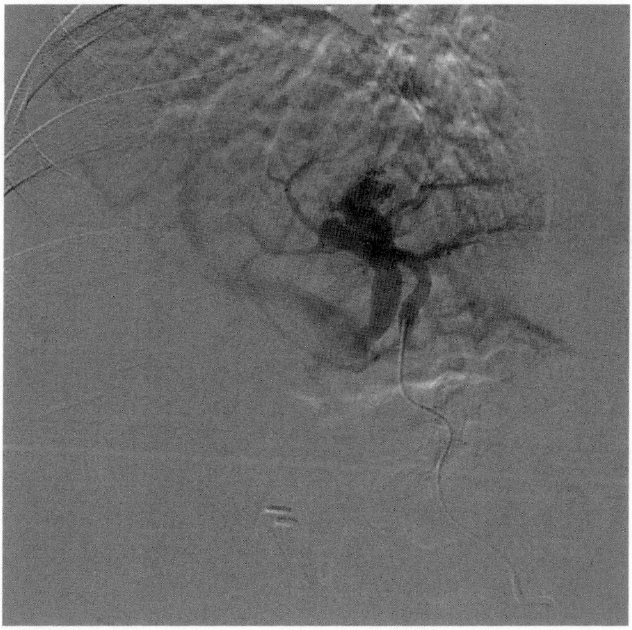

Fig. 55.4 Angiogram

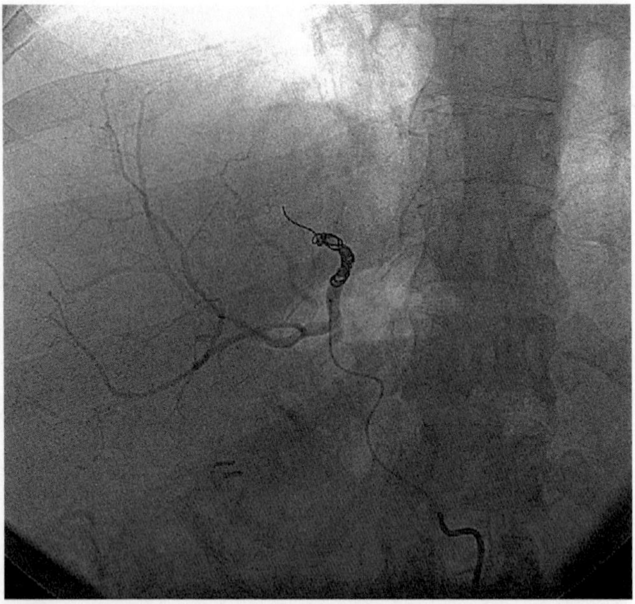

Fig. 55.5 Angiogram

Answer: Hepatic Arterio-Portal Fistula as a Cause of Portal Hypertension

This is a very interesting case that shows not all portal hypertension is due to increased resistance in portal venous flow. The usual classification of portal hypertension is based on the site of the obstruction – prehepatic, intrahepatic, or posthepatic. The normal portal system is under very low pressure and a gradient of <5 mmHg is typical. Clinical consequences arise when the pressure gradient between the portal and hepatic veins reaches 10–12 mmHg. Increases of portal blood flow can be significant in the postprandial state (from 700 to 1,500 ml/min) but due to the passive dilation of low resistance vessels in and around the liver, the portal pressure rises only marginally.

In this patient, the trauma of the motor vehicle accident has led to the formation of a fistula between the hepatic artery and portal vein. The portal blood flow increases dramatically in this situation, beyond the capacity of low resistance vessels to accommodate and portal hypertension ensues. It can also lead to significant fibrosis in the liver and cirrhosis.

The CT images (Figs. 55.1 and 55.2) show the arterial phase and the hepatic artery fills, but a connection can be seen to the portal vein which is seen filling in Fig. 55.2. The angiogram (Figs. 55.3–55.5) shows a catheter in the right hepatic artery and the portal vein can be seen filling rapidly (Fig. 55.3). The magnified second image (Fig. 55.4) shows the catheter in the fistula and coils are being placed, and the third image (Fig. 55.5) shows closure of the fistula without flow into the portal system.

Hepatic (or splenic) arterioportal fistula is a very rare cause of portal hypertension but illustrates the physiology of the portal system very well. It typically can occur after trauma or rupture of an arterial aneurysm, tumor invasion and has been reported as a complication of liver biopsy. Congential causes include hereditary hemorrhagic telangiectasia. There are reports in the older literature of surgical repair of fistulae, but most case reports and case series now detail successful radiologic treatment as in this case. Occasionally, liver transplantation is required.

References

1. Aithal GP, Alabdi BJ, Rose JD et al. Portal hypertension secondary to arterio-portal fistulae: two unusual cases. Liver 1999;19:343–7.
2. Dumortier J, Pilleul F, Adham M et al. Severe portal hypertension secondary to arterio-portal fistula: salvage surgical treatment. Liver Int 2007;27:865–8.
3. Korula J, Fried J, Weissman M et al. Fatal hemorrhage from an arterio-portal-peritoneal fistula after percutaneous liver biopsy. Gastroenterology 1989;96:244–6.

Case 56

A 31-year-old lady presents to the emergency room with hematemesis. She has a history of cirrhosis likely secondary to autoimmune disease that has been complicated in the past by several episodes of variceal bleeding but otherwise she denies ascites or encephalopathy. Her last endoscopy was 3 months ago and revealed grade I esophageal varices and small gastric varices. She has undergone multiple sessions of band ligation in the past and is maintained on secondary prophylaxis for variceal hemorrhage.

Her past medical history is significant for thyroid disease.

Her current medications include levothyroxine and nadolol.

She does not smoke or drink and is married without children and is working as a legal assistant.

The rest of her review of systems is negative.

On exam, she looks well with vital signs showing BP 110/60, pulse 62, and she is afebrile. There is no scleral icterus although she has several spider nevi. She is alert and oriented. Her heart and lungs are normal. Abdomen is soft and nontender with a spleen tip palpable but no ascites.

Laboratory Studies

Hb 10.7 g/dl
Platelets 75,000/μl
INR 1.2
Tbili 1.1 mg/dl
AST 45 iu/l
ALT 32 iu/l
ALP 87 iu/l
Albumin 3.5 g/dl
Creatinine 0.7 mg/dl

After adequate resuscitation and somatostatin, endoscopy is performed and reveals grade II esophageal varices with red wale signs and gastric varices in the fundus. Bands are placed on the esophageal varices.

Questions

1. Should this patient be referred for transplant?
2. Are there other options available?

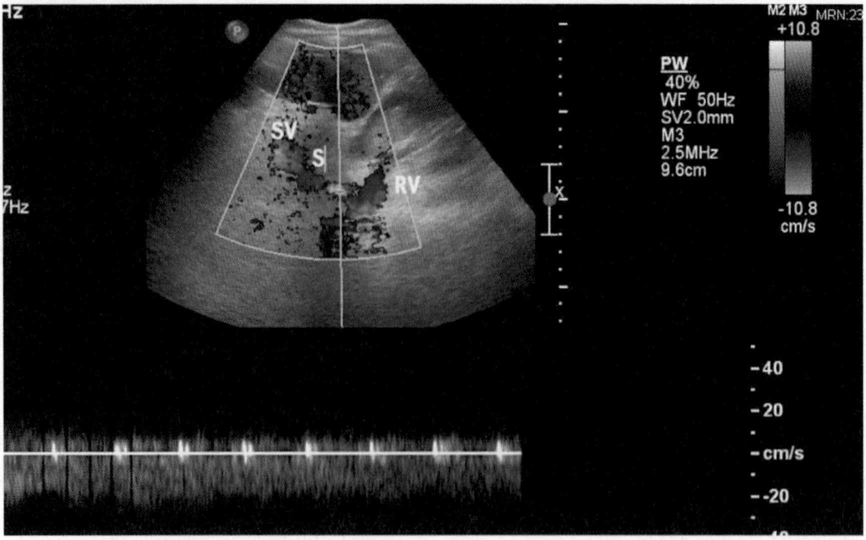

Fig. 56.1 Ultrasound

Answer: Prevention of Recurrent Variceal Hemorrhage with Distal Splenorenal Shunt

This lady presents with another episode of variceal bleeding despite being on a beta-blocker and having undergone multiple endoscopies in the past. Her liver synthetic function is normal and she appears to be active and is still working. Liver transplant would fix the underlying portal hypertension, but she is early based on her MELD score, and most experts would not recommend this.

You could continue with the current strategy but she has bled again despite adequate medical therapy. TIPS would be a consideration in this patient. Another option would be surgical decompression.

In the 1980s, there were several trials comparing endoscopic therapy with portocaval shunting which showed similar efficacy, and this was in the days of sclerotherapy rather than band ligation. In addition, this type of surgery is complex and requires significant expertise and is only available in certain centers. Another study published in 1990 suggested that distal splenorenal shunt (DSRS) was superior to sclerotherapy in bleeding control but the sclerotherapy arm had improved survival, which was still apparent if sclerotherapy failed to control the bleeding and the patient needed salvage DSRS.

However, today a patient would undergo band ligation for esophageal varices rather than sclerotherapy, and TIPS would be a viable option.

A more recent study compared TIPS with DSRS and found that in Child's A and B patients, the control of recurrent bleeding was similar, but the TIPS group needed more intervention for TIPS stenosis or dysfunction. This study was started in the era before covered TIPS which have lower stenosis rates.

The ultrasound image (Fig. 56.1) shows a patent DSRS (the "S") between the splenic vein ("SV") and renal vein ("RV"). Good flow is noted on the Doppler. This lady did well after DSRS and has not bled in the last 2 years. I have followed several other patients from the TIPS vs. DSRS trial that similarly have not bled in 10 years and are still early for transplant suggesting that in patients with well-preserved liver synthetic function and significant portal hypertension, DSRS is a viable alternative if the anatomy is amenable, and the center has the expertise to perform the procedure.

References

1. Cello JP, Grendell JH, Crass RA et al. Endoscopic sclerotherapy versus portacaval shunt in patient with severe cirrhosis and acute variceal hemorrhage. Long-term follow-up. N Engl J Med 1987;316:11.
2. Henderson JM, Kutner MH, Millikan WJ et al. Endoscopic variceal sclerosis compared with distal splenorenal shunt to prevent recurrent variceal bleeding in cirrhosis. Ann Intern Med 1990;112:262.
3. Henderson JM, Boyer TD, Kutner MH et al. Distal splenorenal shunt versus transjugular intrahepatic portal systematic shunt for variceal bleeding: a randomized trial. Gastroenterology 2006;130:1643–51.

Case 57

A 36-year-old man presents to your outpatient office with abdominal distension which has gradually worsened over several weeks. He denies fever, chills, weight loss, or abdominal pain. He denies GI bleeding or encephalopathy.

His only past medical history is knee surgery following his collegiate athletic career.

He takes occasional over the counter analgesics but takes no prescribed medication.

He is married and works in a local advertising agency. He has never been a heavy drinker and does not smoke or drink.

There is no family history of liver disease.

The rest of his review of systems is negative.

On exam he looks well and is alert and oriented.

Vital signs show BP 115/65, pulse 64 and he is afebrile.

There is no scleral icterus and no spider nevi.

Heart reveals normal S1 and S2 without added sounds. Chest reveals clear lung fields.

His abdomen is distended with a fluid thrill. Spleen is easily palpable, and there are dilated abdominal veins. There is a murmur heard best in the epigastric area which grows louder with a Valsalva manouever and seems to diminish when pressure is applied over the umbilical area with the palm of the hand. He has +ankle edema bilaterally.

Laboratory Studies

Hb 14.1 g/dl
Platelets 73,000/μl
WBC 5.3 × 10^3/μl
INR 1.1
Creatinine 1.3 mg/dl
Tbili 0.6 mg/dl
AST 18 iu/l
ALT 16 iu/l
GGTP 83 iu/l
ALP 96 iu/l
Albumin 3.1 g/dl

Questions

1. What is the sound that is heard over the epigastric area?
2. What makes the sound?
3. Does the patient need to have cirrhosis to produce this sound?
4. What might you see on ultrasound?

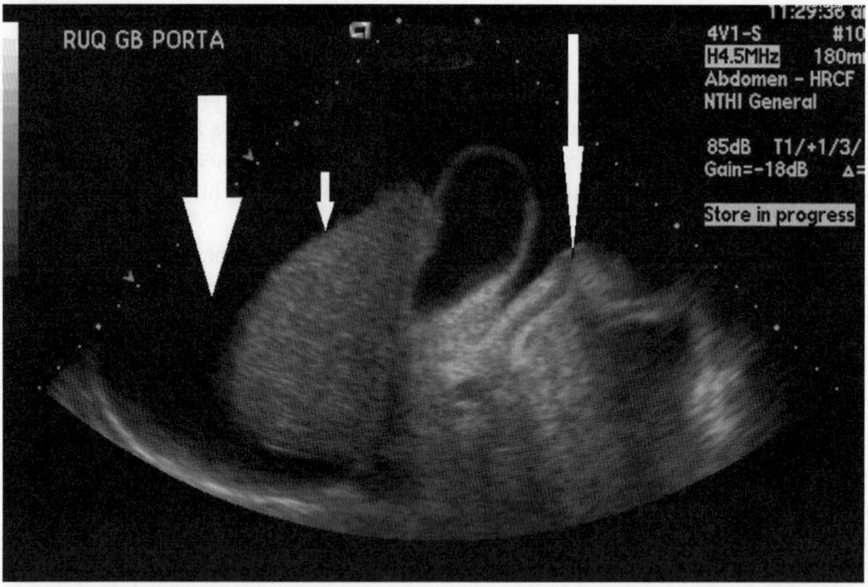

Fig. 57.1 Ultrasound

Answer: Cruveilhier–Baumgarten Disease or Syndrome

This patient obviously has portal hypertension. He has ascites, splenomegaly, and dilated abdominal veins, and the sound in the epigastric area is a venous hum. Some experts suggest that the direction of flow of blood in the dilated abdominal veins is indicative of either portal hypertension or vena caval obstruction, but the presence of valves can make it difficult to distinguish inferior flow (suggesting portal hypertension) or flow superiorly (vena caval obstruction).

The ultrasound image (Fig. 57.1) shows a liver that is echogenic in echotexture (smallest arrow), and on other images was markedly decreased in size, and nodular in contour. A large amount of abdominal ascites is present (large arrow) and there is a patent paraumbilical vein (long arrow). The venous hum results from collateral connections between the portal system and the remnant of the umbilical vein and should increase with the Valsalva and decrease with pressure over the umbilicus.

The term Cruveilhier–Baumgarten syndrome is based on a description by Cruveilhier in 1852 and then Baumgarten in 1908 and is characterized by portal hypertension, splenomegaly, and evidence of excessively prominent umbilical circulation – visible abdominal veins and a venous hum. The disease refers to these findings in a patient who has a patent umbilical vein, an atrophic liver but with little or no fibrosis on pathology, whereas the syndrome most commonly occurs in patients with cirrhosis.

There is some suggestion that the presence of the collaterals in this syndrome makes typical varices in the distal esophagus and proximal stomach smaller (and less likely to bleed).

The classic intrahepatic venous circulation found in the syndrome can be appreciated on Doppler sonography with hepatopetal flow in the segmental portal veins and hepatofugal flow leaving the liver in a paraumbilical vein in the falciform ligament which joins veins in the anterior abdominal wall around the umbilicus (causing the venous hum).

References

1. Valk HL, Horne SF. Cruveilhier–Baumgarten syndrome (splenomegaly, portal hypertension and patent umbilical vein): case report. Ann Surg 1942;116:860–3.
2. Jahnke EH, Palmer ED, Brick IB. The Cruveilhier–Baumgarten syndrome: a review and report of four cases; three treated by direct portacaval shunt. Ann Surg 1954;140:44–55.
3. Morin C, Lafortune M, Pomier G et al. Patent paraumbilical vein: anatomic and hemodynamic variants and their clinical importance. Radiology 1992;185:253–6.

Case 58

A 37-year-old white male with a history of chronic lower back pain is admitted directly to the hospital from his scheduled pain clinic visit with new onset jaundice and abdominal distension. The patient has been experiencing increasing back pain for the last 2 weeks. He states that the pain is higher than his chronic back pain. He also has developed new onset lower extremity edema in the last week. The patient's wife noticed some confusion and disorientation in the last several days. One day prior to admission, she noticed yellowing of his eyes. Review of systems is notable for nausea, constipation with intermittent rectal bleeding in the last month, dyspnea on exertion, and diaphoresis. One month prior, the patient and his wife were in South Carolina on vacation. There is no history of fevers, chills, sick contacts, or antibiotic use. The patient is a former police man and was involved in a work-related injury 3 years ago. Since then, he has been suffering with lower back pain. He is seen regularly in the chronic pain clinic and has been consistent with his physical therapy regimen. In the last several months, he has been able to wean to as needed narcotics, although in the last several weeks, his narcotic use had increased to hydrocodone/acetaminophen 7.5/750 up to 8 pills a day. He also has recently been diagnosed with depression and insomnia and was started on a low dose of amitriptyline. The patient lives with his wife of 4 years. He is monogamous and has never used illicit drugs. He drinks 10–14 beers per week. He does not smoke. He has no tattoos nor has he ever had any blood transfusion. He currently works at the department of motor vehicles. The patient's sister was diagnosed with leukemia at the age of 24. She has been in remission for over 10 years.

Physical exam was notable for a lethargic, ill-appearing white male. Vital signs reveal: temperature 37.2°C, heart rate 110, Blood pressure 98/54, respiratory rate 22, saturation 92%, and BMI 31.7 kg/m^2. Sclerae were icteric. Other than tachycardia, cardiac and pulmonary exam were normal. Abdominal exam was notable for marked distension. Liver edge was palpable 8 cm below right costovertebral angle and was tender. There was no splenomegaly. Fluid wave was easily elicited. Pitting edema was noted from ankles to mid thigh. Rectal exam revealed moderate external hemorrhoids one of which was thrombosed and oozing a small amount of blood, no internal masses were palpated. There was no palpable adenopathy.

A diagnostic tap was performed: hematocrit 22%

A CT scan is performed (see Fig. 58.1). In addition, a note is made of an enhancing lesion in the sigmoid colon.

Laboratory Data

Na 135 mM/l
BUN 39 mg/dl
Creat 3.2 mg/dl
Arterial blood gas: pH 7.20, pCO2 19, pO2 226; lactate 14

WBC 24,000; 93% neutrophils
Hb 7.5 g/dl
Platelets 347,000/μl
Tbili 7.2 mg/dl
AST 2443 iu/l
ALT 2487 iu/l
ALP 500 iu/l
GGTP 2452 iu/l
LDH 2136 iu/l
CPK 800 iu/l
Uric Acid 16 mg/dl
Alb 3.4 g/dl, total protein 6.1 g/dl
NH3 94 μmol/l
PT 94 seconds, INR 11; PTT 48 seconds
Fe 92 ug/dl, TIBC 223 ug/dl, % Sat 41, Ferritin 2,900 ng/dl
Urine tox, acetaminophen level negative
HAV IgM –
HBsAg –, core total/IgM –, HBsAb –
HCV PCR –
CMV/HSV negative
EBV indicates past exposure
ANA, smooth muscle, LKAM, Immunoglob all normal
Ceruloplasmin 39 mg/dl, AIAT 269 mg/dl
AFP 9 ng/ml, CA 19-9 660 iu/ml, CEA 9 ng/ml

Questions

1. What is the differential diagnosis?
2. How do you account for the hematocrit level in the ascites fluid?
3. How would you make a definitive diagnosis in this case?
4. What treatment if any would you recommend?

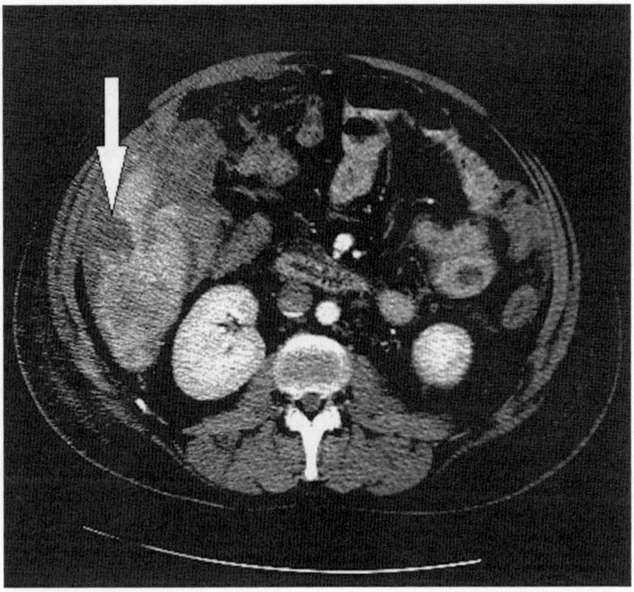

Fig. 58.1 CT scan

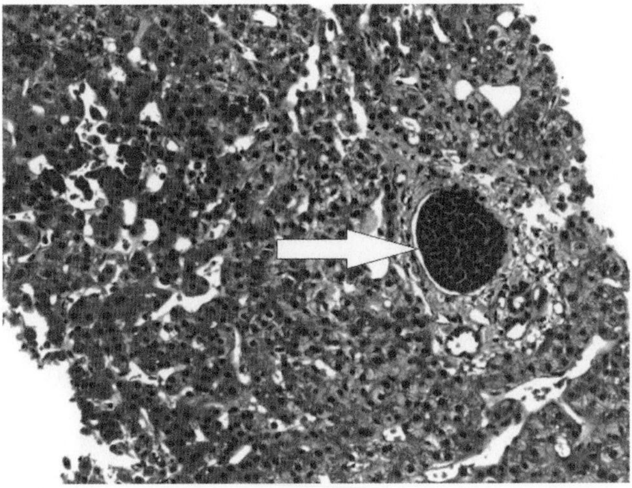

Fig. 58.2 Liver biopsy

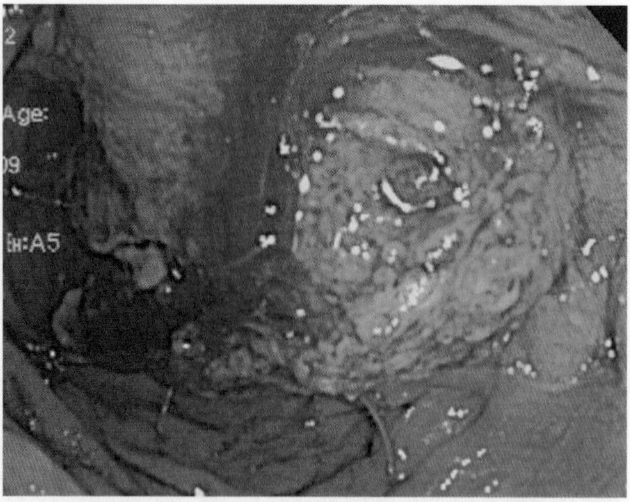

Fig. 58.3 Sigmoidoscopy

Answer: Metastatic Colon Cancer to the Liver presenting as Acute Liver Failure

This case fulfills criteria for acute liver failure (ALF): the rapid deterioration of liver function resulting in coagulopathy and alteration in the mental status of a previously healthy individual. The differential diagnosis in this case includes: acetaminophen/drug induced, viral, veno-occlusive, ischemic, and autoimmune hepatitis. All of these, however, can reasonably be ruled out with history, exam, blood work, and imaging. The extreme elevations in iron studies seen in many cases of acute severe hepatitis can cause some confusion to the unseasoned clinician; however, these constitute a manifestation of hepatocellular damage and likely have no prognostic value. Moreover, hereditary hemochromatosis should never be on the differential of acute liver failure.

The presence of massive hepatomegaly, cholestatic pattern to the liver function tests, and bloody tap in a relatively young person make an infiltrative or malignant process the most likely cause. Prior to histology, given the elevated LDH and high uric acid, lymphoma was at the top of our list of possible causes.

The patient's hemodynamic instability was secondary to intraperitoneal hemorrhage. The equivalent ascites and serum hematocrit measured from the diagnostic paracentesis, in conjunction with inappropriate response to multiple blood transfusions were evidence of active bleeding. The CT scan (Fig. 58.1, white arrow) showed an actively bleeding lesion in the periphery of the right lobe. The patient was sent emergently to angiography where emoblization of a branch of the right hepatic artery was performed resulting in cessation of active bleeding.

Both a transjugular liver biopsy (peformed prior to knowledge of a questionable sigmoid lesion was discovered on CT scan) and flexible sigmoidoscopy were performed. Liver biopsy (Fig. 58.2) revealed normal liver parenchyma with tumor thrombus noted within branches of the portal vein (white arrow). Sigmoidoscopy revealed a 5 cm, bleeding, partially obstructing mass in the recto-sigmoid junction (Fig. 58.3). Pathological evaluation and special stains confirmed a diagnosis of colon cancer with metastatic spread to the liver.

Hematological malignancies (leukemia and lymphoma) aside, metastatic spread of *solid* organ cancers to the liver presenting as ALF is a very rare phenomenon with only a handful of cases described in the literature. Given the unique blood supply of the liver, massive metastatic tumor burden in the liver is not an uncommon occurrence. So, why then did this patient develop acute liver failure? We hypothesize (given the presence of tumor only within the branches of the portal vein and not the hepatic parenchyma) that the tumor metastasis via the portal vein, in conjuction with the intraperitoneal hemorrhage, resulted in an ischemic liver injury; this in conjunction with massive tumor burden resulted in this patient's liver failure.

In every case of ALF with prodromal symptoms or abnormal imaging, hepatic histology should be obtained by liver biopsy as soon as possible to diagnose infiltrative hepatic disease and avoid futile transplantation.

The unfortunate gentleman in this case developed anuric renal failure and worsening mental status. He was made comfort measures only and died 7 days after admission. Microsatellite instability was performed on the pathology of the colon cancer and was negative. Screening colonoscopies were performed on the patient's two sisters and were normal.

References

1. Ostapowicz G, Fontana RJ, Schiødt FV et al. Results of a prospective study of acute liver failure at 17 tertiary care centers in the United States. Ann Intern Med 2002;137:947–54.
2. Rowbotham D, Wendon J, Williams R. Acute liver failure secondary to hepatic infiltration: a single centre experience of 18 cases. Gut 1998;42:576–80.

Case 59

You are called by the ER to come and see a 66-year-old lady who has presented with jaundice. She is from out of state and has been visiting family in the area for the last 2 weeks. No medical records are available.

She denies any fever, abdominal pain, change in urine or stool color, or pruritus. She does not speak English and relatives with her say that she has a history of alcoholic cirrhosis. She has a small scrap of paper with her that looks like a medication list and includes a small dose of furosemide and spironolactone, and she has been taking lactulose.

She was apparently diagnosed with a liver lesion 3 months ago based on surveillance imaging and has been undergoing treatment although it is unclear which type of treatment.

Her physical exam is notable for an elderly woman in no apparent distress. Her vital signs are normal, and she is afebrile. She is obviously icteric with multiple spider nevi, palmar erythema, and an easily palpable left lobe of liver and spleen tip. There is no obvious ascites or ankle edema.

Laboratory Studies

Hb 9.8 g/dl
Platelets 58,000/μl
WBC 4.1 × 10^3/μl
INR 1.6
Creatinine 1.1 mg/dl
Tbili 12.5 mg/dl
AST 67 iu/l
ALT 48 iu/l
GGTP 105 iu/l
ALP 157 iu/l
Albumin 2.4 g/dl
AFP 2.4 ng/ml
Blood ethanol level undetectable

Ultrasound – small shrunken liver, no biliary ductal dilation, ill-defined 6 cm heterogeneous mass in the left lobe.

Questions?

1. What is the differential diagnosis?
2. How would you manage this patient?

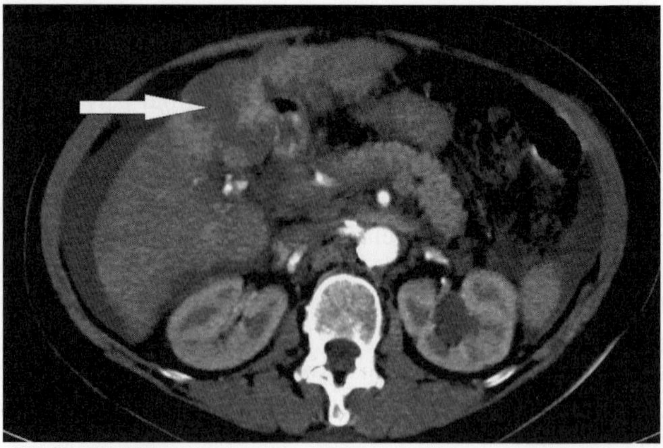

Fig. 59.1 CT scan

Answer: Decompensation After Arterial Chemoembolization

This unfortunate lady has developed worsening liver function manifested by jaundice several weeks after transarterial chemoembolization (TACE) for HCC. The CT scan (Fig. 59.1) shows a lesion that does not enhance after contrast compatible with a treated lesion (arrowed). The liver is cirrhotic, and ascites is apparent. No biliary dilation is seen to suggest obstruction.

The differential diagnosis includes anything that could cause decompensation in a cirrhotic patient such as infection, bleeding, acute alcohol, and medications. However, she looks well and has an undetectable alcohol level. Her enzymes argue against infection or a medication-induced effect. Her tumor could have recurred or perhaps she has developed another lesion at or near the hilum that is causing biliary obstruction but again her numbers and imaging do not correlate with this. The most likely explanation is worsening of her underlying liver disease due to TACE.

Since the bulk of blood supply to HCCs comes from the hepatic artery, the principle behind TACE is to embolize or infuse chemotherapy directly into a hepatic artery branch that supplies the tumor. It is not surprising that some adjacent liver tissue suffers some ischemic damage.

Indeed, some of the contraindications for TACE include situations where an added ischemic insult could push the patient into liver failure such as portal vein thrombosis, elevated bilirubin, high tumor volume, ascites, or high transaminases.

Several large studies and meta-analyses have examined the incidence of complications after TACE and found the most common adverse effect, occurring in 60–80%, is a self-limiting postembolization syndrome that causes pain, fever, and a rise in liver enzymes. The rate of liver failure after TACE depends on the pretreatment liver function but can be as high as 20% and can be irreversible in 2–3%.

References

1. Camma C, Schepis F, Orlando A et al. Transarterial chemoembolization for unresectable hepatocellular carcinoma: meta-analysis of randomized controlled trials. Radiology 2002;224:47.
2. Marelli L, Stigliano R, Triantos C et al. Transarterial therapy for hepatocellular carcinoma: which technique is more effective? A systematic review of cohort and randomized studies. Cardiovasc Intervent Radiol 2007;30:6.
3. Chan AO, Yuen MF, HuiCK et al. A prospective study regarding the complications of transcatheter intraarterial lipiodol chemoembolization in patients with hepatocellular carcinoma. Cancer 2002;94:1747.

Case 60

A 57-year-man presents to the emergency room with fatigue and just not feeling well. He has a history of cirrhosis likely secondary to fatty liver disease. His complications include ascites controlled on diuretics and mild encephalopathy. His last endoscopy was 2 years ago which showed mild portal hypertensive changes.

His other medical problems include diabetes controlled on insulin and a remote cholecystectomy.

He is married and is accompanied to the hospital by his wife. He is on disability but used to work as a chef.

He denies tobacco, alcohol, or drug use.

His father was an alcoholic.

The rest of his review of systems is pertinent for some shortness of breath on exertion but he denies blood in the stool, melena, abdominal pain, or weight loss. He has had no fever or chills.

On exam, he looks tired but is alert and oriented.

Vital signs show BP 100/60, pulse 112 and he is afebrile.

There is mild scleral icterus and several spider nevi.

Heart reveals normal S1 and S2 without added sounds. Chest reveals lung fields.

His abdomen is obese but soft and non-tender with a palpable spleen tip.

Laboratory Studies

Hb 6.7 g/dl
MCV 72 fl (normal 80–95fl)
Platelets 59,000/μl
WBC 3.8 × 10^3/μl
INR 1.3
Creatinine 1.1 mg/dl
Tbili 2.9 mg/dl
AST 68 iu/l
ALT 53 iu/l
GGTP 123 iu/l
ALP 118 iu/l
Albumin 2.6 g/dl
Stool hemoccult positive

After adequate resuscitation he undergoes upper GI endoscopy.

Questions

1. Is the severity of changes seen on endoscopy related to the degree of portal hypertension?
2. If this patient has esophageal varices that are banded/sclerosed, does this affect this condition?
3. What is the appropriate treatment?

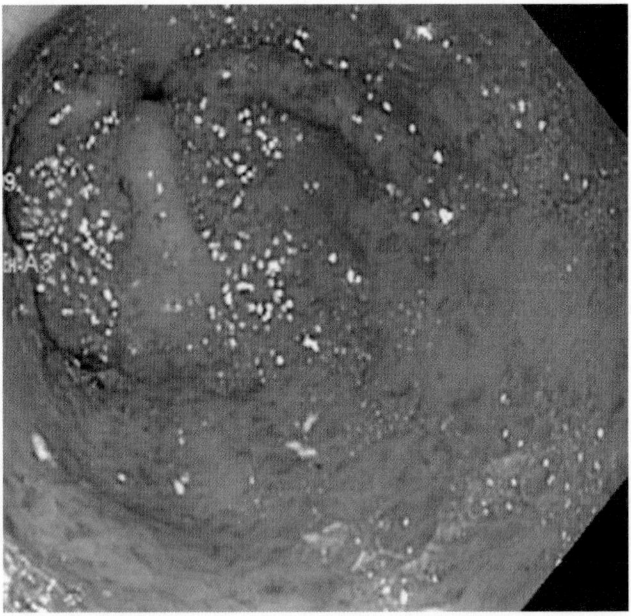

Fig. 60.1 Endoscopic images

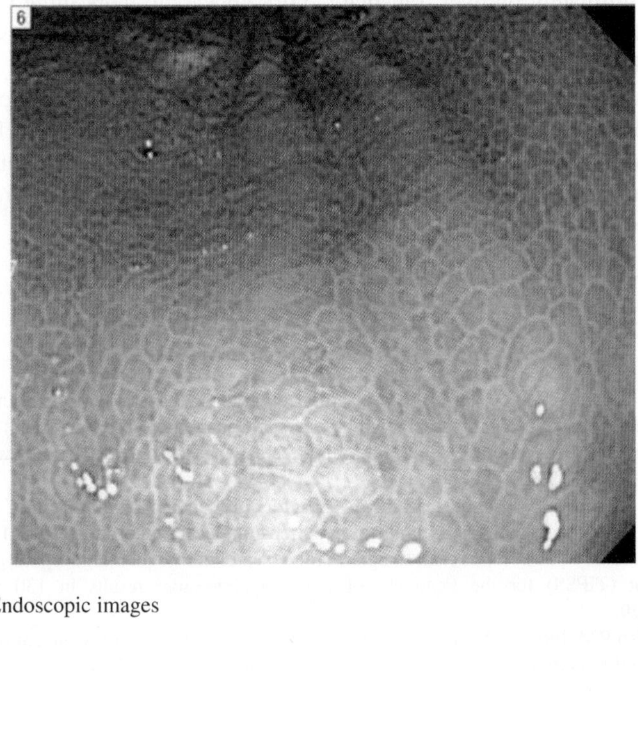

Fig. 60.2 Endoscopic images

Answer: Portal Hypertensive Gastropathy

The endoscopic images (Figs. 60.1 and 60.2) show portal hypertensive gastropathy (PHTG). The first image (Fig. 60.1) shows the gastric antrum where there is severe PHTG with hyperemic mucosa and diffuse oozing on contact with the scope. More proximally in the stomach, the second image demonstrates the "chickenwire" appearance of mild PHTG.

Severe PHTG in the antrum can be confused with gastric antral vascular ectasia (GAVE or watermelon stomach). The latter is characterized by ecstatic mucosal blood vessels and is also seen in patients with cirrhosis. It can present in a similar manner with microcytic anemia but can be treated with cautery or argon plasma coagulation.

PHTG typically is worse in the proximal stomach but can be present anywhere. Biopsy is usually not required to make a diagnosis. Increasing incidence or severity is not always the natural history in cirrhosis and the presence of PHTG is not related to age, sex, cause of cirrhosis, or grade of gastroesophageal varices. However, severe gastropathy is associated with an increase in portal venous pressure gradient and impaired liver metabolic activity. Interestingly, several studies have suggested that sclerotherapy or band ligation of esophageal varices increases the risk of developing portal hypertensive gastropathy.

As with causes of bleeding in portal hypertension, PHTG can be treated by trying to decrease portal pressure through non-selective beta blockers, TIPS, shunt surgery or ultimately by liver transplant. TIPS appears to work quite well for this condition, but in my experience most patients seem to do well with iron supplementation and beta-blockade.

This patient presents with anemia which is presumably from chronic blood loss as his esophageal varices were small (and variceal bleeding typically has a more dramatic presentation). Endoscopy shows severe distal PHTG. Treatment with oral iron and nadolol was started and appeared to decrease the transfusion requirement over the next 6–12 months.

References

1. Payen JL, Cales P, Voigt JJ et al. Severe portal hypertensive gastropathy and antral vascular ectasia are distinct entities in patients with cirrhosis. Gastroenterology 1995;108:138.
2. Iwao T, Toyonaga A, Sumino M et al. Portal hypertensive gastropathy in patients with cirrhosis. Gastroenterology 1992;102:2060–5.
3. Sarin SK, Sreenivas DV, Lahoti D, Saraya A. Factors influencing development of portal hypertensive gastropathy in patients with portal hypertension. Gastroenterology 1992;102:994.
4. Stanley AJ, Jalan R, Forrest EH et al. Longterm follow up of transjugular intrahepatic portosystemic stent shunt (TIPSS) for the treatment of portal hypertension: results in 130 patients. Gut 1996;39:479.
5. Perez-Ayuso RM, Pique JM, Bosch J et al. Propranolol in prevention of recurrent bleeding from severe portal hypertensive gastropathy in cirrhosis. Lancet 1991;337:1431.

Case 61

You are asked by the obstetric service to see a 31-year-old lady for abnormal liver enzymes and nonspecific symptoms. She is in week 37 of her first pregnancy. She had some problems with hyperemesis in the first trimester, but otherwise, the pregnancy has been normal. Her ALT yesterday was 67 iu/l.

She has no other medical problems. Medications include a prenatal vitamin.

She does not smoke or drink. She is married and works as a secretary.

There is no family history of liver disease.

Her review of symptoms is significant for some nausea and vomiting and upper abdominal pain. She has some loose stool over the last 24 h. She denies fever or chills. She has no pruritus.

You are busy in the clinic and send a fellow to see the patient.

The fellow calls back several hours later with his assessment and with new laboratory studies.

The patient's vital signs show a BP 145/95, pulse 100, and she is afebrile.

She is able to answer questions appropriately, but her husband states that she looks sleepier than earlier today.

She has mild scleral icterus and palmar erythema.

Cardiovascular system reveals normal heart sounds. Lungs are clear.

Abdomen demonstrates a gravid uterus consistent with a 37 week pregnancy. There is right upper quadrant tenderness.

Ankles reveal +ankle edema.

Laboratory Studies

Hb 9.7 g/dl
Platelets 62,000/μl
WBC 10.2×10^3/μl
INR 1.4
Creatinine 1.4 mg/dl
Tbili 3.1 mg/dl
AST 367 iu/l
ALT 359 iu/l
GGTP 140 iu/l
ALP 196 iu/l
Albumin 2.8 g/dl
Blood glucose 67 mg/dl

You urgently go over and see the patient and inform the primary service that she likely needs emergent delivery.

Questions

1. What is the characteristic appearance of the liver biopsy in this condition?
2. Is there a risk of this disease recurring in subsequent pregnancies?

Ultrasound: Normal-looking liver without biliary dilation
Liver biopsy: Pathology resident states the hepatocytes have a “foamy cytoplasm”

Answer: Acute Fatty Liver of Pregnancy

This clinical scenario probably occurs a few times a year at a tertiary care liver transplant center.

Liver disease in pregnancy can be separated into diseases that are unique to pregnancy, "normal" liver or biliary diseases occurring in a pregnant woman (viral hepatitis or gallstone disease), and pregnancy occurring in a patient with known liver disease (typically viral hepatitis or cirrhosis).

The approach to liver disease in pregnancy is guided by a few factors, namely, the trimester, the degree of liver enzyme elevation, the presence of itching, and the severity of disease.

Hyperemesis gravidarum occurs in the first trimester and presents with relatively mild elevation of liver enzymes and intractable nausea and vomiting. It can be confused with viral hepatitis. Intrahepatic cholestasis of pregnancy is a disorder of late pregnancy and presents with itching, cholestatic enzymes, and negative imaging for biliary dilation. It often recurs in subsequent pregnancies and is associated with fetal loss. Treatment is delivery. Acute fatty liver of pregnancy (AFLP), HELLP syndrome (hemolysis with a microangiopathic blood smear, elevated liver enzymes, and a low platelet count), and severe preeclampsia cause the most confusion in making a diagnosis since they can have a similar presentation.

This lady presents in the third trimester with nausea, vomiting, and abdominal pain, all of which are common in AFLP. Her laboratory studies show elevated transaminases and hypoglycemia, which together with her mental status, are concerning for significant liver dysfunction. The low platelet count might suggest HELLP, but disseminated intravascular coagulopathy is not infrequent in AFLP.

The pathogenesis of AFLP is not completely understood, but several studies have shown an association with one of the inherited defects in mitochondrial beta-oxidation of fatty acids, long-chain 3-hydroxyacyl CoA dehydrogenase deficiency (LCHAD). This suggests that some affected women and their fetuses might have an inherited enzyme deficiency in beta-oxidation that predisposes the mother to AFLP. LCHAD catalyzes one of the steps in the beta-oxidation of fatty acids in mitochondria (the formation of 3-ketoacyl-CoA from 3-hydroxyacyl-CoA), and deficiency leads to the accumulation of long-chain 3-hydroxyacyl metabolites produced by the fetus or placenta which is toxic to the maternal liver. Not all cases of AFLP have the enzyme deficiency.

The diagnosis of AFLP is based on an appropriate clinical presentation and supportive laboratory tests. Liver biopsy is not necessary and will be risky because of the coagulopathy. However, it is diagnostic, showing a characteristic microvesicular fatty infiltration of the hepatocytes. There is a foamy cytoplasm due to fat droplets surrounding centrally located nuclei, and there is sparing of a sharply defined rim of cells around the portal tracts.

Treatment is based on maternal support and emergent delivery. Maternal and fetal mortality has improved with better recognition of the disease but is still seen. Recurrence in subsequent pregnancies has been documented.

References

1. Knight M, Nelson-Piercy C, Kurinczuk JJ et al. A prospective national study of acute fatty liver of pregnancy in the UK. Gut 2008;57:951–6.
2. Wilcken B, Leung KC, Hammond J et al. Pregnancy and fetal long-chain 3-hydroxyacyl coenzyme A dehydrogenase deficiency. Lancet 1993;341:407–8.
3. Schoeman MN, Batey RG, Wilcken B. Recurrent acute fatty liver of pregnancy associated with a fatty-acid oxidation defect in the offspring. Gastroenterology 1991;100:544–8.

Case 62

A 57-year-old Caucasian male presents to the emergency room with hematemesis. His wife states that he has a history of chronic hepatitis C infection diagnosed 10 years ago. He was never treated and in fact has not seen a doctor for more than 6 years.

He has no other medical history and denies any prescribed or over-the-conuter medications.

He has a remote history of intravenous drug use from age 19 to 25. He does not smoke or drink.

He has otherwise been well recently without abdominal pain or fever. He denies ascites or prior encephalopathy.

In the emergency room, the patient has another episode of hematemesis. His vital signs show him to be hypotensive with blood pressure 90/40 and heart rate 110. He is intubated for airway protection and resuscitated. An upper endoscopy is performed emergently.

Laboratory Parameters

WBC 7×10^3/uL
Hemoglobin 8.0 g/dl
Platelet 68×10^3/ul
PT 25 seconds
Tbili 1.8 mg/dl
AST 154 U/l
ALT 112 U/l
Creatinine 1.2 mg/dl

Questions

1. What are the appropriate management steps?
2. How effective is endoscopic therapy?

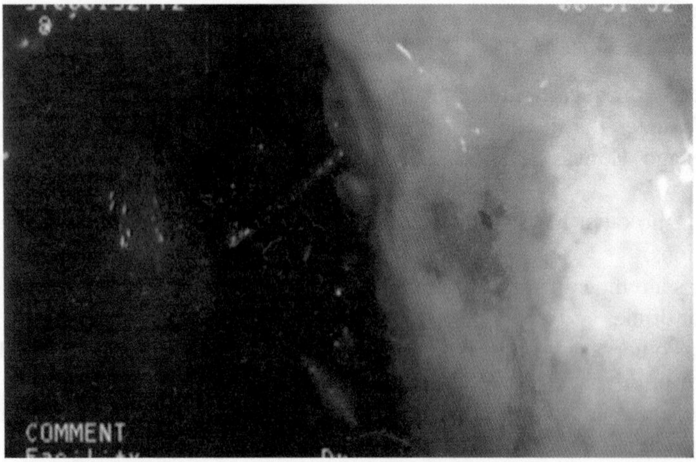

Fig. 62.1 Endoscopic images

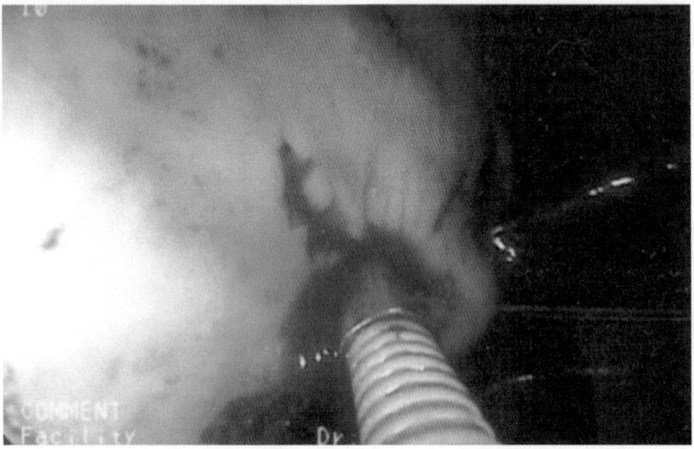

Fig. 62.2 Endoscopic images

Answer: Acute Variceal Bleeding

The EGD pictures (Figs. 62.1 and 62.2) demonstrate a large amount of fresh blood in the fundus and a gastric varix spurting blood along the greater curvature (GOVII). A sclerotherapy needle is being used to inject a sclerosant into the varix and the bleeding stops. The patient has a known history of chronic hepatitis C infection. From his social history, it is likely that he had had the infection for more than 30 years, which increases the likelihood of advanced liver disease such as cirrhosis. About one-third of patients with varices experience variceal hemorrhage, and each episode of hemorrhage can have 20–30% mortality. In patients with acute variceal hemorrhage, diagnostic and therapeutic endoscopy should be done emergently once patients are hemodynamically stable. Intravenous octreotide and antibiotics should be started promptly when variceal hemorrhage is suspected. Type I gastric varices (GOV I) are found along the lesser curve (usually 2–5 cm in length) which are potentially treatable with endoscopic band ligation therapy. Type II (GOV II) are found along the greater curve extending toward the fundus of stomach. Isolated gastric varices are found in the fundus (IGV I) or other parts of the stomach (IGV II). Band ligation is ineffective in GOV II and IGV.
The AASLD guidelines for variceal hemorrhage recommend:

- Acute GI hemorrhage in cirrhotic patients is an emergency that requires prompt intravascular volume support and blood transfusions, being careful to maintain a hemoglobin of approximately 8 g/dl.
- Short-term (max. 7 days) antibiotic prophylaxis should be instituted in any patient with cirrhosis and GI hemorrhage with PO norfloxacin or IV ciprofloxacin.
- In patients with advanced cirrhosis, IV ceftriaxone (1 g/day) may be preferable, particularly in centers with a high prevalence of quinolone-resistant organisms.
- Pharmacological therapy (somatostatin or its analogues octreotide and vapreotide; terlipressin) should be initiated as soon as variceal hemorrhage is suspected and continued for 3–5 days after the diagnosis is confirmed.
- EGD, performed within 12 h, should be used to make the diagnosis and to treat variceal hemorrhage either with band ligation or sclerotherapy.
- TIPS is indicated in patients in whom hemorrhage from esophageal varices cannot be controlled or in whom bleeding recurs despite combined pharmacological and endoscopic therapy.
- Balloon tamponade should be used as a temporizing measure (max. 24 h) in patients with uncontrollable bleeding for whom a more definitive therapy (e.g., TIPS or endoscopic therapy is planned).
- For gastric varices, endoscopic variceal obturation using tissue adhesives such as cyanoacrylate is preferred, where available. Otherwise, EVL is an option.
- TIPS should be considered in patients in whom hemorrhage from fundal varices cannot be controlled or in whom bleeding recurs despite combined pharmacological and endoscopic therapy.

As well as cyanoacrylate (that is not available outside of a study in the United States), intravariceal thrombin injection has also been shown to be useful.

References

1. Garcia-Tsao G, Sanyal AJ, Grace ND et al. Prevention and management of gastroesophageal varices and variceal hemorrhage in cirrhosis. Hepatology 2007;46:922.
2. Datta D, Vlavianos P, Alisa A et al. Use of fibrin glue (beriplast) in the management of bleeding gastric varices. Endoscopy 2003;35:675–8.
3. Yang WL, Tripathi D, Therapondos G et al. Endoscopic use of human thrombin in bleeding gastric varices. Am J Gastroenterol 2002;97:1381–5.

Case 63

A 52-year-old African American male presents with a 4-week history of progressively worsening abdominal pain and distension. Four weeks ago, he began to develop diffuse, crampy abdominal pain which he describes as sharp and jabbing with radiation to his upper chest and back. He also describes increasing abdominal distension and is no longer able to fit into his pants. Over the last 2 weeks, he has reported constant nausea, intermittent nonbloody emesis, and nonbloody diarrhea. His appetite is poor, and he has lost 15 pounds. He also is very short of breath and has developed a new dry cough. The patient has a history of poorly controlled diabetes and schizoaffective disorder and is on sertraline and quetiapine fumarate, although he admits to noncompliance. He has a history of hepatitis C diagnosed 8 years ago but never treated due to his psychiatric history. The patient currently lives with his girlfriend. He has seven children from previous relationships. He works as a construction worker but has been forced to quit given his recent illness. He has drunk most of his adult life, averaging between 6 and 10 beers per day in addition to a pint of rum. He does admit to drinking more heavily in the last month. His last drink was the day of admission. He has a 60 pack year smoking history and currently smokes 2 packs per day. He uses IV drugs in the form of heroin, and his last use was 1 week prior to admission. The patient is adopted and does not know details regarding the medical history of his biological family. On review of systems, he complains of chills, fatigue, light headedness, and darkening of his urine.

Physical exam is notable for an ill-, lethargic-appearing male with a BMI of 21.8 kg/m^2. He is afebrile, with a heart rate of 98, and a blood pressure of 106/48. Respiratory rate is 18 per minute and oxygen saturation is 91% on room air. He has temporal wasting and scleral icterus. His parotid glands are enlarged bilaterally. His mucous membranes are dry. He has decreased breath sounds one-third of the way up on his right side. Heart sounds are distant. His abdomen reveals dilated umbilical veins, a firm liver palpable 3 cm below the right costal margin. There is no audible hepatic bruit. He has full flanks and shifting dullness. He is tender diffusely. Extremities reveal multiple needle tracks and trace lower extremity edema. He has palmar erythema, Duputryen's contractures bilaterally and a few scattered spider nevi. He answers questions appropriately and is oriented but does have a liver flap.

Laboratory Data

WBC 25,0 × 103/μl00 with 19% bands
Hg 9 g/dl, MCV 111 f/l
Platelet count 71,000/μl

Tbili 7 mg/dl (conjugated 2.5 mg/dl)
AST 488 iu/l
ALT 200 iu/l
ALP 215 iu/l

GGTP 681 iu/l
Alb 2.3 g/dl

Serum NH_3 77 μmol/l
INR 2.2 (PT 25 seconds)

HCV Ab +, Genotype 1
Viral load 1,344,990 iu/ml
HAV Total +
HBsAg −, HBc +, sAb +

Ascites tap: Alb < 1.0, TP < 1.5; WBC 125 × 103/μl with 58% Neutrophils
RBC 490K
Cytology: abundant RBCs, mesothelial cells, macrophages, neutrophils and lymphocytes; negative for malignant cells

Questions

1. What is the differential diagnosis?
2. What additional testing if any would you recommend?
3. What treatment if any would you recommend?

AFP 28450 ng/ml

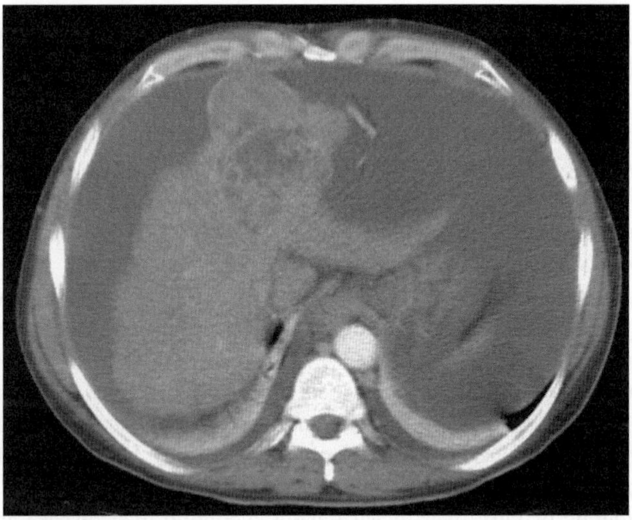

Fig. 63.1 CT scan abdomen

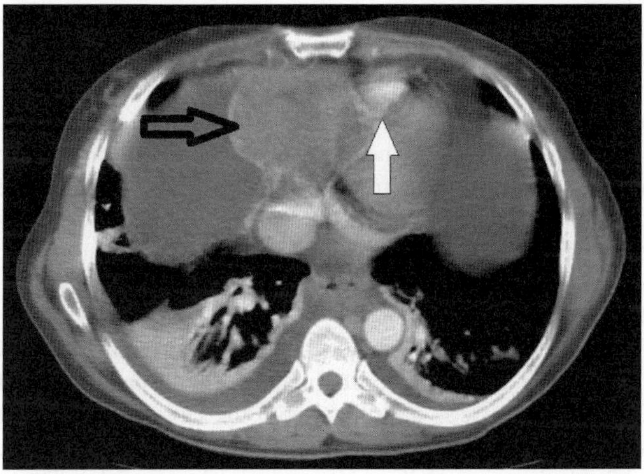

Fig. 63.2 CT scan abdomen

Answer: HCV/ETOH Cirrhosis with Superimposed Acute Alcoholic Hepatitis and Multifocal HCC

The acute deterioration in this patient can be accounted for by both the development of HCC with hepatic/portal vein thrombus and superimposed acute alcoholic hepatitis.

The symptoms of weight loss, night sweats, and new onset abdominal pain with radiation to the back are all concerning for malignancy. In the setting of a cirrhotic liver with classic characteristics (hypervascular lesion with washout in the portal venous phase) and marked elevation in AFP, a liver biopsy is not needed to establish the diagnosis of HCC.

Although markedly elevated in this case, and solidifying the diagnosis, AFP is a notoriously poor marker for screening of HCC. The sensitivity of AFP is 41–65%, with a specificity of 80 to 94%.

The acute onset of jaundice, elevated INR, WBC, 2:1 pattern of elevation of AST/ALT and marked elevation in GGT in the setting of excessive consumption of alcohol are consistent with acute alcoholic hepatitis. Acute alcoholic hepatitis occurs superimposed on cirrhosis in approximately 40% of individuals.

The epidemic of fatty liver disease aside, alcoholic liver disease and HCV are the two most common causes chronic liver disease in the country and many times coexist in the same individual. The combination of insults seems to work in synergy in both the progression of fibrosis and the development of HCC. A daily uptake of >80 g of alcohol alone increases HCC risk fivefold while the presence of HCV alone increases HCC 20-fold. The combination of both factors increases the risk of HCC development over 100-fold.

Men are far more likely to develop HCC. Although not completely understood, these differences in sex distribution are thought to be due to variation in viral hepatitis carrier states, exposure to environmental toxins, and the trophic effect of androgens. In addition, the incidence of HCC is greater in black Americans than white Americans. Other risk factors for HCC present in the case, but more controversial and less definitive in their association include smoking, diabetes, and the positive hepatitis B core antibody.

The differential for frankly bloody ascites include: traumatic tap, cirrhosis, or malignancy. Ascites is bloody in approximately 50% of patients with HCC.

The HCC in this case was multifocal with the largest lesion being 7 cm. The lesion was invading the right diaphragm and was actually abutting the right heart (see Fig. 63.2; black arrow: HCC, white arrow right ventricle). There was subocclusive thrombosis of the inferior vena cava, middle hepatic, right and main portal veins. Per the patient's wishes, he was made palliative care, sent home on hospice and died 8 days after his presentation.

References

1. Mueller S, Millonig G, Seitz HK. Alcoholic liver disease and hepatitis C: a frequently underestimated combination. World J Gastroenterol 2009;15:3462–71.
2. Gupta S, Bent S, Kohlwes J. Test characteristics of alpha-fetoprotein for detecting hepatocellular carcinoma in patients with hepatitis C. A systematic review and critical analysis. Ann Intern Med 2003;139:46–50.

Case 64

You are asked to see a 71-year-old man who is on the non-teaching service by the medical resident.

The patient has a history of cryptogenic cirrhosis complicated by ascites that was refractory to diuretics. He has been undergoing regular large volume paracentesis. There is no history of encephalopathy or GI bleeding although endoscopy 3 months ago had shown small esophageal varices.

He was admitted for observation following placement of a TIPS yesterday afternoon. The procedure was uncomplicated, and the initial hepatic venous pressure gradient was 22 mmHg and dropped to 5 mmHg following the TIPS.

This morning he is combative and was put in restraints by the covering housestaff.

On exam, he is confused and uncooperative. Vital signs show BP 135/80, pulse 92 regular, and he has a normal axillary temperature.

He has palmar erythema and several spider nevi. There is mild scleral icterus.

He will not cooperate to look for asterixis.

Heart reveals normal S1 and S2 without added sounds. Chest reveals clear lung fields.

His abdomen is mildly distended with dull flanks. There is no tenderness, and bowel sounds are heard. There is +ankle edema bilaterally.

Laboratory Studies

Hb 11.5 g/dl
Platelets 61,000/μl
WBC 8.1 × 10^3/μl
INR 1.8
BUN 32 mg/dl
Creatinine 1.8 mg/dl
Tbili 3.1 mg/dl
ALT 32 iu/l
Albumin 2.2 g/dl

Questions

1. What test(s) are required to make a diagnosis?
2. What treatment options are available apart from medical therapy?
3. If the current laboratory parameters were similar prior to TIPS, should the patient have undergone TIPS?

Venous ammonia: 16 μmol/l
MELD score: 23

Answer: Hepatic Encephalopathy Following TIPS

This elderly patient has developed altered mental status after placement of a TIPS, likely related to hepatic encephalopathy (HE).

This is a diagnosis that can be difficult to make since it is defined by a variety of neuropsychiatric abnormalities seen in patients with liver disease, after *excluding* other unrelated neurologic and/or metabolic abnormalities. The severity of HE can be graded from stages I through IV with stage I representing mild symptoms and stage IV coma. More recently, there have been attempts to reclassify HE to enable better clinical studies. This new system uses the following:

Type A – HE associated with acute liver failure

Type B – HE associated with porto-systemic bypass and no liver disease

Type C – HE associated with cirrhosis and portal hypertension and/or shunts.

Type C is subdivided into episodic, persistent and mild. This last subdivision of minimal HE has gained attention since the diagnosis is based on psychometric testing and patients have no signs or symptoms (stage 0), and several studies have suggested that these patients are at increased risk of accidents while driving.

The diagnosis of HE should be made clinically and does not require an ammonia level. Ammonia levels do not correlate well with the degree of HE and are difficult to measure accurately. Ammonia is produced in the gut from several sources including the breakdown of nitrogenous material by bacteria and also from glutamine in enterocytes. It enters the portal vein, and the liver metabolizes it back to glutamine or urea. In liver dysfunction, ammonia clearance is impaired, and shunting also occurs if there is portal hypertension.

Accurate measurement of venous (or preferably arterial) ammonia requires the sample to be placed on ice and analyzed quickly. The partial pressure of ammonia is a better test since it is in this state that ammonia crosses the blood brain barrier, but again is difficult to measure directly.

The pathogenesis of HE is still unclear but likely involves ammonia as well as other neurotransmitters such as gamma-aminobutyric acid (GABA) in the central nervous system.

After TIPS, HE is seen in up to 30% of patients and is more likely to occur in older patients, more severe liver disease and in patients with HE prior to the TIPS. Prior to being used to prioritize organ allocation for liver transplant in the US, the MELD score was developed to predict mortality after TIPS. A score of greater than 18 predicts poor outcome and this patient should not have undergone TIPS for this nonemergent indication.

The treatment of post-TIPS HE is the same as HE in other situations. Precipitating factors should be reversed if present such as constipation, GI bleeding, dehydration, electrolyte abnormalities, infections, and medications, and worsening hepatic function. Lactulose should be titrated to 3–4 soft bowel movements daily. Protein restriction is generally not recommended. Other agents used include neomycin, metronidazole, and zinc although the data for their efficacy is limited. Recently, oral rifaximin has been shown to be effective but is very expensive in the US. As a last resort, the TIPS can be occluded or downsized, but this will very likely cause the ascites to reaccumulate.

References

1. Ferenci P, Lockwood A, Mullen K et al. Hepatic encephalopathy – definition, nomenclature, diagnosis, and quantification: final report of the working party at the 11th World Congresses of Gastroenterology, Vienna, 1998. Hepatology 2002;35:716–21.
2. Sanyal AJ, Freedman AM, Shiffman ML et al. Portosystemic encephalopathy after transjugular intrahepatic portosystemic shunt: results of a prospective controlled study. Hepatology 1994;20:46–55.
3. Malinchoc M, Kamath PS, Gordon FD et al. A model to predict poor survival in patients undergoing transjugular intrahepatic portosystemic shunts. Hepatology 2000;31:864–71.

Case 65

A 61-year-old lady is brought to the emergency room by her husband with several hours of confusion. She has a history of alcoholic liver disease that has been complicated in the past with encephalopathy. She has esophageal varices detected on endoscopy but no history of GI bleeding. Her ascites has been controlled on diuretics in the past, but she has not been seen for almost a year. Her last imaging was an ultrasound at that time that showed portal hypertension but no mass.

She is usually alert and oriented, and her husband states that he thinks she has been compliant with her lactulose and appeared to be well last night. There has been no nausea or vomiting. Her bowels have been moving normally without blood.

Her past medical history is significant for diabetes controlled on diet and depression.

Medications include lactulose, nadolol, and a multivitamin.

She lives with her husband and they have no children. She smokes a packet of cigarettes a day. She has not been evaluated for transplant because of continued alcohol use. Her husband confirms that she drinks a bottle of vodka every few days and several beers a night. There is no history of drug use and no family history of liver disease.

The rest of her review of systems is negative.

On exam, she is confused and appears disheveled. Vital signs show BP 105/60, pulse 68 regular and she has a low grade temperature of 100.1°F.

There is palmar erythema, scleral icterus and multiple spider nevi.

Heart reveals normal S1 and S2 without added sounds. Chest reveals clear lung fields.

Her abdomen is distended with a fluid thrill. Palpation of the upper abdomen elicits a grimace. Bowel sounds are sparse. Her liver and spleen are impalpable. She has +ankle edema bilaterally.

Laboratory Studies

Hb 10.4 g/dl
Platelets 41,000/μl
WBC 12.1 × 10^3/μl (74% neutrophils)
INR 2.4
Sodium 122 mmol/l
Creatinine 1.3 mg/dl
Tbili 18.2 mg/dl
AST 159 iu/l
ALT 86 iu/l
GGTP 207 iu/l
ALP 175 iu/l
Albumin 2.3 g/dl

Questions

1. What should you do next?
2. What should you do straight after that?
3. Does she need albumin/octreotide/hypertonic saline?

Ascitic fluid tap

Blood tinged fluid

Cell count	50,000 red cells 700 white cells 60% polymorphonuclear
Gram stain	negative for any organisms
Albumin	0.9 g/dl

After 48 h

Ascitic fluid culture no growth

Answer: Spontaneous Bacterial Peritonitis (SBP)

This lady presents with a relatively acute onset of change in mental status, low-grade fever, and ascites in the setting of ongoing alcohol use. She has not been seen for some time, and we are not told her baseline bilirubin. However, she is coagulopathic, has an elevated white-cell count with abdominal tenderness in the setting of jaundice. She very likely has hepatic encephalopathy, but the question is what is the etiology? The main differential diagnosis is between alcoholic hepatitis and SBP, but the development of HCC or another infection is also possible. Apart from SBP, which is defined as infection in the ascitic fluid without evidence of an intraabdominal surgically treatable source, the possibility of secondary bacterial peritonitis (from a ruptured viscus – gallbladder, colon, or peptic ulcer) should be considered and abdominal imaging is advisable.

The first test that should be performed is a diagnostic ascitic tap. Despite the thrombocytopenia and elevated INR, she does not need blood products prior to the tap. Several studies have documented that a tap in this situation is very safe and guidelines from the AASLD do not recommend prophylactic platelet or plasma/cryoprecipitate transfusion. Apart from the tap, blood cultures and a sepsis workup are warranted, and abdominal imaging with ultrasound would not be unreasonable.

The ascitic tap should be performed at the bedside, and antibiotics can be started while waiting for the result if the suspicion for SBP is high (as is the case in this patient). The diagnosis of SBP is made on a positive culture and an elevated absolute polymorphonuclear leucocyte (PMN) cell count of >250 cells/mm^3. A small amount of the fluid should be sent for chemistry to determine the albumin content. In this case, the difference between the serum albumin and ascites albumin (serum ascites albumin gradient or SAAG) was 1.4 g/dl, indicative of portal hypertension. Another 10 ml should be inoculated into blood culture bottles at the bedside (rather than sent to the laboratory in a syringe since this reduces the sensitivity). The gram stain can be ordered but has a very low sensitivity in determining if bacteria are present.

The cell count should be available within 1–2 h. In this case, the tap was bloody and needs to be corrected by subtracting one PMN for every 250 red cells. The PMN count was 300, positive for SBP. The choice of antibiotic should cover gut organisms, as well as streptococcal species and the possibility of staphylococcal infection and a third generation cephalosporin such as cefotaxime 2 g intravenous every 8 h is reasonable, with 5–7 days of treatment usually sufficient. We also give intravenous albumin (1.5 g/kg of body weight on day 1 and 1 g/kg of body weight on day 3) on the basis of a study that showed very low mortality in SBP patients treated in this manner.

There are several SBP variants based on cell count and culture. In this patient, the ascitic fluid culture was negative, so she falls into the category of culture negative neutrocytic ascites, which may be related to poor culture technique. The opposite variant is monomicrobial, nonneutrocytic bacterascites where the culture is positive but the PMN count is <250. Both should be treated as SBP, particularly if the clinical setting is convincing. It is also possible to get polymicrobial bacterascites from trauma to the bowel during paracentesis.

Prophylaxis for SBP is also important in patients with prior episodes or in those with a low protein concentration (<1.5 g/dl) in the ascitic fluid. Daily norfloxacin 400 mg or double strength bactrim, or weekly ciprofloxacin 750 mg are acceptable dosing schedules.

References

1. Sort P, Navasa M, Arroyo V et al. Effect of intravenous albumin on renal impairment and mortality in patients with cirrhosis and spontaneous bacterial peritonitis. N Engl J Med 1999;341:403–9.
2. Runyon BA. Management of adult patients with ascites due to cirrhosis: an update. Hepatology 2009;49:2087–2107.

Part III
Transplant Hepatology

Cases 66–90

Case 66

A 72-year old gentleman presents with abnormal liver enzymes on routine testing. Two months ago his liver enzymes had been essentially normal. He had undergone orthotopic liver transplant 2 years ago for alcoholic liver disease that had been complicated by ascites and a 2-cm hepatocellular carcinoma (HCC). He received a 63-year-old allograft with a duct-to-duct anastomosis. He was maintained on tacrolimus and prednisone immunosuppression. His posttransplant course has been unremarkable other than an episode of acute rejection several months after transplant that responded completely to a steroid recycle. He has remained abstinent of alcohol.

He denied fever, chills, weight loss, abdominal pain, or change in stool color although his urine was a little darker than usual.

Physical exam revealed a well-looking male, with normal vital signs. Sclerae were anicteric. The liver allograft was palpable but no ascites or edema was noted.

CT scan of the abdomen 2 months earlier showed a normal looking allograft without biliary dilation and patent vessels.

Laboratory Parameters

Tbili 1.9 mg/dl
AST 92 iu/l
ALT 123 iu/l
GGTP 1003 iu/l
FK level 10.3 ng/ml (normal 4–16 ng/ml)
Creatinine 1.6 mg/dl

Questions

1. What are the diagnostic considerations?
2. What are the next appropriate tests?

DOI 10.1007/978-1-4419-7085-5_3,

Ultrasound – patent vessels, normal arterial resistive indices. No masses and minimal intrahepatic biliary dilation.

Liver biopsy – showed mild-to-moderate portal edema, mixed portal inflammation indeterminate for rejection (RAI score 3/9), and 10% steatosis.

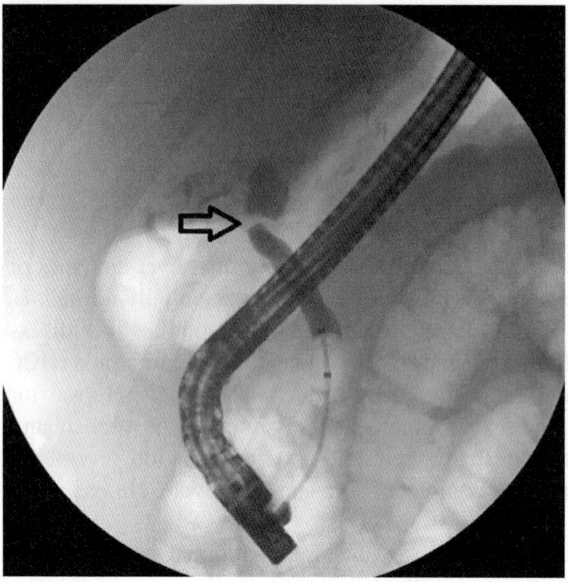

Fig. 66.1 Cholangiogram

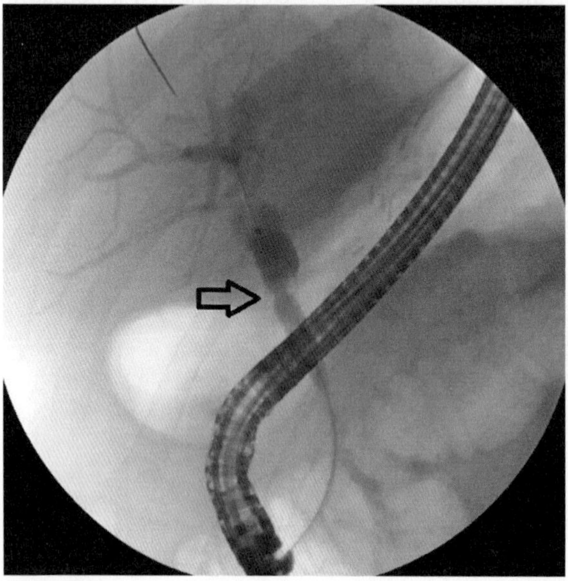

Fig. 66.2 Cholangiogram

Answer: Anastomotic Stricture After Orthotopic Liver Transplant

The differential diagnosis in a patient presenting several years after transplant with abnormal liver tests is wide. It is helpful that the patient was not transplanted for hepatitis C as recurrent hepatitis C would be a leading consideration and can present with only mild elevations in transaminases and occasionally cholestatic enzymes.

The interesting feature in this case is the very high GGT which is nonspecific but indicates that something relatively acute has happened, particularly in light of the normal liver tests recently. Possibilities include a vascular issue such as hepatic artery thrombosis (HAT) or stenosis. Rejection is still possible but his tacrolimus level is normal and he is still on prednisone. He had a history of HCC in the native liver and this may have recurred but he had a CT scan recently that did not show a lesion. He could be drinking again despite his denials and he is still at risk for conditions that can affect a nontransplanted liver such as viral hepatitis or fatty liver. A biliary stricture has to be a leading consideration despite the normal CT scan 2 months ago. This typically will be at the biliary anastomosis.

In this case, the imaging ruled out an issue with hepatic artery stenosis (HAS) or thrombosis, and a liver biopsy was performed. No significant rejection was seen but portal edema can be seen with biliary obstruction and hence ERCP was indicated. MRCP could have been obtained prior to ERCP but an experienced liver transplant pathologist is usually very good at picking up biliary problems. The cholangiogram is shown in Figs. 66.1 and 66.2. Duct-to-duct mismatch is common where the donor and recipient ducts are of different sizes and this can sometimes be confused with a stricture. Since ERCP is a dynamic procedure, the speed at which contrast drains from the intrahepatic radicles can help in determining the degree of obstruction. In addition, a balloon can be inflated and passed through the narrowed segment and the extent to which the balloon is deformed or held up is a good indication of the severity of the stricture. In this case, the arrow points to the strictured anastomosis and the biliary tree proximal to the stricture is significantly dilated and contrast does not appear to be draining well. The second figure shows a dilating balloon being inflated in the area of the anastomosis and still demonstrates a waist (arrowed) in the balloon from the tight stricture. A plastic stent was deployed through the stricture and the patient's liver enzymes normalized. The patient will likely require several repeat ERCPs and stents over the next year to try and dilate open the stricture and prevent restenosis. Failure to provide biliary drainage will lead to secondary biliary cirrhosis. If repeated ERCP and stent placement do not lead to durable drainage then surgical correction with a biliary enteric anastomosis will be required.

References

1. Graziadei IW, Schwaighofer H, Koch R et al. Long-term outcome of endoscopic treatment of biliary strictures after liver transplantation. Liver Transpl 2006;12:718–25.
2. Holt AP, Thorburn D, Mirza D et al. A prospective study of standardized nonsurgical therapy in the management of biliary anastomotic strictures complicating liver transplantation. Transplantation 2007;84:857–63.

Case 67

As a hepatology consultant you are asked to see a 69-year-old female for possible hepatic encephalopathy.

She underwent bilateral cadaveric lung transplant 2 weeks ago for worsening shortness of breath due to rapidly progressive idiopathic pulmonary fibrosis. She received a 23-year-old allograft.

She had initially done well but was difficult to wean off the ventilator and was on antibiotics for *Klebsiella* pneumonia. She had become lethargic and unresponsive. Head CT scan showed no evidence of acute changes. EEG showed possible partial seizure activity and she was started on phenytoin.

She was not known to have underlying liver disease and had no significant alcohol consumption.

On exam she is intubated and unresponsive.

She has normal vital signs.

There are no localizing neurological signs and no stigmata of chronic liver disease.

Her abdomen is soft and nontender, without hepatosplenomegaly and no ascites.

Laboratory Parameters

Hb 8.6 g/dl
Platelets 20,000/μl
INR 3.4
Creatinine 0.3 mg/dl
Tbili 0.6 mg/dl
AST 35 iu/l
ALT 38 iu/l
ALP 80 iu/l
Albumin 1.1 g/dl

Abdominal USS normal

Questions

1. What test would you order next?
2. What is the prognosis?

Arterial ammonia level 363 μmol/l (normal 10–40).

Answer: Idiopathic Hyperammonemia Post Lung Transplant

This unfortunate lady has developed idiopathic hyperammonemia after a lung transplant and the prognosis is typically very poor and usually fatal.

The cause is unclear although it can occur in up to 4% of lung transplant recipients. It usually presents within the first few weeks after transplant and appears to be associated with the development of major gastrointestinal complications, use of total parenteral nutrition and lung transplantation for primary pulmonary hypertension. One study suggested that deficiency of liver glutamine synthetase may be responsible but the exact mechanism is unclear but importantly can occur in the absence of liver disease.

Ammonia levels can be elevated if there is overproduction but typically if there is impaired clearance through hepatic dysfunction or porto-systemic shunting. Ammonia readily crosses the blood–brain barrier leading to functional and structural abnormalities which are manifested as neuropsychiatric dysfunction.

This is one case where the ammonia level was useful but typically in a cirrhotic patient, ammonia is an abused test. I am forever telling residents and fellows not to order it yet it continues to be ordered ad nauseam. One of the problems is the way in which it is collected. Ideally an arterial sample should be collected but a venous sample is satisfactory if collected on ice and analyzed quickly. Suffice it to say, this hardly ever happens and the result is usually a falsely elevated level. In addition, the ammonia level is not necessary to make a diagnosis of hepatic encephalopathy which is a diagnosis made on clinical grounds. Using ammonia to guide therapy is similarly not useful since response can be determined clinically.

References

1. Tuchman M, Lichtenstein GR, Rajagopal BS et al. Hepatic glutamine synthetase deficiency in fatal hyperammonemia after lung transplantation. Ann Intern Med 1997;127:446–9.
2. Lichtenstein GR, Yang YX, Nunes FA et al. Fatal hyperammonemia after orthotopic lung transplantation. Ann Intern Med 2000;132:283–7.
3. Ong JP, Aggarwal A, Krieger D et al. Correlation between ammonia levels and the severity of hepatic encephalopathy. Am J Med 2003;114:188–193.

Case 68

A 57-year-old male presented with a right pleural effusion that had required large volume thoracentesis on two occasions. He had developed some shortness of breath on exertion and a chest X-ray revealed the effusion. Diagnostic studies demonstrated the effusion to be a transudate. It reaccumulated several weeks after the initial tap and he was placed on diuretics. A CT of his chest showed some small non-specific areas of calcification.

He was otherwise well without fever, cough, or weight loss.

He had undergone orthotopic liver transplantation 9 years ago for cirrhosis secondary to chronic hepatitis C. His main complications prior to transplant had been related to portal hypertension including ascites and a right pleural effusion. He received a 12-year-old allograft and developed recurrent hepatitis C, genotype 1 that was treated successfully with pegylated interferon and ribavirin 3 years after the transplant. His pre-treatment liver biopsy showed minimal fibrosis. He was maintained on tacrolimus-based immunosuppression.

His other medical problems included diabetes on insulin and hypertension.

He denied tobacco or alcohol use.

Physical exam demonstrated a healthy-looking male with normal vital signs, BMI 22.5, and no scleral icterus.

He had a stony dull percussion note with decreased tactile vocal fremitus at the right lung base consistent with a moderate right pleural effusion. Abdomen was soft without ascites. There was no ankle edema.

Laboratory Parameters

Tbili 0.5 mg/dl
AST 29 iu/l
ALT 22 iu/l
ALP 98 iu/l
Albumin 4.3 g/dl
INR 1.1
Platelets 171,000/μl
Creatinine 1.1 mg/dl
HCV RNA negative
Chest X-ray – moderate right pleural effusion
Imaging – Ultrasound showed patent vessels and a normal looking allograft

Questions

1. What tests would you do next and why?
2. What is the long-term prognosis?

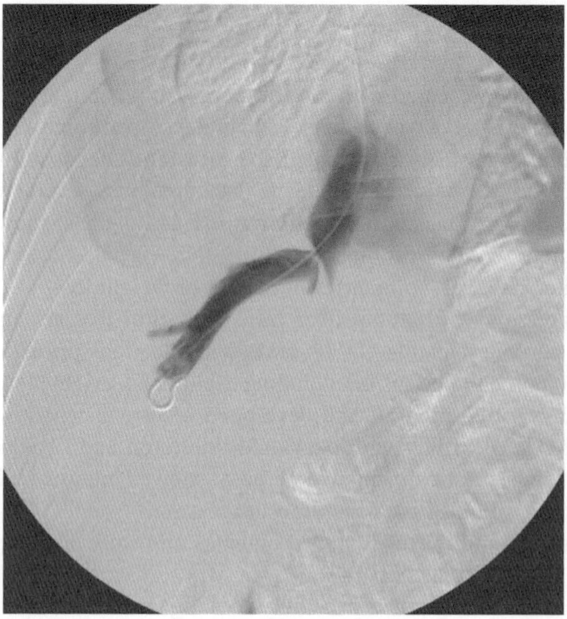

Fig. 68.1 Venogram

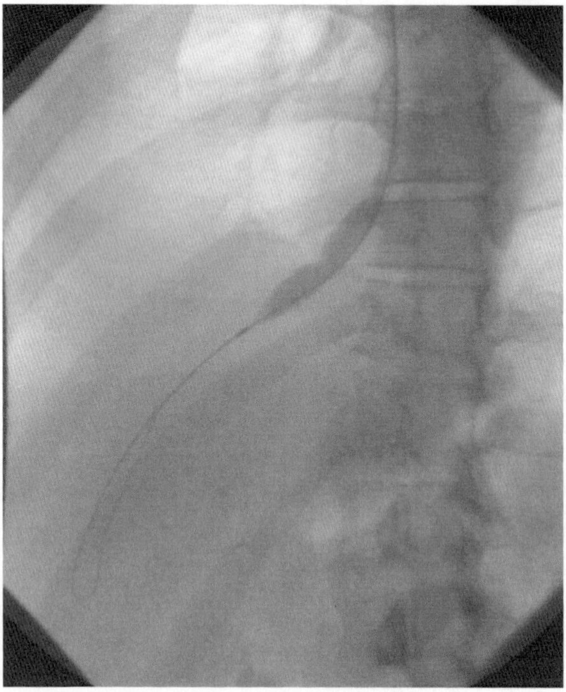

Fig. 68.2 Venogram

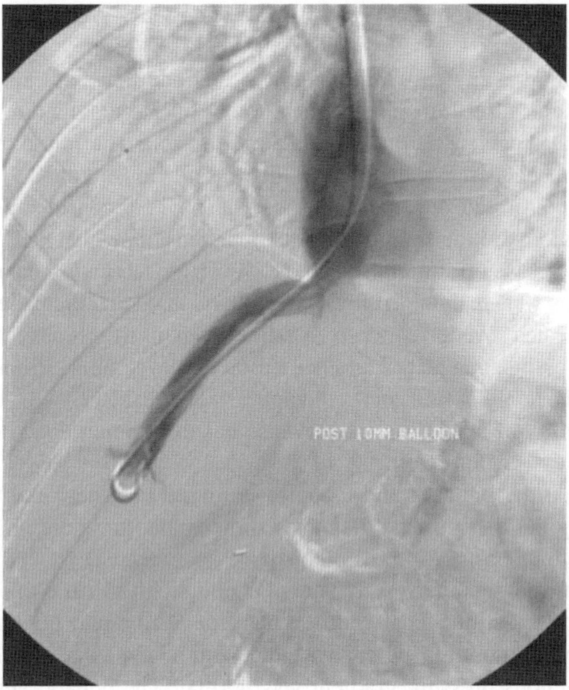

Fig. 68.3 Venogram

Answer: Stenosis of Hepatic Vein-Inferior Vena Cava Anastomosis

This is a very interesting case that illustrates the importance of being exhaustive in managing patients after transplant if they do not fit into classic diagnoses.
The differential diagnosis is that of a pleural effusion. The initial test should be a diagnostic thoracentesis. We are told that this was previously found to be a transudate and this was confirmed on repeat testing. The obvious consideration would be a hepatic hydrothorax in the setting of portal hypertension, which had complicated the patient's liver disease prior to transplant. However, the laboratory data would suggest he currently has well-maintained liver synthetic function and the patient's hepatitis C had been eradicated several years ago, at a time when his liver biopsy showed minimal fibrosis. It is possible that he had another reason for developing cirrhosis such as fatty liver disease. His only risk factor would appear to be diabetes.

The possibility of a lung malignancy also has to be entertained despite the transudative nature of the effusion.

The fact that the imaging and Doppler study did not show any vascular issues was reassuring but the ultimate diagnosis showed that these are unreliable to look for hepatic venous obstruction (as others have documented).

The patient went on to have a transjugular study with a liver biopsy. This showed no evidence of rejection, focal centrilobular congestion and no significant active hepatitis. Only mild portal fibrosis was noted and no evidence of bridging fibrosis. The hepatic venous pressure gradient was normal. The hepatic veins were determined to be patent. On closer discussion with the radiologist, however, the right hepatic vein was not seen. We sent him back for another transjugular study and this time they were able to place a catheter into the right hepatic vein. Right hepatic venogram was performed demonstrating a severe stenosis at the venous anastomosis (Fig. 68.1). Pressure measurements were obtained yielding a hepatic venous pressure of 28 mmHg and a pressure above it of 8 mmHg for a gradient of 20 mmHg. A 10 mm balloon was used to dilate the stenosis (Fig. 68.2) and a repeat venogram (Fig. 68.3) was performed demonstrating better flow through the stenosis. Repeat pressure measurements were obtained yielding a gradient of approximately 4 mmHg. A further dilation was performed using a 12 mm balloon. The patient's effusion has not reaccumulated over the next 18 months.

References

1. Kubo T, Shibata T, Itoh K et al. Outcome of percutaneous transhepatic venoplasty for hepatic venous outflow obstruction after living donor liver transplantation. Radiology 2006;239: 285–90.
2. Lee SS, Kim KW, Park SH et al. Value of CT and Doppler sonography in the evaluation of hepatic vein stenosis after dual-graft living donor liver transplantation. AJR Am J Roentgenol 2007;189:101–8.

Case 69

A 43-year-old woman presents with 1 week of nausea vomiting, diarrhea, and abdominal distention, and an 8 pound weight gain. The patient had a history of liver transplant 7 years ago for fulminant hepatic failure secondary to autoimmune hepatitis and had been maintained on tacrolimus and prednisone. Imaging 2 years ago showed a normal looking liver without portal hypertension.

She denied any alcohol or substance abuse.

Exam demonstrates a patient in no apparent distress. Vital signs are all normal and she is afebrile. There is no scleral icterus and no palmar erythema.

Abdominal exam demonstrates a soft abdomen with shifting dullness. Bowel sounds are present and there is +ankle edema.

Laboratory Studies

Hb 10.9 g/dl
Platelets 168,000/μl
INR 1.1
WBC 9.2×10^3/μl (normal differential)
Tbili 0.3 mg/dl
AST 8 iu/l
ALT 22 iu/l
ALP 98 iu/l
Albumin 3.7 g/dl
Creatinine 1.0 mg/dl
LDH 665 iu/l

A CT scan is performed and a colonoscopy shows evidence of patchy colitis with a thickened ileocecal valve. Multiple biopsies are taken and show mildly active chronic colitis and the terminal ileal biopsies demonstrate atypical lymphoid proliferation and ulceration. No viral inclusions are seen.

Quantitative Epstein–Barr virus by PCR – not detected

Questions

1. What is the diagnosis?
2. What are the treatment modalities?
3. What is the prognosis?

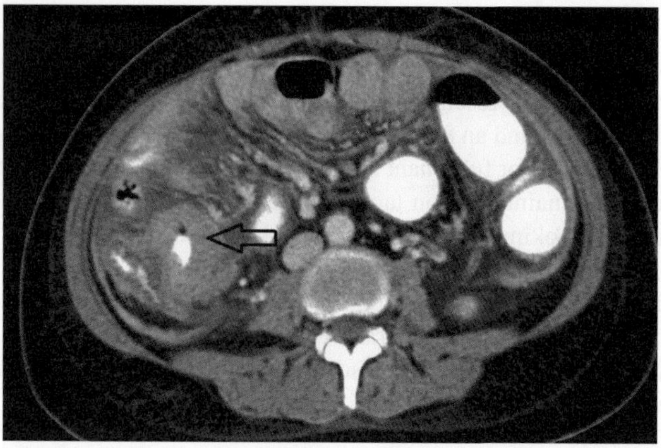

Fig. 69.1 CT scan abdomen

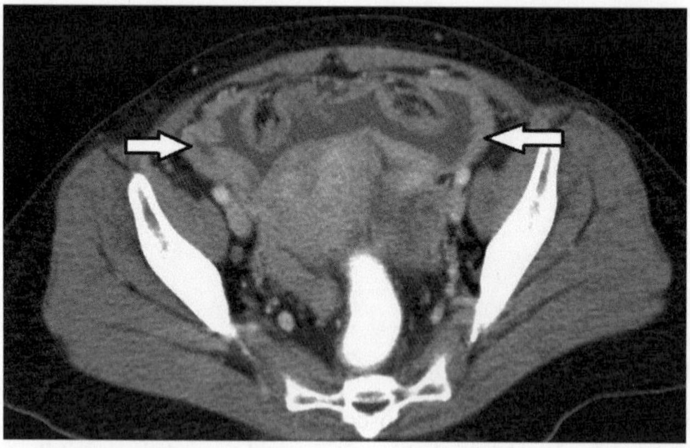

Fig. 69.2 CT scan abdomen

Answer: Posttransplant Lymphoproliferative Disorder

The imaging (Figs. 69.1 and 69.2) shows thickening of the terminal ileum (arrowed in Fig. 69.1) and a prominent omentum (arrowed in Fig. 69.2). The colonoscopy report is very suggestive of lymphoma. The differential diagnosis here would be infectious causes (tuberculosis or viral including CMV) and malignancy, and Crohn's disease could also give a similar CT image. Lymphoma has to be a consideration and since this is a transplant patient, posttransplant lymphoproliferative disorder (PTLD) is high up on the differential.

The diagnosis was clinched by immunohistochemical stains of the enteric biopsies. The lymphoid cells were positive for CD20 (B-cell marker) and CD79 and negative for CD3 (T-cell marker). There was a "starry sky" pattern consistent with PTLD (Burkitt-type). Stains for CMV were negative.

Lymphoproliferative disorders are common after solid organ transplant. The vast majority are non-Hodgkin lymphomas and almost always B-cell type. The pathogenesis appears to be related to B-cell proliferation induced by EBV infection under conditions of chronic immunosuppression. An EBV-associated protein (LMP-1) mimics members of the tumor necrosis factor (TNF) receptor family, and growth factor signals are transmitted from the cell membrane to the nucleus leading to cell growth and transformation. However, as in this case, EBV can be negative. The lymphoproliferative cells can come from the donor or recipient but in the former, the disease is limited to the allograft. EBV-negative disease usually appears much later (5–10 years) and has a worse prognosis.

The incidence of PTLD is higher when more immunosuppression is used so lung and multivisceral transplants have the highest incidence (5–30%) and only 1–2% in liver recipients. Hence, prolonged immunosuppression or induction therapies that deplete B and T cells increase the risk.

Treatment relies on reducing immunosuppression, systemic chemotherapy, and more recently rituximab which is an anti-B-cell antibody (anti-CD20 monoclonal antibody). Reducing immunosuppression does increase the risk of allograft rejection and doses need to be carefully monitored. Antiviral therapy for EBV is usually not successful.

The prognosis is poor with overall survival rates of only 25–35% and is even worse if monoclonal or T-cell based. Survival is worse in older patients, multiple sites, and particularly involvement outside the allograft.

References

1. Liebowitz D. Epstein-Barr virus and a cellular signaling pathway in lymphomas from immunosuppressed patients. N Engl J Med 1998;338:1413–21.
2. Leblond V, Davi F, Charlotte F et al. Posttransplant lymphoproliferative disorders not associated with Epstein-Barr virus: a distinct entity? J Clin Oncol 1998;16:2052–9.
3. Starzl TE, Nalesnik MA, Porter KA et al. Reversibility of lymphomas and lymphoproliferative lesions developing under cyclosporin– steroid therapy. Lancet 1984;1(8377):583–7.
4. Leblond V, Dhedin N, Mamzer Bruneel MF et al. Identification of prognostic factors in 61 patients with posttransplantation lymphoproliferative disorders. J Clin Oncol 2001;19:772–8.

Case 70

A 69-year-old lady presents with fever, chills, and jaundice. She had undergone liver transplant 9 months ago. Her liver disease was secondary to cryptogenic cirrhosis and had been complicated by hepatic encephalopathy and refractory ascites requiring intermittent large volume paracentesis and occasional thoracentesis for hepatic hydrothorax. She had not been considered for TIPS due to her age and history of encephalopathy.

She was not a candidate for a live donor transplant and had been listed for almost 2 years. She had experienced several episodes of spontaneous bacterial peritonitis.

Her other medical problems include diabetes and hypertension.

She had not received any suitable donor offers and then agreed to undergo transplant when the transplant team offered her an organ that had been procured from a 73-year-old donor who had had a stroke. The offer was only received after the patient suffered cardiac death (as opposed to brain death). The organ had been turned down at the local level and the cold ischemia time (CIT) was close to 10 h.

She has been on tacrolimus and mycophenolate based immunosuppression.

On exam she looks ill and is febrile to 101°F. She is mildly tachcardic. She has scleral icterus but her abdomen is soft with minimal right upper quadrant tenderness.

Laboratory Studies

Hb 10.6 g/dl
Platelets 118,000/μl
INR 1.5
WBC 14.6 × 10^3/μl (left shift)
Tbili 3.4 mg/dl
AST 109 iu/l
ALT 154 iu/l
ALP 254 iu/l
Albumin 2.4 g/dl
Creatinine 1.4 mg/dl

Questions

1. What is the next test to perform?
2. What is the significance (if any) of the donor organ?
3. What is the prognosis?

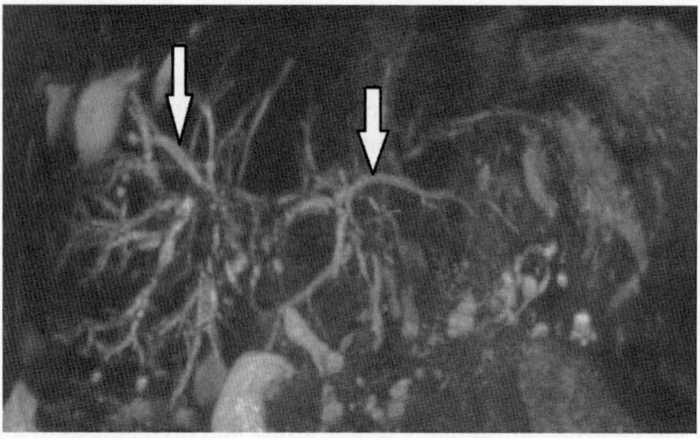

Fig. 70.1 MRCP biliary tree

Answer: Biliary Complication from Donation After Cardiac Death (DCD) Donor

This lady and her family took a difficult decision to get a transplant from a donor that would be considered marginal (or expanded criteria), although there is no clear definition of this entity. She had been listed for a long time and was very unlikely to get a transplant with a "good quality organ" any time soon. She had a very poor quality of life and took a calculated gamble.

The presentation and liver enzymes fit with a picture of cholangitis. Imaging would be the next test of choice and ultrasound would not be unreasonable, to look at the biliary tree and also to ensure hepatic artery patency. MRI can give a detailed cholangiogram and Fig. 70.1 shows evidence of diffuse intrahepatic biliary structuring and dilation particularly peripherally. This is consistent with an ischemic cholangiopathy type picture, even though the hepatic artery was patent.

The use of DCD donors in the USA has been advocated to try and increase the pool of donor organs. Several centers have published their experience performing such transplants with some conflicting results. The most recent studies suggest that DCD organs are associated with worse outcome in terms of the incidence of primary nonfunction and a 5-year graft survival of fewer than 60% in one of the largest series. Factors predictive of a worse outcome with the use of DCDs includes older donor age (>60 years), warm ischemia time of more than 20 min and CIT of more than 8–9 h.

As well as mortality, morbidity is a concern from ischemic cholangiopathy. The mechanism is unclear but appears to be related to ischemic damage to the biliary tree even though some studies have shown no difference in hepatic artery patency between DCD and donation after brain death transplants. Treatment of this complication is very difficult since the strictures are diffuse and not really amenable to endoscopic therapy.

Interestingly, many centers seemed to use DCD donors for patients with lower MELD scores, perhaps in the belief that sicker patients may not tolerate these organs. The most recent studies would seem to suggest that since sicker patients have the most survival benefit to gain from transplant, that even a marginal organ is better in this situation.

References

1. de Vera ME, Lopez-Solis R, Dvorchik I et al. Liver transplantation using donation after cardiac death donors: long-term follow-up from a single center. Am J Transplant 2009;9:773–81.
2. Chan EY, Olson LC, Kisthard JA et al. Ischemic cholangiopathy following liver transplantation from donation after cardiac death donors. Liver Transpl 2008;14:604–10.
3. Selck FW, Grossman EB, Ratner LE et al. Utilization, outcomes, and retransplantation of liver allografts from donation after cardiac death: implications for further expansion of the deceased-donor pool. Ann Surg 2008;248:599–607.

Case 71

A 61-year-old lady presents with abnormal liver enzymes. She had undergone orthotopic liver transplant 6 weeks earlier for end-stage liver disease secondary to hepatitis C complicated by HCC. The cancer had been treated with transarterial chemoembolization prior to transplant and was within Milan criteria (one lesion less than 5 cm or three lesions less than 3 cm and without vascular invasion or metastatic disease).

She had received a 57-year-old allograft with 20–30% macrosteatosis. Her postoperative course had been uneventful and symptomatically she felt well.

Her immunosuppression consisted of tacrolimus, mycophenolate mofetil (mycophenolate mofetil), and a tapering dose of prednisone. Her exam was unremarkable.

Ultrasound and MRI/MRCP of the abdomen demonstrated a patent hepatic artery and no evidence of any biliary ductal dilation.

Laboratory Studies

Hb 11.9 g/dl
Platelets 173,000/μl
INR 1.1
WBC 9.3 × 10^3/μl (normal differential)
Tbili 1.7 mg/dl
AST 316 iu/l
ALT 377 iu/l
ALP 446 iu/l
Albumin 3.0 g/dl
Creatinine 1.2 mg/dl
Tacrolimus level 12.8 ng/ml

You perform a liver biopsy that demonstrates mild chronic portal inflammation with rare eosinophils and lobular activity including scattered acidophilic bodies. There is mild macrovesicular steatosis with ballooning degeneration. There is no evidence of acute cellular rejection (ACR). You decide she needs hepatitis C treatment but want to wait a few more weeks to let her recover from the surgery.

Tbili 20.2 mg/dl (direct 19.0 mg/dl)
AST 756 iu/l
ALT 385 iu/l
ALP 451 iu/l
Tacrolimus level 18.1ng/ml

Questions

1. What should you do next?
2. What other blood test is important to draw to clarify the diagnosis?
3. What is the treatment for this condition?

HCV RNA viral load –

64,000,000 iu/ml

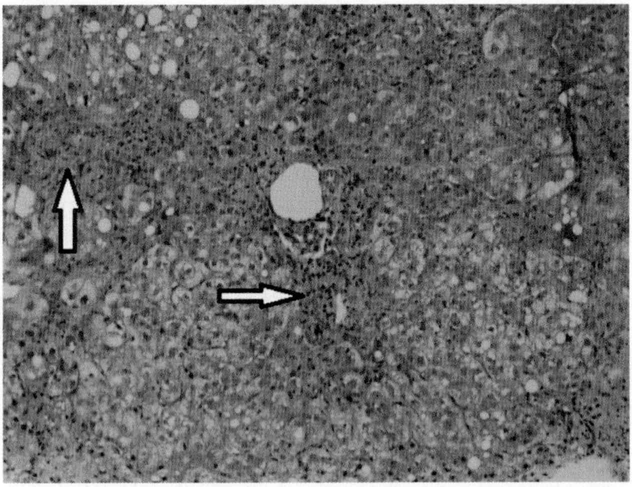

Fig. 71.1 Liver biopsy trichrome 100×

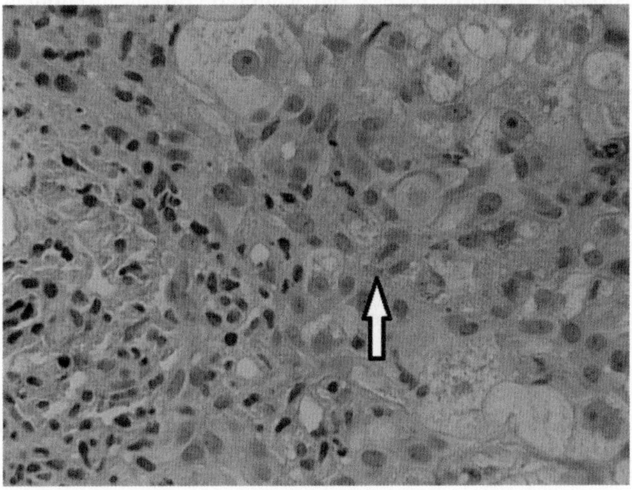

Fig. 71.2 Liver biopsy H&E 250×

Answer: Fibrosing Cholestatic Hepatitis C

This lady has developed fibrosing cholestatic hepatitis C. This is a rare condition characterized by cholestasis, fibrosis, and a very elevated HCV RNA typically occurring early after liver transplant. It has a very aggressive course without treatment and can lead to early graft loss.

The main differential diagnosis can be divided into biliary problems due to hepatic artery thrombosis/stenosis, acute rejection, or recurrent hepatitis C. Other possibilities do exist including a drug reaction or acute hepatitis from atypical viruses including CMV. The imaging suggests that the hepatic artery is open and it would be unusual to get acute rejection with her tacrolimus level. The next step would be a biopsy which illustrates a nonspecific pattern but consistent with hepatitis C. It is reassuring that no rejection was seen.

It would be reasonable to wait for a few more weeks to treat the hepatitis C as she is only 6 weeks from transplant and studies in the 1990s showed that early treatment of hepatitis C after transplant (before 3 months) is not associated with good outcomes. The very elevated HCV RNA and the worsening liver enzymes with jaundice, together with the high tacrolimus level are very concerning for fibrosing cholestatic hepatitis C. Since there is still concern about the diagnosis, a repeat liver biopsy is the next best test and as shown demonstrates that the lobules are remarkable for hepatocytic cholestasis (Fig. 71.2 arrowed) with feathery degeneration. The portal tracts are expanded by proliferating bile ductules accompanied by neutrophils. Occasional acidophilic bodies and scattered chronic inflammatory cells are seen. The trichrome stain in Fig. 71.1 shows periportal fibrosis. The blood test that clinches the diagnosis is the very elevated HCV RNA level.

Treatment for this condition is difficult. Standard therapy with pegylated interferon and ribavirin is usually not successful but several case series have suggested that regular interferon three times a week with ribavirin may be helpful.

In this case, she was started on low-dose interferon alpha-2b at 1.5 million units three times a week and low-dose ribavirin. Within 2 months, her jaundice resolved along with her liver enzymes and her HCV RNA dropped to 200,000 iu/ml. Some reports suggest that this treatment may need to be continued indefinitely although anecdotally I have successfully treated two patients with less than a year of this treatment.

References

1. Dixon LR, Crawford JM. Early histologic changes in fibrosing cholestatic hepatitis C. Liver Transpl 2007;13:219–26.
2. Gopal DV, Rosen HR. Duration of antiviral therapy for cholestatic HCV recurrence may need to be indefinite. Liver Transpl 2003;9:348–53.

Case 72

A 35-year-old presents to the ER with nausea, vomiting, and diarrhea that has been going on for several days. He denies fever or abdominal pain. He has also noticed that he has become jaundiced over the last week with dark urine, pale stool, and some pruritus. He denies weight loss.

He underwent liver transplant 3 years ago for cirrhosis secondary to alcohol. He was maintained on tacrolimus and mycophenolate with prednisone tapered over several months. His postoperative course was significant for an episode of acute rejection 6 months after transplant that was felt to be related to noncompliance.

He had otherwise only been seen in the clinic on one occasion since and had only called the office intermittently to refill his medications.

He denies other medical problems.

He states he is only taking tacrolimus and mycophenolate. He is single and not working.

Exam demonstrates an anxious man. His vital signs show a weight of 170 pounds, BP 140/90, pulse 110, and he is afebrile.

He is icteric and has a palpable liver edge. No ascites is noted.

Laboratory Studies

Hb 14.1 g/dl
Platelets 195,000/μl
INR 1.2
WBC 5.4 × 10^3/μl (normal differential)
Tbili 13.7 mg/dl
Direct bili 9.8 mg/dl
AST 179 iu/l
ALT 194 iu/l
ALP 349 iu/l
Albumin 4.1 g/dl
Creatinine 1.8 mg/dl
Tacrolimus level 10.9 ng/ml

Ultrasound shows no biliary dilation. Hepatic artery has normal resistive indices.

Questions

1. What should you do next?
2. What is the incidence of this condition in adults?
3. Is it treatable, and if so, with what?

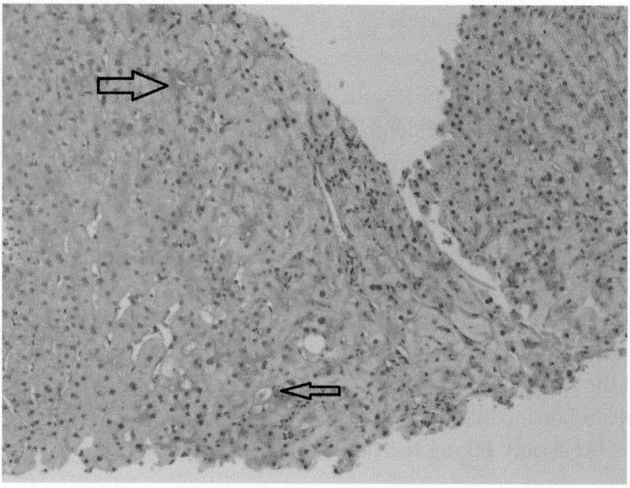

Fig. 72.1 Low power liver biopsy H&E 100×

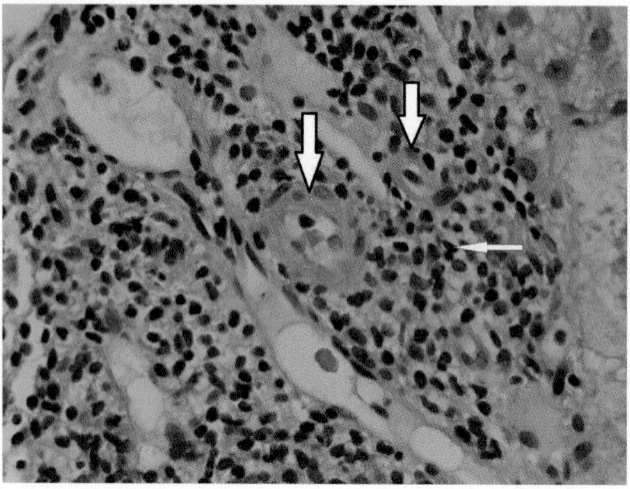

Fig. 72.2 High power liver biopsy H&E 250×

Answer: Chronic Rejection

This gentleman has developed chronic rejection almost certainly due to noncompliance. A liver biopsy is indicated since the imaging shows no ductal dilation making obstruction less likely. The first image (Fig. 72.1) is at low power and demonstrates a mild chronic nonspecific inflammatory infiltrate in the portal tract and the lobules are remarkable for severe canalicular and hepatocytic cholestasis (arrows). On higher power it is apparent that bile ducts are either damaged or missing. The two thicker arrows in Fig. 72.2 point to hepatic artery branches. The thinner arrow points to an area where the bile duct used to be and all that is left is some inflammatory cells. This is a very important fact about liver pathology – in the portal tract the bile duct and hepatic artery should be adjacent to one another. A CK7 (cytokeratin 7) stain is usually done in this situation to stain for bile ducts. In this patient, five of seven portal tracts were missing bile ducts, indicative of ductopenia. Other features of chronic rejection include a foam cell (obliterative) arteriopathy and biliary epithelial atrophy.

This patient had very erratic follow-up in the transplant clinic and probably was not taking his immunosuppression. The elevated tacrolimus level may indicate that he decided to take more than the prescribed dose when he became jaundiced. Alternatively, it may reflect decreased clearance due to his elevated creatinine.

The current incidence of chronic rejection of 3–4% in adults has decreased over the last 15–20 years due to the introduction of stronger immunosuppressive drugs. In children, the incidence of 8–12% has not changed, perhaps related in part due to compliance. Several factors are associated with the development of chronic rejection including the number of acute rejection episodes and the histological severity of acute rejection episodes, underlying liver disease, HLA donor-recipient matching, positive lymphocytotoxic cross-match, CMV infection, recipient age, donor-recipient ethnic origin, and male donor into female recipient. Obviously, not taking the immunosuppression (evidenced by a low tacrolimus or cyclosporine level) is also a risk factor.

Unlike acute rejection, the chronic variety often leads to graft failure, although some studies have suggested that an increased dose of tacrolimus may lead to improvement in histology and occasionally complete reversibility. Tacrolimus can be used as rescue therapy in patients previously on cyclosporine, particularly if chronic rejection is diagnosed before the bilirubin gets to 10 mg/dl.

References

1. Wiesner RH, Batts KP, Krom RA, Evolving concepts in the diagnosis, pathogenesis, and treatment of chronic hepatic allograft rejection, Liver Transpl Surg 1999;5:388.
2. Sher LS, Cosenza CA, Michel J et al. Efficacy of tacrolimus as rescue therapy for chronic rejection in orthotopic liver transplantation: a report of the U.S. Multicenter Liver Study Group. Transplantation 1997;64:258–63.

Case 73

A 25-year-old lady presents to the outpatient clinic with abdominal distension and abnormal liver enzymes. She speaks English poorly and is accompanied by her brother. Her abdomen has gradually increased in size over the last 2 years and she has some dull abdominal pain and fatigue. She denies fever or chills and her weight has been stable. She is otherwise asymptomatic with normal bowel movements and no change in urine or stool color.

Her past medical history is unremarkable and she takes no prescribed medications but occasional over-the-counter analgesics.

She smokes a packet of cigarettes a day and drinks socially.

She is single without children and works as a waitress. She recently arrived in this country from South America.

Her family history is notable for heart disease in her father and diabetes in her mother.

On exam she is alert and oriented. Her vital signs show BP 110/65, pulse 74 and regular, and she is afebrile. She weighs 110 pounds. There is no palmar erythema or spider nevi. There is no scleral icterus. Her heart and lungs are normal.

Her abdomen is massively distended, hard, and irregular but nontender. It appears that the liver edge is palpable in the right and left lower quadrants. There is no obvious ascites. There is no ankle edema.

Laboratory Studies

Hb 10.8 g/dl
WBC 3.7 × 10^3/μl
Platelets 361,000/μl
INR 0.9
Creatinine 0.5 mg/dl
Tbili 0.2 mg/dl
AST 21 iu/l
ALT 18 iu/l
GGTP 60 iu/l
ALP 135 iu/l
Albumin 4.5 g/dl

Questions

1. What is the differential diagnosis?
2. What test(s) are appropriate?
3. Is this lady a candidate for liver transplant?

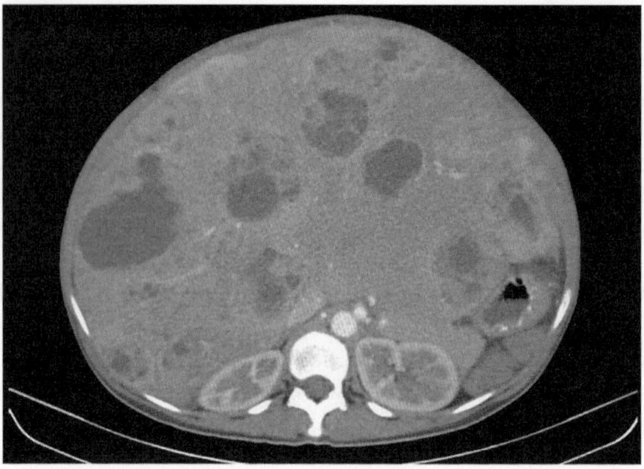

Fig. 73.1 CT scan

Answer: Metastatic Neuroendocrine Tumor

This unfortunate lady presents with a slowly enlarging abdomen and a hard irregular liver that is massively enlarged. The concern has to be for a malignant process, but she is very young and this has been going on for at least 2 years. A primary hepatic neoplasm is a consideration, but she has no obvious liver disease. Fibrolamellar HCC typically occurs in the absence of liver disease and affects young people but would not cause such a huge abdomen. Lymphoma can infiltrate the liver but typically the patient would not present over 2 years.

Metastatic neuroendocrine tumor (NET) has to be a leading diagnosis. The CT scan (Fig. 73.1) shows innumerable hypervascular masses throughout the hepatic parenchyma with only a small amount of intervening normal hepatic parenchyma between them. Many lesions have a central necrotic or cystic component. The liver is massively enlarged and the rest of the abdominal contents are compressed and displaced. Endoscopy showed a duodenal lesion which was confirmed to be a NET.

NETs can be divided into two groups according to poor or well-differentiated histology. The latter typically has indolent biologic behavior and commonly arise in the gastrointestinal tract (but carcinoid tumors can arise in the lung and ovary), and collectively, they are referred to as gastroenteropancreatic NETs. They include carcinoid tumors, pancreatic islet cell tumors, paragangliomas, pheochromocytomas, and medullary thyroid carcinomas.

Patients with functioning metastatic islet cell tumors can have symptoms caused by the specific type of hormone being produced by the tumor such as serotonin with metastatic carcinoid and other vasoactive substances, which cause the carcinoid syndrome (episodic flushing, wheezing, diarrhea, and eventual right-sided valvular heart disease). This patient is only symptomatic from tumor burden and hormone levels (serum gastrin, somatostatin, serotonin, and urinary 5-hydroxyindoleacetic acid) were only mildly elevated.

Treatment with liver transplant has been reported. However, many of these patients have indolent disease and can live for several years and so the 5-year overall survival rate of 70% among patients with metastatic carcinoid who undergo transplant has to be measured against the 40% long-term survival in patients who are just observed, especially considering the risk of recurrent disease after transplant in a majority of patients.

In addition, these patients have well-maintained liver synthetic function and require an appeal to a regional review board to get enough MELD points to have a viable chance of deceased donor transplant or otherwise need a live donor.

References

1. Le Treut YP, Delpero JR, Dousset B et al. Results of liver transplantation in the treatment of metastatic neuroendocrine tumors. A 31-case French multicentric report. Ann Surg 1997;225:355–64.
2. van Vilsteren FG, Baskin-Bey ES, Nagorney DM et al. Liver transplantation for gastroentero-pancreatic neuroendocrine cancers: Defining selection criteria to improve survival. Liver Transpl 2006;12:448–56.
3. Bilimoria K, Talamonti MS, Tomlinson JS et al. Prognostic score predicting survival after resection of pancreatic neuroendocrine tumors: analysis of 3851 patients. Ann Surg 2008;247:490–500.

Case 74

A 52-year-old man presents with abdominal pain and fever that started relatively suddenly yesterday. He had undergone orthotopic liver transplant 4 months earlier. His liver disease was secondary to hepatitis C and had been complicated by HCC. He received a 72-year-old allograft from a female donor who had died of a cerebrovascular event and had longstanding diabetes and hypertension.

He had a complicated postoperative course and had to be taken back to the operating room twice for several small collections and debridement of some necrotic liver due to preservation injury at the dome of the liver.

He has been on tacrolimus, mycophenolate mofetil, and prednisone-based immunosuppression.

On exam he looks ill with a temperature of 101°F, BP of 90/60, and a heart rate of 108 beats per minute.

He is mildly icteric and his abdomen is distended with minimal bowel sounds and right upper quadrant tenderness.

Imaging studies 2 weeks ago had shown no evidence of recurrent malignancy and a patent hepatic artery and his laboratory studies then were remarkable only for mild pancytopenia but his bilirubin had been normal.

Laboratory Parameters Now

Hb 9.3 g/dl
Platelets 94,000/μl
WBC 15.1 × 10^3/μl
INR 1.4
Creatinine 1.7 mg/dl
Tbili 3.4 mg/dl
AST 45 iu/l
ALT 38 iu/l
GGTP 290 iu/l
ALP 334 iu/l
Albumin 2.7 g/dl
Tacrolimus trough level 12.8 ng/ml

Questions

1. What is the most likely diagnosis?
2. How would you manage this patient?

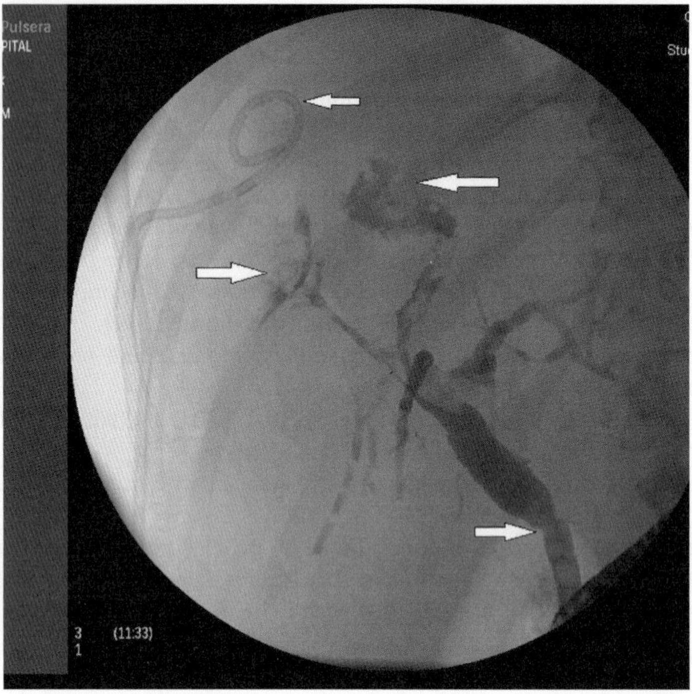

Fig. 74.1 ERCP

Answer: Bile Leak Leading to Abscess Secondary to an Anastomotic Stricture

This patient's prior history of problems after the transplant with the need to debride necrotic tissue and now the onset of pain and fever is very suggestive of an abscess. He looks toxic and is hypotensive with an elevated white cell count and right upper quadrant pain.

The differential diagnosis includes causes of cholestatic enzymes after transplant including rejection and hepatic artery issues but is less likely due to the normal ultrasound 2 weeks ago and the therapeutic tacrolimus trough level.

The elevated bilirubin and cholestatic enzymes in this case were a reflection of an anastomotic stricture that had caused a rise in the pressure in the intrahepatic biliary radicles and subsequent bile leak from the area that had previously been debrided.

The appropriate management in this case would have been to obtain imaging (an ultrasound or noncontrast CT scan would have been sufficient) to look for any perihepatic collections. Blood cultures should have been taken and broad spectrum antibiotics should have been started. Any sizeable collection should have been drained percutaneously in radiology using a pigtail catheter. In the presence of a bile leak the collection would have been bilious and then the patient should undergo ERCP.

The preceding ERCP images show leakage of contrast from the right system and a narrowing at the biliary anastomosis. This was treated with sphincterotomy and biliary stent placement. The idea is to reduce the pressure gradient across the biliary orifice of the ampulla so that less bile flows across the leak which will hopefully spontaneously heal over several days or weeks. This should be apparent since less bile will collect in the drain.

Biliary complications are common after liver transplant and should always be on the differential in patients with abnormal enzymes or jaundice.

References

1. Greif F, Bronsther OL, Van Thiel DH et al. The incidence, timing, and management of biliary tract complications after orthotopic liver transplantation. Ann Surg 1994;219:40–5.
2. Welling TH, Heidt DG, Englesbe MJ et al. Biliary complications following liver transplantation in the model for end-stage liver disease era: effect of donor, recipient, and technical factors. Liver Transpl 2008;14:73–80.

Case 75

A 27-year-old lady presents with acute onset of abdominal pain, nausea and vomiting that developed after eating last evening. She has felt cold and had some chills. She denies diarrhea and in fact has been constipated which is usual for her. She has otherwise been well without chest pain, shortness of breath, cough, or dysuria.

She has a history of orthotopic liver transplant for acute liver failure secondary to acetaminophen 4 months ago. She had an uneventful postoperative recovery and has been taking tacrolimus and mycophenolate immunosuppression.

She has no past medical history other than depression and denies any change in her medications. She does not smoke or drink and there have been no sick contacts at home.

Examination reveals a young lady who is anxious and in moderate distress. She is alert and oriented. Her vital signs are BP 150/85, pulse 108 and regular, and she is febrile to 101°F.

She has mild scleral icterus. Cardiovascular system reveals normal heart sounds and her chest reveals clear lung fields. She has a normal liver transplant scar. There is mild epigastric tenderness and a liver edge is palpable 2 cm below the right costal margin. There is no rebound tenderness and bowel sounds are heard and are normal. There is no ascites or splenomegaly. Extremities reveal no edema.

Laboratory Parameters

pH 7.4
Lipase normal
Hb 12.2 g/dl
WBC 10.7 × 10^3/μl

	Now	Last month
Tbili	2.7 mg/dl	0.5 mg/dl
AST	738 iu/l	12 iu/l
ALT	441 iu/l	13 iu/l
GGTP	365 iu/l	20 iu/l
ALP	305 iu/l	46 iu/l
FK level	11 ng/ml	9 ng/ml

Questions

1. What is the likely explanation for the liver enzymes?
2. What other blood tests are indicated?
3. What is the treatment and prognosis?

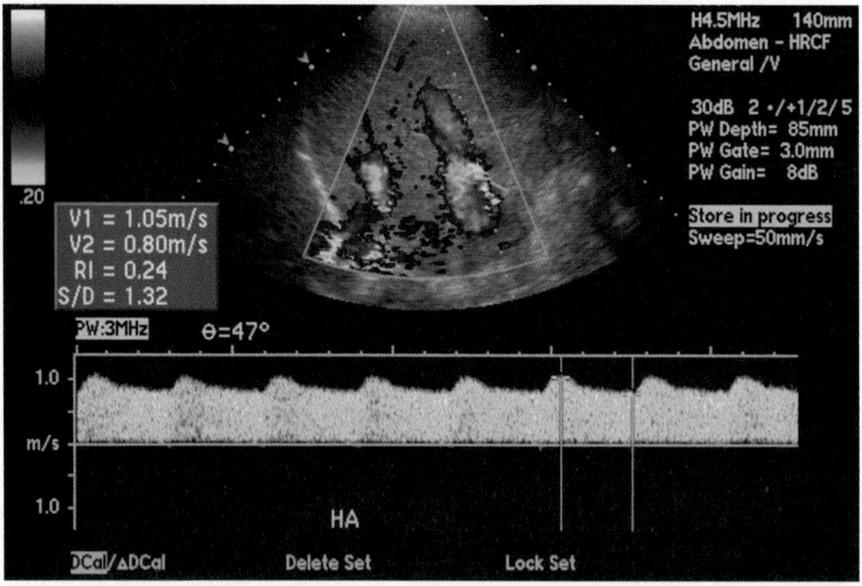

Fig. 75.1 Ultrasound with Doppler study

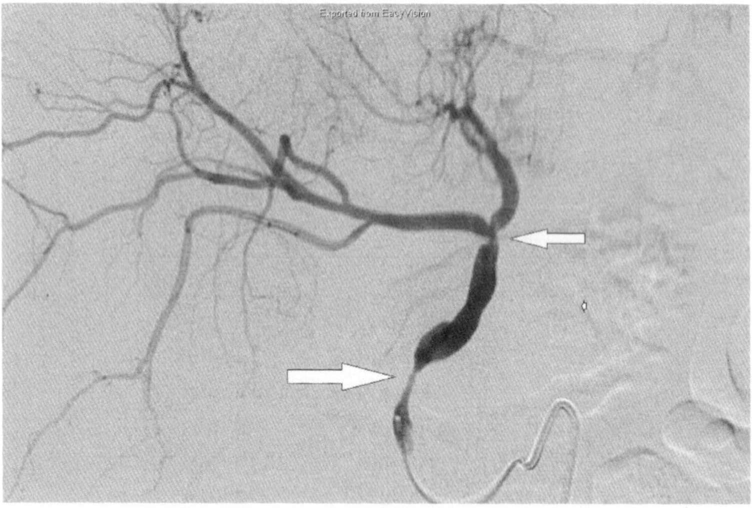

Fig. 75.2 Angiogram

Answer: Hepatic Artery Stenosis (HAS)

This lady has an acute onset of abdominal pain and fever 4 months after transplant and a significant rise in her transaminases. Diagnostic considerations include acute rejection, infection (CMV), biliary obstruction, or hepatic artery obstruction. Rejection is unlikely given the therapeutic FK level. Infection is a definite possibility as she is febrile and within the first few months of transplant when immunosuppression is still high. She needs blood cultures to be sent and empiric antibiotics should be started. She needs imaging which should include an ultrasound to look at the biliary tree and the hepatic vessels. She should have a CMV DNA test sent. The markedly elevated transaminases might suggest an ischemic insult and indeed this lady has developed HAS, a relatively common complication after liver transplant.

The first image (Fig. 75.1) is an ultrasound with Doppler study that demonstrates a patent hepatic artery but a classic tardus parvus waveform with a low resistive index (RI) of 0.24. The hepatic artery had a more normal waveform on a prior study with an RI measuring 0.58 a month ago. The portal vein and hepatic veins were patent with normal Doppler color flow and direction. The tardus parvus refers to the Doppler linear flow velocity vs. time spectrum obtained in an arterial flow system in which there is proximal occlusive disease with a poststenotic pressure drop. The RI is an indicator of resistance of an organ to perfusion. In ultrasonography, it can be calculated from the peak systolic velocity and the end diastolic velocity of blood flow (1-end-diastolic velocity divided by peak systolic velocity) and a value of 0.6–0.8 is considered normal.

The angiogram (Fig. 75.2) demonstrates the hepatic artery with a proximal segment of severe stenosis/stricture and a second stricture at the level of the bifurcation of the right and left hepatic arteries. These strictures underwent balloon angioplasty with improved flow noted immediately afterwards.

The incidence of HAS after OLT is 5–6% and it is a risk factor for HAT. Treatment initially was surgical but there are several case series describing the results of interventional radiology.

Risk factors for HAS include poor hepatic artery flow at the time of OLT but this presents early. Later HAS has no apparent risk factor. Surgical treatment results in initial patency rates of 70–80% but biliary strictures can develop in 25–30% of patients and retransplantation can be required.

Angioplasty and stenting of the hepatic artery can be effective in about 50% of patients but there is a significant restenosis rate and a risk of HAT (although lower than if HAS is not treated).

In this patient there was initial improvement, but she subsequently developed biliary strictures and is currently relisted for liver transplant.

References

1. Ueno T, Jones G, Martin A et al. Clinical outcomes from hepatic artery stenting in liver transplantation. Liver Transpl 2006;12:422–7.
2. Saad WE, Davies MG, Sahler L et al. Hepatic artery stenosis in liver transplant recipients: primary treatment with percutaneous transluminal angioplasty. J Vasc Interv Radiol 2005;16:795–805.
3. Abbasoglu O, Levy MF, Vodapally MS et al. Hepatic artery stenosis after liver transplantation – incidence, presentation, treatment, and long term outcome. Transplantation 1997;63:250–5.

Case 76

A 33-year-old lady presents with abnormal liver enzymes. She had undergone orthotopic liver transplant 9 months ago for cirrhosis secondary to autoimmune hepatitis. She had an uneventful postoperative course and has been maintained on tacrolimus, mycophenolate, and a small dose of prednisone.

Her only complaints are of some dark urine, which she states is due to dehydration and occasional right upper quadrant discomfort after eating. She denies fever or chills and has a normal bowel habit without weight loss.

She is married and working fulltime as a teacher. She denies alcohol, tobacco, or drugs.

Her liver enzymes 3 months ago were essentially normal other than a mildly elevated GGT.

Laboratory Studies

Hb 12.7 g/dl
Platelets 167,000/μl
INR 1.2
Creatinine 1.1 mg/dl
Tbili 1.6 mg/dl
AST 85 iu/l
ALT 59 iu/l
ALP 158 iu/l
GGT 242 iu/l
Albumin 3.4 g/dl

Ultrasound shows a 10 mm bile duct and mild intrahepatic duct dilation. Hepatic artery is patent.

Questions

1. What is the next best test?
2. What treatment is indicated?
3. What is the presumed etiology of this condition?

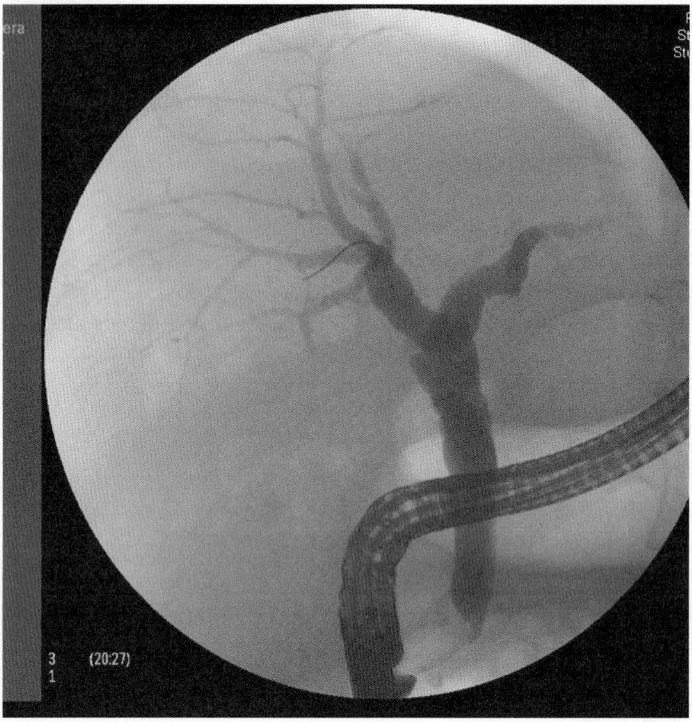

Fig. 76.1 ERCP

Answer: Sphincter of Oddi Dysfunction

The ERCP image (Fig. 76.1) demonstrates a post-OLT cholangiogram. The scope measures 12 mm in diameter and hence the extrahepatic duct is dilated to 10–12 mm and the right and left intrahepatic ducts are also dilated. The dilation extends all the way to the ampulla. No filling defects are seen and the anastomosis is barely seen. The cystic duct is seen superimposed over the extra-hepatic duct. A wire has been inserted through a catheter and the tip is seen in the right intrahepatics.

The differential diagnosis is that of cholestatic enzymes after transplant. The hepatic artery is patent which is reassuring. Recurrent autoimmune disease occurs but typically should have higher transaminases. Stone disease is uncommon after transplant, particularly for this etiology. Rejection is a consideration, but the dilated biliary tree has to be addressed before a liver biopsy. There still has to be concern for biliary obstruction so an anastomotic stricture is the obvious cause. Ultrasound can miss this quite easily and hence I prefer MRI/MRCP in this setting. However, MRI is not a dynamic study and the anastomosis can look narrow when there is duct-to-duct mismatch even though this may not be significant. Since the ducts are dilated in this instance on ultrasound the next best test should be ERCP, particularly as the enzymes are cholestatic and rising.

The cholangiogram demonstrates findings consistent with Sphincter of Oddi Dysfunction (SOD) with dilation all the way down to the ampulla. The contrast did not drain well even after several minutes of watching and hence the treatment of choice should be a sphincterotomy.

SOD is thought to have an incidence of 2–7% after transplant, significantly more common than in the normal population. The pathogenesis is unclear but may be related to denervation of the sphincter muscle around the biliary orifice at the time of transplant leading to sphincter hypertension. This will lead to biliary stasis and cholestatic liver enzymes.

It should be remembered that biliary complications are very common after liver transplant, hence the term "the Achilles heel of transplant."

References

1. Greif F, Bronsther OL, Van Thiel DH et al. The incidence, timing, and management of biliary tract complications after orthotopic liver transplantation. Ann Surg 1994;219:40–5.
2. Pascher A, Neuhaus P. Biliary complications after deceased-donor orthotopic liver transplantation. J Hepatobiliary Pancreat Surg 2006;13:487–96.

Case 77

A 45-year-old man presents to the emergency room with abdominal pain, cough, fever, and shortness of breath. He had undergone orthotopic liver transplant 1 year earlier for end-stage liver disease secondary to hepatitis C, genotype 1a.

His past medical history was significant for diabetes and hypertension.

He had received a 62-year-old allograft with less than 5% steatosis. Both the recipient and donor were CMV positive. His postoperative course was complicated by prolonged intubation and respiratory failure requiring tracheostomy. He eventually recovered and has been maintained on cyclosporine and mycophenolate mofetil immunosuppression as he developed a diffuse neuropathy soon after transplant while on tacrolimus. He had undergone a liver biopsy 6 months ago after his liver enzymes were elevated that demonstrated recurrent chronic hepatitis C with periportal fibrosis and 25% mixed macro- and microvesicular steatosis. There was no evidence of ACR.

His exam was remarkable for a low-grade fever and scleral icterus, but his abdomen was soft and nontender.

Ultrasound and MRI/MRCP of the abdomen demonstrated a patent hepatic artery and no evidence of any biliary ductal dilation. HCV RNA level was 560,000 iu/ml.

Laboratory Studies

Hb 12.1 g/dl
Platelets 228,000/μl
INR 1.0
WBC 9.2 × 10^3/μl (normal differential)
Tbili 21.8 mg/dl
Direct bili 20.1 mg/dl
AST 158 iu/l
ALT 85 iu/l
ALP 666 iu/l
GGT 1252 iu/l
Creatinine 1.7 mg/dl
Cyclosporine level 185.9 ng/ml

2 months ago his laboratory studies showed
Tbili 0.7 mg/dl
Direct bili 0.1 mg/dl
AST 35 iu/l
ALT 29 iu/l
ALP 124 iu/l
GGT 389 iu/l

Questions

1. What is the next test?
2. How should he be treated?

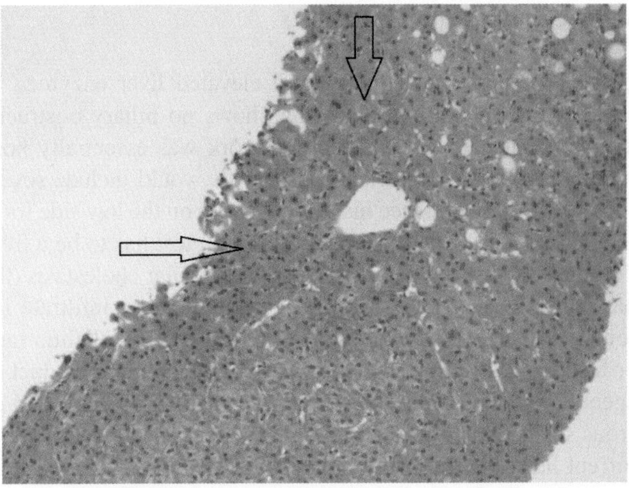

Fig. 77.1 Liver biopsy – low power H&E stain

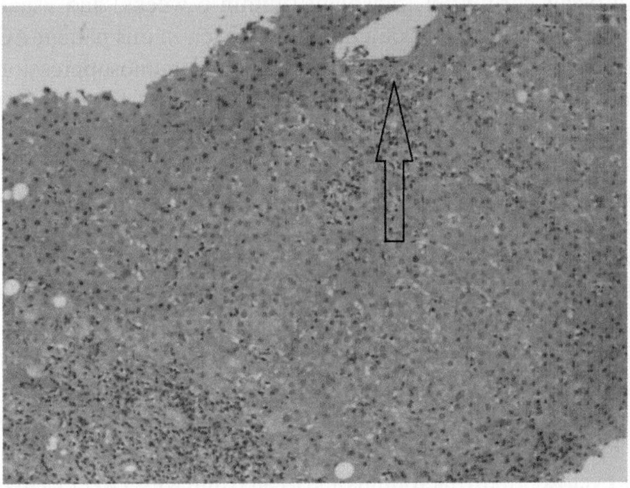

Fig. 77.2 Liver biopsy – low power H&E stain

Answer: Acute Cellular Rejection (ACR)

This gentleman presents with jaundice and elevated liver enzymes 1 year after transplant. It is reassuring that his imaging shows no biliary obstruction and his hepatic artery is patent. However, his blood work was essentially normal only a couple of months ago so the differential diagnosis would include severe recurrent hepatitis C but this is unlikely since his HCV RNA is on the low side for a transplant patient. The other concern has to be ACR. The next test has to be a liver biopsy.

Figure 77.1 shows marked hepatocytic and canalicular cholestasis (the brownish infiltrate that is arrowed). There is a mixed inflammatory infiltrate in the portal tracts (bottom left of Fig. 77.2) but also some mild endothelialitis (arrow in Fig. 77.2). Other features that can be seen on high power include bile duct damage and feathery degeneration. The trichrome stain (not shown) demonstrated portal fibrosis with fibrous septa. This is consistent with moderate ACR (and also some background recurrent hepatitis C). Pathological criteria for ACR have been developed and often an RAI (rejection activity index) is given with a score between 1–9. In this example the RAI was 6, consistent with moderate rejection and an indication for treatment.

ACR can occur early after transplant (within 6 weeks) and usually does not adversely affect graft or patient outcomes. However, in this patient ACR occurred later and this is often associated with low blood immunosuppression levels and is associated with reduced graft survival. Risk factors for early ACR include lower recipient age, fewer HLA-DR matches, longer CIT (more than 15 h), higher donor age (>30 years). Etiology of liver disease may also play a role with lower ACR incidence in viral and alcoholic liver disease, and higher in autoimmune diseases.

The treatment of ACR involves increasing immunosuppression. High dose methylprednisolone is usually first line therapy for ACR at a dose of 500–1,000 mg given daily for 1–3 days as a bolus. This is effective in 70–80% of cases and can be repeated if necessary. This patient did not improve after two courses of steroids and several options are then available to treat steroid-resistant ACR. Drugs that have been used include OKT3 (Muromonab), thymoglobulin, anti-interleukin receptor antibodies, mycophenolate mofetil, sirolimus, and tacrolimus. In this patient, we switched his cyclosporine to tacrolimus and treated him with a week of thymoglobulin. Within a month his liver enzymes and bilirubin almost normalized.

Care has to be taken in treating patients for ACR since the increased immunosuppression increases susceptibility to infection such as oral candidiasis, cytomegalovirus (CMV), Aspergillus, and Pneumocystis carinii. Antimicrobial prophylaxis is usually required.

The other concern in this patient is his HCV. Several studies have demonstrated that treatment of ACR with corticosteroids or with T-cell depletion is associated with acceleration of HCV progression and increased mortality. In addition, ACR and HCV can show similarities on biopsy making a definitive diagnosis difficult, although the HCV RNA level is very helpful in distinguishing the two.

References

1. Wiesner RH, Demetris AJ, Belle SH et al. Acute hepatic allograft rejection: incidence, risk factors, and impact on outcome. Hepatology 1998;28:638–45.
2. Banff schema for grading liver allograft rejection: an international consensus document. Hepatology 1997;25:658–63.
3. Volpin R, Angeli P, Galioto A et al. Comparison between two high-dose methylprednisolone schedules in the treatment of acute hepatic cellular rejection in liver transplant recipients: a controlled clinical trial. Liver Transpl 2002;8:527–34.
4. Charlton M, Seaberg E. Impact of immunosuppression and acute rejection on recurrence of hepatitis C: results of the National Institute of Diabetes and Digestive and Kidney Diseases Liver Transplantation Database. Liver Transpl Surg 1999;5(4 Suppl 1):S107–14.

Case 78

A 65-year-old man presents for a routine outpatient visit to the posttransplant clinic. He has a history of liver transplant 15 years ago for cirrhosis and HCC secondary to hepatitis B.

He has had an uneventful posttransplant course and his only other current medical problems include hypertension, which is well controlled on medication, and hypercholesterolemia. He does not smoke or drink and lives with his wife. He is a retired accountant.

Medications include tacrolimus, entecavir, simvastatin, and amlodipine.

His review of systems is unremarkable other than some intentional weight loss.

He follows regularly with a dermatologist after a small squamous cell carcinoma was removed from his face last year. His PCP follows his blood pressure and lipids which have been within normal limits. He saw a cardiologist last year prior to the facial surgery due to an abnormal EKG but had a normal stress test and cardiac catheterization. His PSA is checked regularly.

On exam he looks comfortable and is alert and oriented.

Pulse is 65 beats per minute, regular, and blood pressure 135/70. Weight is 132 pounds.

His heart and lungs are normal and his abdomen is soft and nontender. Extremities reveal mild ankle edema.

Laboratory Studies

Hb 12.3 g/dl
Platelets 134,000/μl
INR 1.1
Creatinine 1.4 mg/dl
Tbili 0.7 mg/dl
AST 31 iu/l
ALT 27 iu/l
Albumin 3.7 g/dl
Tacrolimus level 6 ng/ml

Question

1. What other studies should this patient undergo?

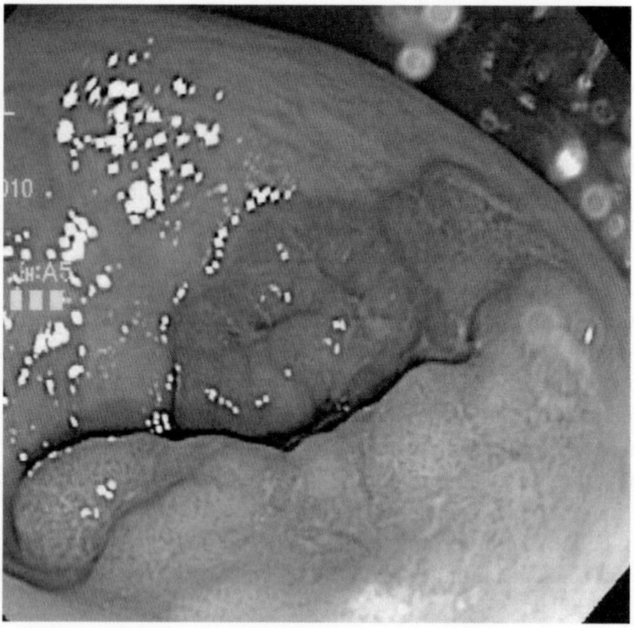

Fig. 78.1 Colonoscopy

Answer: Malignancy Post-transplant

This gentleman has done very well after transplant, which is typically the case for patients with liver disease from hepatitis B.

He has experienced some of the complications after liver transplant, namely skin cancer, hypertension, and hyperlipidemia.

The other tests he should undergo include a colonoscopy. He had undergone a routine colonoscopy about 10 years ago that was normal, but current opinion is that patients over the age of 50 years should undergo screening colonoscopy every 6–10 years, and this would especially be the case in a transplant patient. Figure 78.1 shows a 3 cm irregular lesion in the rectum that was noted to be an adenocarcinoma on histology. He underwent a resection and is doing well.

Malignancy is increased after liver transplant. Skin cancers are the most common, occurring in up to 40% of patients after solid organ transplant and hence regular follow-up with dermatology is recommended. Other malignancies are also more common, even excluding post transplant lymphoproliferative disorder.

As with nontransplant patients, increasing age, smoking, and alcohol appear to increase the risk. Disease etiology is also important with higher risk in patients with primary sclerosing cholangitis (for colon cancer) and alcohol for head and neck cancer.

Lymphoma is common and related to the use of higher doses of immunosuppression and T-cell depleting regimens such as OKT3.

The other test that may be considered would be a measure of bone density. Bone loss is an important source of morbidity in liver transplant recipients, but this patient lacks some of the risk factors including prolonged steroid use and cholestatic diseases such as primary biliary cirrhosis.

In women, routine pelvic examination and Papanicolaou smears are recommended as is an annual breast examination and mammogram after age 40 or 50, and may be considered earlier in women who are more than 10 years after transplant if prior to age 40.

References

1. Penn I. Posttransplantation de novo tumors in liver allograft recipients. Liver Transpl Surg 1996;2:52–9.
2. Yao FY, Gautam M, Palese C et al. De novo malignancies following liver transplantation: a case-control study with long-term follow-up. Clin Transplant 2006;20:617–23.
3. Tan-Shalaby J; Tempero M. Malignancies after liver transplantation: a comparative review. Semin Liver Dis 1995;15:156–64.

Case 79

A 57-year old white female who underwent orthotopic liver transplantation for end-stage liver disease secondary to non alcoholic steatohepatitis (NASH) 4 years ago returns to the transplant clinic for her annual check up. Her cirrhosis at the time of transplant was complicated by refractory hydrothorax and encephalopathy and she had a MELD score of 21. She received a 47-year-old female donor. Cold ischemic time (CIT) was 560 min, warm ischemic time (WIT) was 23 min, operative time was 6 h, and she received a total of ten units of blood. Examination of the explant revealed 35% steatosis with cirrhosis with no evidence of HCC. She did well posttransplantation and was discharged home on day 9. Currently she is doing well, although she has gained 18 pounds since her transplant and has been diagnosed with diabetes. She has a past medical history significant for hypertension, hyperlipidemia, and osteoarthritis. Her surgical history is significant for a remote cholecystectomy and a right knee replacement 2 years ago. Her current medications include tacrolimus, amlodipine, and pioglitazone. She takes occasional acetaminophen and ibuprofen for arthralgias. The patient is married and lives with her husband of 38 years. They have two grown children. She formerly worked as a secretary for the department of welfare but has been on disability since her transplant. The patient has no history of alcohol, pre- or posttransplant. She does not smoke, and there is no other high risk behavior. Her only blood transfusions were during the transplant.

Physical exam reveals a pleasant female in no distress. Vital signs show BMI 34.1 kg/m^2. There is no scleral icterus, but she does have a few scattered spider angiomas and palmar erythema. Her heart and lung exam are normal. Abdomen reveals a well-healed "mercedes" scar. There is a moderate size incisional hernia. Liver allograft is palpable 4 cm below the costal margin and is smooth. Spleen tip is palpable. There is no shifting dullness. She has trace lower extremity edema. There is no asterixis.

Lab Values

Creatinine 1.2 mg/dl
Total cholesterol 200 mg/dl (HDL 32, TG 212)
Hemoglobin A1c 6.4
Platelets 142,000/μl
Tbili 0.7 mg/dl
AST 24 iu/l
ALT 37 iu/l
ALP 82 iu/l
GGT 70iu/l

Her yearly ultrasound shows increased hepatic echogenicity consistent with fatty liver. Vessels are patent with appropriate flow.

Questions

1. Would you recommend any further testing to further evaluate the findings on US?
2. Would you institute any treatment?
3. What would you recommend for follow-up?

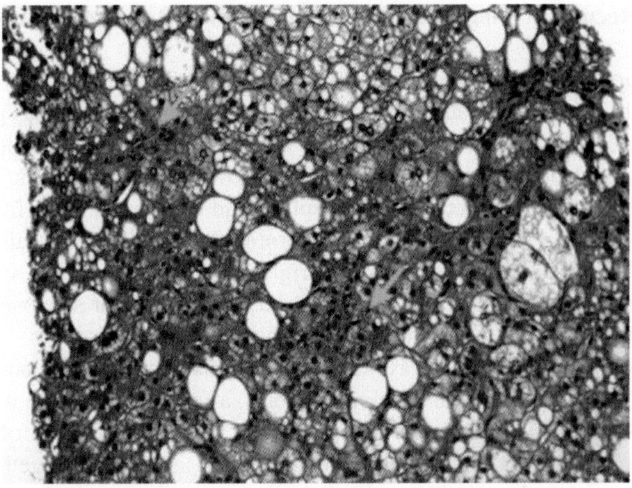

Fig. 79.1 Liver biopsy H&E 200×

Answer: Recurrent Nonalcoholic Steatohepatitis After Liver Transplant

This lady appears to be doing very well after liver transplant. She is 4 years out and has normal liver enzymes and normal liver synthetic function. She has gained some weight and has features of the metabolic syndrome which have become apparent after the transplant. However, her ultrasound shows fatty liver and the concern has to be whether this can recur after transplant and whether normal liver enzymes preclude this. This patient underwent a protocol biopsy that reveals ballooning degeneration of the hepatocytes (middle right arrow, Fig. 79.1) and spotty lobular inflammation in addition to mixed micro-and macrovesicular steatosis, consistent with recurrent NASH. The trichrome stain showed portal fibrosis.

Nonalcoholic fatty liver disease (NALFD) has become the most common cause of chronic liver disease in the developing world, affecting nearly one in every three individuals. NASH is considered the progressive form of NALFD affects nearly 10 million Americans and can eventually lead to cirrhosis and end-stage liver disease. It is not surprising that NASH cirrhosis is projected to overtake hepatitis C virus (HCV) as the leading indication for liver transplantation in the next 10 years.

Recurrent disease post-liver transplantation is an important problem and can be a common cause of allograft failure. Recurrent disease is very common after LT for NASH cirrhosis. The largest study on this subject demonstrated that the incidence of recurrent steatosis at a mean follow-up of 1.5 years was 70%. Recurrent NASH was also not uncommon, with an incidence of 25%. Although a significant number of patients with recurrent disease developed stage II fibrosis, no patients developed recurrent cirrhosis or allograft failure.

There do not appear to be any significant pre-LT factors that predict recurrence. However, similar to the presentation in this case, those who develop recurrent disease are more prone to develop weight gain, diabetes, dyslipidemia, and the metabolic syndrome. There has been some suggestion that the use of high-dose steroids correlates with the development of post-LT fatty liver.

Like the patient in the above case, the largest study on this subject demonstrated that one in every three patients with recurrent NASH had normal liver function tests at the time of diagnosis posttransplant. Nearly 75% of patients with recurrent NASH had AST/ALT ratios less than 1, similar to what is seen in the pre-LT population. The poor correlation of liver enzymes with the diagnosis of NASH is well-documented in the pre-LT population and the same seems to be true post-LT. Because of the lack of reliability of blood work, yearly protocol biopsies are recommended in order to better monitor patients with more progressive disease. Longer follow-up is needed in this group in order to determine if recurrent disease will lead to recurrent cirrhosis and allograft failure.

Large, randomized studies with protocol biopsies post LT are needed to determine if medications (vitamin E, metformin, pioglitazone, and ursodiol) can help improve or slow progression of recurrent NAFLD, as has been recently shown in the nontransplant setting. For the time being, we encourage patients to control their weight and metabolic syndrome and use vitamin E 800 units daily.

References

1. Contos, MJ, Cales W, Sterling RK et al. Development of nonalcoholic fatty liver disease after orthotopic liver transplantation for cryptogenic cirrhosis. Liver Transpl 2001;7:363–373.
2. Malik SM, deVera ME, Fontes P et al. Recurrent disease following liver transplantation for nonalcoholic Steatohepatitis cirrhosis. Liver Transpl 2009;15:1843–51.

Case 80

A 56-year-old white male is admitted to the hospital for increasing abdominal swelling over the last 2 months. He has a medical history significant for a native left nephrectomy at 3 months of age for an "infected" kidney. He was diagnosed with hypertension at the age of 18 and eventually developed renal failure. He underwent a cadaveric renal transplant in 1988. His first allograft failed secondary to chronic rejection and he underwent a second kidney transplant 10 years later. He also has a history of coronary artery disease and underwent a four vessel coronary artery bypass grafting in 2000. His other medical history includes diabetes and gout. His current medications include clopidogrel, allopurinol, mycophenolate mofetil, azothrioprine, and insulin. The patient states that over the last 2 months he has begun to notice increasing abdominal girth. He has gained 13 pounds and his pants no longer fit him. He also complains of dyspnea on exertion and new onset lower extremity swelling. He otherwise denies any confusion, bleeding, or jaundice. His creatinine over the last several months has begun to rise and is currently 2.3 mg/dl. He underwent an allograft biopsy showing some borderline changes. His urine output, however, has remained adequate and he has not required dialysis since his last renal transplant. The patient has been married for 30 years and has two grown sons. He was a smoker prior to his first kidney transplant. He drinks seldomly. He does have a 2-year history of hemodialysis before his first transplant and 6 months before his second. He has received multiple blood transfusions before 1992. He is a former vending machine repair man. His father and mother are alive and healthy in their late seventies.

Physical exam reveals a pleasant gentleman in no apparent distress. Vital signs are stable with a BMI of 31.4 kg/m^2. There is no evidence of scleral icterus or stigmata to suggest chronic liver disease. Cardiac exam is notable for a 2/6 systolic murmur with radiation to the left axilla. His JVP is normal. Pulmonary exam is normal. Abdominal exam reveals moderate distension; liver is palpable 3 cm below the right costo vertebral angle and is firm. He has a palpable spleen tip and shifting dullness is elicited. He has some dilated abdominal veins. He has trace lower extremity edema. There is no asterixis.

Lab Tests

Total bilirubin 1.8 mg/dl (direct 0.9)
AST 40 iu/l
ALT 29 iu/l
ALP 191 iu/l
GGT 98 iu/l
Albumin 3.7 g/dl
Hb 11 g/dl
Platelet count 111,000/μl
INR 1.0

MRI: A "questionably" cirrhotic liver, with evidence of portal hypertension (recanalized paraumbilical vein and splenomegaly to 17 cm).

Vessels on RUQ US with Doppler are all patent.

A diagnostic and therapeutic tap is performed. Six liters of clear, translucent yellow ascites is removed. Ascites tap: ascites protein 1.3 g/dl (serum albumin 3.8 g/dl); total protein 2.0 g/dl.

Cardiology is consulted and a right heart catheterization (RHC) is performed revealing a pulmonary artery pressure (PAP) of 24 mmHg with normal left-sided filling pressures and normal cardiac output.

Chronic liver workup reveals: HCV Ab negative

HBsAg neg, core total +, HBsAb 118 miu/ml

Autoimmune markers negative

Questions

1. What is your differential diagnosis for the ascites?
2. What further testing would you recommend?
3. Would you "clear" this patient for a second kidney transplant?

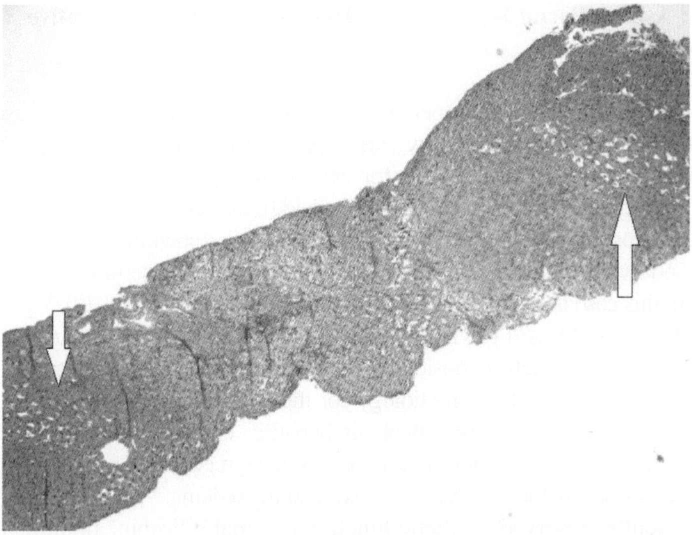

Fig. 80.1 Liver biopsy H&E ×50

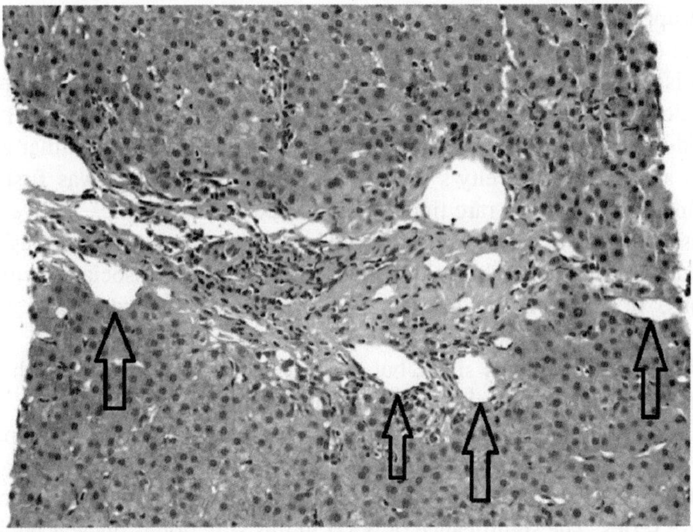

Fig. 80.2 Liver biopsy H&E ×200

Answer: Ascites/Portal Hypertension Due to Nodular Regenerative Hyperplasia

The first test which should be performed in a patient with new onset ascites is a diagnostic paracentesis. It is a very safe procedure with a low incidence of serious complications. Fluid should be sent for cell count and differential, gram stain and culture (with culture bottles inoculated at bedside), ascites albumin, and total protein. LDH and glucose levels, although not routinely sent, can sometimes help in the diagnosis of a "secondary" peritonitis or ascites of malignant origin. The serum albumin to ascites (SAAG) in this case is calculated by subtracting the ascites albumin of 1.3 g/dl from the serum albumin of 3.8 g/dl to yield a value of 2.5. A value greater than 1.1 is "high" (as opposed to <1.1 which is considered "low") and is an extremely accurate means of diagnosing a portal hypertension etiology for the ascites. The differential for a "high" SAAG ascites includes: cirrhosis, alcoholic hepatitis, cardiac (congestive heart failure, constrictive pericarditis), hepatic metastases, nodular regenerative hyperplasia (NRH), vascular occlusion (including myelofibrosis), and myxedema.

The patient's preserved synthetic function (normal bilirubin, albumin, and INR) speak against decompensated cirrhosis. Most of the other listed etiologies of "high SAAG" ascites can be adequately ruled out clinically with a combination of history, physical exam, blood tests, and imaging. The "cirrhotic"-appearing liver on imaging, immunosuppression regimen including azathioprine in a post transplant, make NRH a possible diagnosis.

NRH is a histological diagnosis, demonstrating micronodular transformation of the hepatic parenchyma without fibrous septa between the nodules. NRH was first described in 1953 by Ranstrom under the name "miliary hepatocellular adenomatosis" in a patient with Felty's syndrome and the term NRH was first used by Steiner in 1959. NRH is a rare finding, diagnosed in less than 3% of liver biopsies in autopsy series. The pathogenesis of NRH is not known, but it hypothesized to be related to abnormalities in hepatic blood flow. It has been associated with over 25 conditions, in particular autoimmune, hematological disorders and has more recently been associated with HIV infection and anti-retrovirals.

NRH is usually clinically silent, but as it progresses it can present with signs and sequelae of portal hypertension including ascites and variceal bleeding. Although NRH is infrequent, it is the most common cause of noncirrhotic portal hypertension in the western world, comprising up to 27% of cases.

NRH has been reported after solid organ and bone marrow transplantation in small case series. The significance of NRH in this situation is unclear but can be of concern, particularly after liver transplantation, since it can mimic cirrhosis on imaging and present with portal hypertension, suggesting graft failure.

A small study published in *Hepatology* in 1994 reviewed 9 patients who had undergone orthotopic liver transplant with postoperative NRH. All patients were on azathioprine, and six of the nine presented with signs of portal hypertension. Four patients developed graft failure and required retransplantation. More recently a series of 14 patients with NRH post-liver transplant was described. Patients were categorized into early (within 4 years of transplant) and late occurrence. "Early" patients were more likelihood to present with signs and symptoms of portal hypertension. Azathioprine, although used in a handful of the 14 patients, was felt not to be related to the development of NRH in a majority of patients.

The largest case series of NRH posttransplantation reviewed one-hundred patients who were diagnosed with NRH post-solid organ transplant between (1.1% of 9,172 total transplants). These were divided into post-LT 76 and 24 non-liver (majority post-kidney, but also included heart, lung, and multivisceral). This study concluded that although NRH occurs rarely in the postoperative period, it should be on the differential as a cause of portal hypertension in patients posttransplantation. Liver biopsy is crucial in these patients as it may change management.

The patient in this case was ordered a transjugular liver biopsy (Fig. 80.1 and 80.2). The hepatic venous pressure gradient (HVPG) was recorded at 15 mmHg. The biopsy shows focal sinusoidal dilatation (arrowed, Fig. 80.1) alternating with hepatocyte compression and atrophy on low power. At higher power, focal portal sclerosis (center) and shunt-type portal vein branching (single black arrows, Fig. 80.2) is seen, consistent with NRH with minimal fibrosis. With concerns of controlling ascites and continued development of complications related to portal hypertension, the patient is being considered for combined kidney/liver transplantation.

References

1. Naber AH, Van Haelst U, Yap SH. Nodular regenerative hyperplasia of the liver: an important cause of portal hypertension in non-cirrhotic patients. J Hepatol 1991;12:94–9.
2. Gane E, Portmann B, Saxena R et al. Nodular regenerative hyperplasia of the liver graft after liver transplantation. Hepatology 1994;20:88–94.
3. Devarbhavi H, Abraham S, Kamath PS. Significance of nodular regenerative hyperplasia occurring de novo following liver transplantation. Liver Transpl 2007;13:1552–6.
4. S Malik, D Sass, J Behari et al. Nodular regenerative hyperplasia post solid organ (non-liver) transplant. Hepatology 2007;46:503A.

Case 81

A 46-year-old lady presents to the emergency room with jaundice, abdominal distension, and lower extremity edema. She is known to have cirrhosis secondary to hepatitis C and alcohol but has been sober for more than a year. She is currently listed for liver transplant with a MELD score of 26 and has blood type A but has not yet received any offers. She denies fever, chills, weight loss or abdominal pain, GI bleeding, or encephalopathy. Her liver disease has been complicated by spontaneous bacterial peritionitis in the past and she is on antibiotic prophylaxis.

Her past medical history is significant for diabetes and hypertension.

Current medications include metoprolol, metformin, and norfloxacin.

She is divorced with grown-up children. She does not work.

There is no family history of liver disease.

The rest of her review of systems is negative.

On exam she looks ill but is alert and oriented.

Vital signs show BP 105/55, pulse 74, and she is afebrile.

There is scleral icterus and multiple spider nevi.

Heart reveals normal S1 and S2 without added sounds. Chest reveals clear lung fields.

Her abdomen is distended with a fluid thrill and dilated abdominal veins. Liver and spleen are easily palpable. She has ++ankle edema bilaterally.

Laboratory Studies

Hb 8.2 g/dl
Platelets 39,000/μl
WBC 14.3 × 10^3/μl
INR 1.9
Creatinine 2.8 mg/dl
Tbili 13.9 mg/dl
AST 47 iu/l
ALT 49 iu/l
GGTP 103 iu/l
ALP 127 iu/l
Albumin 2.0 g/dl

Ultrasound shows a patent portal vein and ++ascites. Diagnostic tap confirms SBP with 350 neutrophils. She is made inactive for transplant and is started on broad spectrum antibiotics and albumin. Her infection improves but her renal function worsens requiring renal replacement therapy.

She is reactivated for transplant after 7 days with a MELD score of 38 and three donor offers come in immediately.

Offer 1: 73-year-old male donor who died in a motor vehicle accident. Biopsy shows 30% steatosis and the cold ischemia time (CIT) will likely be less than 12 hours.

Offer 2: 22-year-old female who was found unconscious in the street and likely died of a drug overdose. Hepatitis C serology is positive and she is in a neighboring state and has been offered as there are no local potential recipients. Her serum sodium was 159 mmol/l.

Offer 3: 51-year-old diabetic male who is a non-heart-beating donor in a local hospital. Biopsy shows 10% steatosis.

Questions

1. Which organ should be used?
2. Is there a way of quantifying the risk of graft failure?

Answer: Donor Selection for Liver Transplant

This is an artificial case but the patient and her presentation is a common scenario in busy transplant centers, particularly those in areas of the USA where transplant typically does not occur until the MELD score gets to the high 20s or low 30s.

This lady has a very high MELD score and was recently infected and now appears to have a small window in which she can get transplanted. Her risk of dying in the next 90 days is very high so she does not have the luxury of waiting for an optimal organ.

Multiple studies have shown that outcome after transplant is affected by donor factors and the length of CIT.

Older donors are now common practice but can be associated with higher rates of ischemia-reperfusion injury and delayed nonfunction, although some recent studies have suggested carefully selected older organs work very well. In hepatitis C patients, in particular, older organs should be avoided if possible as these organs are associated with worse outcome and the risk of severe recurrent hepatitis C. Interestingly, the surgeon's assessment of the organ is a good predictor of outcome, even allowing for donor age.

Severe fat on a liver biopsy is a strong risk factor for primary nonfunction and organs with >60% fat should not be used. A figure of <30% steatosis is mild and not a concern and 30–60% (moderate) carries an increased risk but these organs can still be used.

Hypernatremia of >155 mmol/l carries an increased risk of early graft dysfunction but is likely an indicator of other factors that can affect outcome so hypernatremia in itself should exclude a donor unless the Na level is >160 or definitely 170 mmol/l.

A prolonged CIT affects outcome after transplant. Donor organs are kept in a cooled (<4°C) University of Wisconsin solution but a CIT of >12 h is associated with graft injury, particularly in an older donor. These organs can still be used.

Using organs from a donor with hepatitis C would appear to be counter-intuitive but several studies have shown that these organs can be used in hepatitis C positive recipients but a pretransplant biopsy is necessary to ensure no significant fibrosis. In extreme circumstances, these organs can even be used in non-hepatitis C recipients.

Using organs from donation after cardiac death (DCD) donors is now common practice but is associated with an increased risk of primary nonfunction and the development of biliary complications from ischemic cholangiopathy.

The concept of a donor risk index (DRI) has recently been advocated. The DRI is derived from several factors including donor age, DCD, use of split/partial grafts, African-American race, less height, cerebrovascular accident, and "other" causes of brain death. A higher DRI is associated with increased risk of graft loss.

This patient has a tough choice. She has hepatitis C and should avoid an older donor as in offer 1. Offer 3 is a DCD and likely should be avoided. Offer 2 would be the best choice if the biopsy shows little or no fibrosis (which should be the case in such a young donor).

References

1. Moore DE, Feurer ID, Speroff T et al. Impact of donor, technical, and recipient risk factors on survival and quality of life after liver transplantation. Arch Surg 2005;140:273–7.
2. Hoofnagle JH, Lombardero M, Zetterman RK et al. Donor age and outcome of liver transplantation. Hepatology 1996;24:89–96.
3. Figueras J, Busquets J, Grande L et al. The deleterious effect of donor high plasma sodium and extended preservation in liver transplantation. A multivariate analysis. Transplantation 1996;61:410–3.
4. Feng S, Goodrich NP, Bragg-Gresham JL et al. Characteristics associated with liver graft failure: the concept of a donor risk index. Am J Transplant 2006;6:783–90.

Case 82

As a hepatology consultant, you are asked to see a 41-year-old man on the hematology service for abnormal liver enzymes. He had undergone allogeneic hematopoetic stem cell transplantation 10 days ago for acute myelogenous leukemia. He had initially done well, but 6 days after the transplant he started to complain of right upper quadrant pain and his vitals shows that he has gained 11 pounds since the transplant. Over the last 3 days his liver enzymes have risen and he is now jaundiced.

There has been no fever or chills. He does complain of nausea and has had some nonbloody emesis. There has been some diarrhea, although his *C. difficile* toxin was negative.

He has no relevant past medical history and no history of underlying liver disease.

His current medications include prednisone, allopurinol, ursodeoxycholic acid, and percocet. He denies any herbal supplements.

He is married and has three young children. He works as a medical technician.

He has never been a heavy drinker and does not smoke or drink.

There is no family history of liver disease.

The rest of his review of systems is negative.

On exam he looks uncomfortable. He is alert and oriented.

Vital signs show BP 125/75, pulse 112, and he is afebrile.

There is mild scleral icterus.

Heart reveals normal S1 and S2 without added sounds. Chest reveals a few crackles at both lung bases.

His abdomen is distended with dullness in the flanks. His liver is enlarged 6 cm below the costal margin and is tender. He has ++ankle edema bilaterally.

Ultrasound at the bedside shows a heterogeneous liver and ascites but patent hepatic and portal veins and no ductal dilation.

Laboratory Studies

Hb 9.2 g/dl
Platelets 38,000/μl
WBC 1.3×10^3/μl
INR 1.4
Creatinine 2.0 mg/dl
Tbili 4.6 mg/dl (conjugated 3.4 mg/dl)
AST 193 iu/l
ALT 242 iu/l
GGTP 301 iu/l
ALP 158 iu/l

Questions

1. Where is the pathology in this condition?
2. How is the diagnosis made?
3. Where would the earliest changes be seen on a liver biopsy?
4. What treatment options are available?

Answer: Hepatic Sinusoidal Obstruction Syndrome or Veno-Occlusive Disease (Following Hematopoietic Cell Transplant)

This gentleman presents with classic symptoms and signs of hepatic sinusoidal obstruction syndrome (HSOS). He has just undergone stem cell transplant and within a week has gained weight, complains of right upper quadrant pain and has an enlarged tender liver on exam. He has subsequently become jaundiced.

The diagnosis of HSOS is a clinical one and is very similar to Budd–Chiari syndrome. The severity of the disease varies widely as does the incidence, but more severe liver synthetic dysfunction portends a worse prognosis. In this patient, the early rise in bilirubin and mild elevation in INR are concerning. Imaging is not usually helpful in making a diagnosis. Helpful laboratory tests include a low anti-thrombin, protein C, and increased plasminogen activator inhibitor-1 levels.

HSOS affects the terminal hepatic venules and sinusoids and the primary injury is in the endothelium. As well as after stem cell transplant, similar changes can be seen with ingestion of pyrrolizidine alkaloids which can be found in certain herbal teas, after liver transplant and after high dose radiation to the liver. On liver biopsy hepatic sinusoids are dilated and can be congested with red cells. The earliest changes will be seen in zone 3 but can spread to include the whole lobule. Later changes include sinusoidal fibrosis and occlusion of terminal venules.

Multiple risk factors have been suggested for HSOS including pre-existing liver disease, especially with an elevated AST level, the type of pre-transplant cytoreductive therapy or radiation dose and polymorphisms of the glutathione S-transferase gene. Prophylactic low-dose heparin and ursodeoxycholic acid may be protective.

Treatment for HSOS is mainly supportive with diuretics and analgesics in mild cases. More severe cases have been treated with agents that try to reverse the hypercoagulability that is the hallmark of HSOS but the data is based on case series. Recombinant tissue-type plasminogen activator or tPA and defibrotide (a polydeoxyribonucleotide with multiple antithrombotic and fibrinolytic actions) have been used with some success but mortality remains high in patients with severe disease.

References

1. Kumana CR, Ng M, Lin HJ et al. Herbal tea-induced hepatic veno-occlusive disease: Quantification of toxic alkaloid exposure in adults. Gut 1985;26:101.
2. McDonald GB, Hinds MS, Fisher LD, Schoch HG, Wolford JL, Banaji M, Hardin BJ, Shulman HM, Clift RA Veno-occlusive disease of the liver and multiorgan failure after bone marrow transplantation: a cohort study of 355 patients. Ann Intern Med 1993;118:255–67.
3. McDonald GB, Sharma P, Matthews DE, Shulman HM, Thomas ED Venocclusive disease of the liver after bone marrow transplantation: diagnosis, incidence, and predisposing factors. Hepatology 1984;4:116–22.
4. DeLeve LD, Valla DC, Garcia-Tsao G. Vascular disorders of the liver. Hepatology 2009;49:1729.

Case 83

As the transplant hepatology consultant you are asked to see a 56-year-old lady on the renal transplant service for diarrhea.

She had undergone renal transplant 6 months ago for stage V chronic kidney disease secondary to renal vasculopathy due to hypertensive nephropathy and renal artery stenosis. She was not on dialysis prior to the transplant and received a kidney from a daughter.

She had done well after the transplant but 1 week ago developed nonbloody diarrhea, which she describes as loose and frequent but not voluminous. Her bowels were moving normally prior to this. She has a lost a few pounds in weight but denies abdominal pain, fever or chills. Initial laboratory studies on admission revealed a creatinine of 4.1 mg/dl, up from a baseline of 1.4 mg/dl, which improved with hydration.

Her other medical problems include dyslipidemia, hypertension, secondary hyperparathyroidism, and gout.

Current medications include metoprolol, levothyroxine, simvastatin, amlodipine, mycophenolate mofetil 1 g bid, aspirin, prednisone 5 mg qd, and tacrolimus 1 mg bid.

She denies tobacco or alcohol.

On exam she looks well with stable vital signs.

Heart and lungs are normal. Her abdomen is soft and nontender. The renal allograft is easily felt in the right lower quadrant.

Laboratory Studies

Hb 9.2 g/dl
Platelets 134,000/μl
WBC 2.1×10^3/μl
BUN 51 mg/dl
Creatinine 2.9 mg/dl
Tbili 0.2 mg/dl
AST 13 iu/l
ALT 16 iu/l
GGTP 23 iu/l
ALP 35 iu/l
Albumin 3.0 g/dl
FK level 12 ng/ml

Stool studies: negative for ova and parasites, negative for *C. difficile*, negative for *Salmonella*, *Shigella*, *Yersinia* and *Campylobacter*.
CMV early antigen test is negative.

Questions

1. What should you do next?
2. What causes this condition?
3. Is it reversible?
4. What is/are the treatment options?

Findings at colonoscopy:
The colonic mucosa was hyperemic and mildly granular in the right colon with a gradual transition to normal looking mucosa in the mid-transverse and left colon. No ulcers or frank inflammation seen.
Random colonic biopsies:
Colorectal mucosa with edema and gland dropout.

Answer: Mycophenolate Mofetil (MMF) Colitis

This lady has developed severe enough diarrhea after renal transplant to cause acute kidney injury due to dehydration. The first concern in a transplant patient has to be an infectious cause but she looks well and her stool studies and CMV tests are negative. Stool electrolytes are used to distinguish between a secretory and osmotic diarrhea in general gastroenterology, but I usually do not find this a useful test in the transplant population. She could have a viral infection which should be self-limited but typically a colonoscopy and biopsy is required in this situation.

Medication induced diarrhea has to be a consideration in a transplant patient and the leading culprit is mycophenolate mofetil. This immunosuppressive agent is often used in transplantation as a maintenance drug as it is not nephrotoxic and has less bone marrow toxicity than azathioprine. It works by impairing lymphocyte function by blocking purine biosynthesis via inhibition of the enzyme inosine monophosphate dehydrogenase. The main complaint patients have with this drug are its gastrointestinal adverse effects.

Diarrhea is very common but can be managed with anti-diarrheal agents. However, in severe cases, the drug has to be stopped.

The mechanism behind the diarrhea is unclear although a recent study has demonstrated frequent histologic changes which can resemble self-limited colitis, graft vs. host disease and inflammatory bowel disease leading to diagnostic difficulties. Another study found that erosive enterocolitis, which was similar to Crohn's type changes, was seen in 40% of patient and 60% had infectious changes. Since reducing or stopping mycophenolate mofetil was the only effective therapy, the drug or its metabolites may be the cause. However, this increases the risk of allograft rejection.

Another method of alleviating the adverse gastrointestinal effects is to use an enteric coated formulation of mycophenolate (myFortic) but some studies have shown no reduction in the side effect profile.

This patient improved with a reduction in the mycophenolate mofetil dose to 750 mg bid.

References

1. Selbst MK, Ahrens WA, Robert ME et al. Spectrum of histologic changes in colonic biopsies in patients treated with mycophenolate mofetil. Mod Pathol 2009;22:737–43.
2. Maes BD, Dalle I, Geboes K et al. Erosive enterocolitis in mycophenolate mofetil-treated renal-transplant recipients with persistent afebrile diarrhea. Transplantation 2003;75:665–72.

Case 84

You are called to the emergency room to see a 47-year-old lady who presents with 2 days of nausea and mild abdominal pain and her sister noticed that she looked jaundiced.

She underwent liver transplant 2 years ago for fulminant liver failure secondary to autoimmune hepatitis. She was listed as a status 1 for almost a week and had to accept an extended criteria organ. She did well afterwards but has not been seen in the office for over a year although states that she has been taking most of her medications and blood work 2 months ago showed normal liver enzymes and a therapeutic tacrolimus level. Liver biopsy 1 year after transplant showed some mild portal inflammation with some scattered plasma cells but minimal fibrosis.

She denies fever or chills and has had no change in urine or stool color. She has lost a few pounds in weight.

She has thyroid disease but otherwise no other medical problems.

She does not smoke or drink and has not used illicit drugs. She is single and not sexually active. She works as a hairdresser and also runs a local dance instruction class.

Her prescribed medications include tacrolimus, prednisone, mycophenolate mofetil, lamivudine, and levothyroxine.

On exam she looks well but is obviously jaundiced. Vital signs are stable.

There is no palmar erythema or asterixis.

She has scleral icterus but no spider nevi.

Heart and lung exam is unremarkable. Abdomen is soft and nontender without ascites and a liver edge is palpable but no splenomegaly. There is no ankle edema.

Laboratory Studies

Hb 11.4 g/dl
Platelets 192,000/μl
WBC 6.5 × 10^3/μl
Creatinine 0.8 mg/dl
Tbili 12.3 mg/dl
Direct 9.9 mg/dl
AST 425 iu/l
ALT 476 iu/l
GGTP 209 iu/l
ALP 167 iu/l
Albumin 3.2 g/dl
FK level 8 ng/ml

Questions

1. What additional tests are required?
2. What is the significance of lamivudine?

Ultrasound – no ductal dilation
Patent hepatic artery
HBsAg positive
HBV DNA 18 million iu/ml
Liver biopsy – no rejection

Answer: Hepatitis B from Core Antibody (Anti-HBc) Positive Donor

This lady presents with acute hepatitis and jaundice 2 years after liver transplant. Her tacrolimus level is therapeutic and ultrasound shows no biliary obstruction and the hepatic artery is open, making rejection and biliary problems less likely.

She underwent multiple serological studies to look for viral hepatitis and her hepatitis B surface antigen (HBsAg) is positive and she has a very elevated HBV DNA level indicating presumably acute hepatitis B infection, but she has no real risk factors for acute infection.

The clue to this case is the fact she has been prescribed lamivudine despite having been transplanted for autoimmune disease. This would suggest that she received an organ from a donor who was positive for anti-HBc. She admitted that she had not taken the lamivudine for several months after the last prescription ran out. Despite the fact that these donors did not have HBV DNA in serum at the time of transplant, the fact that they had anti-HBc means they likely had some HBV in the liver which is at risk of reactivation under immunosuppression.

Several studies have shown that in donors who are anti-HBc positive, there is a risk of transmitting hepatitis B to recipients who are hepatitis B surface antibody (anti-HBs) negative. The risk runs between 40–80%, and although most patients had mild disease, long-term survival was decreased in these patients compared with donors who were anti-HBc negative.

Since elimination of anti-HBc donors from the donor pool would significantly reduce the number of organs available, a strategy of putting anti-HBc donors in recipients who have a positive anti-HBs has been suggested. In this lady, she was status 1 for a week and had to accept an extended criteria organ which was anti-HBc positive. These patients should be treated indefinitely with an oral antiviral agent such as lamivudine, entecavir, or tenofovir. Since she stopped the lamivudine, she likely had reactivation of hepatitis B. Alternatively, if she had continued taking the lamivudine, she may have developed resistance. The patient was started on entecavir (although resistance studies did not show a mutant) and her hepatitis and jaundice gradually resolved over several weeks.

In patients transplanted for hepatitis B, extrahepatic reservoirs of virus mean that they need an oral antiviral agent but also hepatitis B immune globulin (HBIG), which is infused monthly to maintain an adequate anti-HBs level. This is very expensive and recent studies have suggested that it may be safe to stop HBIG after 1–2 years post-transplant and continue therapy with single or combination oral agents.

References

1. Dodson SF, Issa S, Araya V et al. Infectivity of hepatic allografts with antibodies to hepatitis B virus. Transplantation 1997;64:1582–4.
2. Dickson RC, Everhart JE, Lake JR et al. Transmission of hepatitis B by transplantation of livers from donors positive for antibody to hepatitis B core antigen. The National Institute of Diabetes and Digestive and Kidney Diseases Liver Transplantation Database. Gastroenterology 1997;113:1668–74.
3. Yu L, Koepsell T, Manhart L, Ioannou G. Survival after orthotopic liver transplantation: the impact of antibody against hepatitis B core antigen in the donor. Liver Transpl 2009;15:1343–50.

Case 85

A 56-year-old lady presents to the transplant clinic after a routine set of liver enzymes was noted to be abnormal. She had undergone liver transplant 6 years ago for alcoholic liver disease and has remained abstinent. She received a 24-year-old, CMV negative, anti-HBc negative allograft, with a cold ischemia time (CIT) of 8 hours. She had an uneventful postoperative course and is back at work as a real estate agent. She is accompanied by her husband who confirms her denials about alcohol use and she is still involved in the local alcohol rehabilitation facility.

She takes a calcium antagonist for hypertension but otherwise has no medical problems. She is up to date with health maintenance issues.

Immunosuppressive medications include tacrolimus and mycophenolate mofetil.

She does not smoke or use drugs.

Her review of systems is completely negative.

On exam she looks well with stable vital signs.

There is no scleral icterus.

Her heart and lungs are normal. Abdomen reveals a soft nontender abdomen with impalpable liver and spleen. There is no ankle edema.

Laboratory Studies

Hb 12.5 g/dl
Platelets 149,000/μl
WBC 2.6 × 10^3/μl
INR 1.0
Creatinine 1.3 mg/dl
Tbili 0.7 mg/dl
AST 73 iu/l
ALT 85 iu/l
GGTP 67 iu/l
ALP 97 iu/l
Tacrolimus level 6 ng/dl

Questions

1. What is the differential diagnosis?
2. What other blood tests are important to order?

Ultrasound:

Normal liver
Patent vessels
Anti-HCV negative
Anti-HBs positive
HBsAg negative
HBV DNA negative
HCV RNA negative
HSV IgG positive
CMV IgG positive
EBV IgG positive

Liver biopsy:

Mild mixed portal infiltrate (mainly lymphocytes).
No interface activity.
No evidence of acute rejection.
Portal fibrosis on trichrome stain.
Pathologist's interpretation-chronic hepatitis, favor viral etiology.

Answer: Chronic Hepatitis E After Liver Transplant

This appears to be an odd situation: a lady who is many years out from transplant and completely asymptomatic who presents with mildly elevated liver enzymes. She does not have risk factors for viral hepatitis and did not receive a hepatitis B core antibody positive liver. She has been taking her immunosuppression and has a therapeutic tacrolimus level. Workup should include serology for viral hepatitis which in this case is negative and imaging which showed no evidence of biliary obstruction or hepatic artery stenosis/thrombosis.

The next step is a biopsy which favors a viral etiology but all the typical viruses have been excluded. The scenario of a chronic hepatitis in patients post-liver transplant has been recognized for many years and is sometimes considered a type of autoimmune hepatitis. A predominance of plasma cells in an inflammatory infiltrate would support this and can also be considered a type of atypical rejection. Treatment would be similar with prednisone or increased immunosuppression. In this patient, plasma cells are not seen and the pathologist favors a viral etiology.

One virus that we do not routinely test for is hepatitis E (HEV). This is a cause of acute hepatitis in endemic areas but does not cause chronic hepatitis in immunocompetent hosts. Recently, reports have emerged from Europe that at least some of these cases of chronic hepatitis after transplant are related to chronic HEV infection. In addition, there are case reports of chronic HEV infection in patients immunosuppressed for other reasons including HIV and chemotherapy.

The long-term effects of chronic HEV infection in liver transplant recipients are unclear but some cases of unexplained hepatitis do lead to allograft failure. In the initial report from France, the incidence of acute HEV infection was 6.5% (14/217 patients) and a few of these patients developed chronic infection, which presented as in this patient with mildly elevated transaminases and a compatible biopsy having excluded other causes. Lymphopenia was also more common (particularly T cells – CD3 and CD4). Another report suggests that chronic HEV may exist in transplant patients as a carrier state. The diagnosis is made by checking HEV RNA in serum and a positive anti-HEV antibody. There is no treatment for this condition.

References

1. Kamar N, Selves J, Mansuy JM et al. Hepatitis E virus and chronic hepatitis in organ-transplant recipients. N Engl J Med 2008;358:811–7.
2. Haagsma EB, van den Berg AP, Porte RJ et al. Chronic hepatitis E virus infection in liver transplant recipients. Liver Transpl 2008;14:547–53.

Case 86

A 49-year-old man presents for routine follow-up in the transplant clinic. He has a history of liver transplant a year ago for alcoholic cirrhosis that was complicated by HCC. He was treated with radiofrequency ablation 3 months prior to transplant. He received a 56-year-old allograft with a cold ischemia time (CIT) of 6 hours. The explant showed a 2.5 cm treated lesion in the right lobe of the liver that showed no evidence of vascular invasion. He had an uneventful postoperative course and regular imaging has shown no recurrence of tumor.

He has been maintained on tacrolimus and mycophenolate mofetil immunosuppression.

He had no other medical problems prior to the transplant except for knee surgery.

He is married and has returned to work.

He does not smoke and still attends a weekly rehabilitation meeting to reinforce alcohol abstinence.

On exam he is alert and oriented. His BP is 140/90, pulse 74, BMI 26 kg/m^2, and he is afebrile.

There is no scleral icterus.

Cardiac, lung and abdominal exams are essentially unremarkable. His scar has healed well. There is no ankle edema.

Laboratory Studies

Hb 13.4 g/dl
Platelets 147,000/μl
WBC 5.9 × 10^3/μl
INR 1.0
Creatinine 1.7 mg/dl
Tbili 0.7 mg/dl
AST 35 iu/l
ALT 31 iu/l
GGTP 37 iu/l
ALP 89 iu/l
Albumin 3.4 g/dl
Tacrolimus level 6.1 ng/ml

Recent ultrasound – patent vessels, no mass in liver, normal kidneys
Urinalysis – no proteinuria

Questions

1. How should this patient's blood pressure be treated?
2. What is the likely cause of his elevated creatinine and how should it be managed?

1 month later
BP 140/92

Laboratory Studies

Creatinine 1.9 mg/dl
Tbili 0.8 mg/dl
AST 31 iu/l
ALT 29 iu/l
Tacrolimus level 5.0 ng/ml

Answer: Adverse Effects of Calcineurin Inhibitors on Blood Pressure and Renal Function

This patient presents with a common problem after liver transplant – an elevated blood pressure and creatinine that has persisted presumably after conservative measures were taken for a month.

The hypertension is likely related to his tacrolimus as he did not have hypertension prior to the transplant and is not obese. The mechanism of calcineurin inhibitor (CNI) related hypertension is not well understood but cyclosporine increases both systemic and renal vascular resistance (mainly affecting the afferent arteriole), probably mediated through an increased release of vasoconstrictors such as endothelin. Multiple studies have shown that an elevated BP is a major problem after liver transplant and can be seen in up to 70% of recipients. The management of BP after transplant is similar to the nontransplant setting in that salt intake should be minimized and obese patients encouraged to lose weight. Reducing CNI dose would help but runs the risk of rejection. Most experts would suggest using calcium channel blockers or beta-blockers as first-line agents due to less drug interactions, and ACE inhibitors as a second-line option.

The other concern is the elevated creatinine. In this patient there is no evidence of proteinuria and the ultrasound shows no obstruction. CNIs can cause an acute renal insult that is reversible but they can also lead to a progressive chronic renal failure in 10–30% of patients depending on the dose and length of treatment. The mechanism behind the chronic injury is multifactorial but renal biopsy shows an obliterative arteriolopathy and ischemic damage to the glomeruli with associated global and focal glomerulosclerosis, and patchy areas of interstitial fibrosis and tubular atrophy. This would suggest that vasoconstriction plays a major role.

The management of CNI nephrotoxicity relies on minimizing contributing factors such as hypertension, diabetes, and other nephrotoxic drugs. The effect of CNIs is dose dependent so reducing the dose whenever possible is prudent. Unlike the situation with kidney transplant where chronic rejection is a major concern, allograft failure in liver transplant is more a function of recurrent disease so several recent studies have illustrated that switching patients to alternative (less potent) immunosuppressive agents, such as sirolimus or mycophenolate mofetil monotherapy, can lessen renal injury while preventing rejection.

References

1. Stegall MD, Everson G, Schroter G et al. Metabolic complications after liver transplantation. Diabetes, hypercholesterolemia, hypertension, and obesity. Transplantation 1995;60:1057–60.
2. Gonwa TA, Mai ML, Melton LB et al. End-stage renal disease (ESRD) after orthotopic liver transplantation (OLTX) using calcineurin-based immunotherapy: risk of development and treatment. Transplantation 2001;72:1934–9.
3. Dharancy S, Declerck N, Schneck AS et al. Mycophenolate mofetil monotherapy for severe side effects of calcineurin inhibitors following liver transplantation. Am J Transplant 2009;9:610–3.
4. Morard I, Dumortier J, Spahr L et al. Conversion to sirolimus-based immunosuppression in maintenance liver transplantation patients. Liver Transpl 2007;13:658–64.

Case 87

A 26-year-old lady presents to your posttransplant office complaining of 1 week of fever and some nonspecific symptoms including joint pains, nausea, and some abdominal discomfort. Over the last 2 days she has developed diarrhea.

She had undergone liver transplant 4 months ago for acute liver failure secondary to acetaminophen. She had an uneventful postoperative course but needed dialysis for 2 weeks before her kidney function returned to normal. She is still struggling to come to terms with her condition, particularly in light of her underlying depression.

Her immunosuppression includes tacrolimus and mycophenolate mofetil. She also takes an antidepressant and was prescribed several other medications after transplant that she has not been taking.

Two months after transplant she developed elevated liver enzymes and a liver biopsy was performed that demonstrated acute rejection, which failed to clear with steroid therapy and she required a 1-week course of anti-thymocyte globulin about a month ago. Her liver enzymes improved and a repeat biopsy showed marked improvement.

She states that she has been taking all of her medicines although doubts persist as to her compliance.

She continues to smoke and has had a couple of drinks in the last few weeks.

Her exam is notable for a temperature of 100°F but otherwise normal vital signs. She is not icteric and her abdomen shows a well-healed scar and no tenderness is elicited.

Laboratory Studies

Hb 8.6 g/dl
WBC 1.8 × 10^3/μl
Platelets 43,000/μl
Creatinine 1.6 mg/dl
Tbili 1.3 mg/dl
AST 213 iu/l
ALT 257 iu/l
Tacrolimus level 14.5 ng/ml
Fecal occult blood positive

Questions

1. What should be included in the workup of this patient?
2. How is this condition treated?

Blood cultures
No growth after 48 h
CT scan chest and abdomen
No pulmonary infiltrate
No ascites or lesion in liver
Mild thickening of left colon
Stool studies
Negative for *Salmonella*, *Shigella*, *Campylobacter*, *E. coli*, *Yersinia*
C. difficile toxin negative
Allograft-19-year old DCD liver
Cold ischemia time (CIT) of 7 hours
Warm ischemia time 26 min
Duct-to-duct anastomosis
CMV positive (recipient CMV negative)

Answer: Cytomegalovirus Infection After LT

This young lady has developed a febrile illness within a few weeks of receiving treatment for acute cellular rejection (ACR) making infection a very likely diagnosis. She has some nonspecific symptoms but has also developed diarrhea and her blood work shows pancytopenia, a clue toward CMV infection. She needs a full infectious workup including blood and urine cultures, *C. difficile* toxin and imaging of her chest and abdomen. Stool studies are required and she likely will need a colonoscopy. If a diagnosis is not made quickly, a liver biopsy would also be indicated due to her elevated liver enzymes (which should be done by the transjugular route due to the thrombocytopenia).

The fact that she was CMV negative prior to transplant and she received a CMV positive allograft greatly increases her risk of reactivation of CMV and she would have been placed on prophylaxis after transplant (and this would have reinforced when she received anti-thymocyte globulin for rejection, along with prophylaxis for Pneumocystis). Several studies have demonstrated that without prophylaxis, CMV will reactivate in more than 50% of donor positive, recipient negative (D+R–) patients, with lower rates in D+R+ and the lowest risk in D–R– patients.

CMV disease in transplant recipients usually presents as a mononucleosis-like syndrome with fever, myalgias, and arthralgias and a pronounced leucopenia. Liver enzymes can be mildly elevated or overt CMV hepatitis can also occur with significantly elevated transaminases (see CMV hepatitis case elsewhere in this book). Organ involvement can occur including interstitial pneumonitis, esophagitis, and colitis. In contrast retinal involvement is rare in transplant patients.

The diagnosis of CMV is based on serology, early antigen tests, and DNA assays. Culture is possible but takes weeks. CMV can be rapidly detected in peripheral blood leukocytes using assays of tagged monoclonal antibodies specific to the pp65 lower matrix protein of CMV. The most sensitive test is a CMV DNA assay by a variety of polymerase chain reaction tests. These provide a quantitative viral load and can be used to monitor response to therapy.

Treatment of active disease involves lowering immunosuppression if possible and using intravenous ganciclovir or oral valganciclovir. Both drugs can cause leucopenia and pancytopenia. A recent study has shown these agents are equally effective.

Prophylactic or pre-emptive therapy in liver transplant recipients is also important. The greatest risk for reactivation of CMV is the first few months after transplant when immunosuppression is at its highest. However, several studies have suggested that the risk of CMV infection is still present and using a strategy of only treating patients with ganciclovir or valganciclovir for a few months immediately after transplant and then stopping only delays reactivation of disease.

References

1. Asberg A, Humar A, Rollag H et al. Oral valganciclovir is noninferior to intravenous ganciclovir for the treatment of cytomegalovirus disease in solid organ transplant recipients. Am J Transplant 2007;7:2106–13.
2. Kalil AC, Levitsky J, Lyden E et al. Meta-analysis: the efficacy of strategies to prevent organ disease by cytomegalovirus in solid organ transplant recipients. Ann Intern Med 2005;143:870–80.

Case 88

A 46-year-old African-American man presents to the emergency room with several days of nonbloody diarrhea, mild abdominal pain, and low-grade fever. He had undergone liver transplant 3 months earlier for cirrhosis secondary to hepatitis C. He received a 62-year-old allograft with a cold ischemia time (CIT) of 7 hours. The donor was CMV positive and the recipient CMV negative. He had an uneventful postoperative course.

His past medical history is significant for diabetes and hypertension which had been under good control.

Medications include tacrolimus, mycophenolate mofetil, prednisone, amlodipine, insulin, bactrim, and valganciclovir.

Exam shows a middle-aged male in no distress. Vital signs are remarkable for a temperature of 100°F. There is no scleral icterus and heart and lungs are normal. Abdomen is soft with a 2–3 cm liver edge palpable, no ascites, and no splenomegaly.

Initial Laboratory Studies Reveal

Hb 10.2 g/dl
Platelets 131,000/μl
WBC 0.3×10^3/μl
INR 1.0
Creatinine 1.0 mg/dl
Tbili 0.8 mg/dl
AST 17 iu/l
ALT 19 iu/l
ALP 107 iu/l
Tacrolimus level 11 ng/ml

Question

1. What is the differential diagnosis at this time?

Subsequently, his medications are altered and he undergoes several procedures including a colonoscopy, which shows some scattered erythema and shallow ulceration. He spikes a fever and antibiotics are started. He develops a fine macular, erythematous rash over his entire body.

Laboratory Studies 1 Week Later

Hb 8.1 g/dl
Platelets 13,000/μl
WBC 0.1 × 10^3/μl

Questions

1. What is the diagnosis and how is it made?
2. What is the treatment and prognosis?

Bone marrow biopsy:
Bone marrow with marked patchy hypocellularity with a few foci of granulocytic or erythroid precursors. Megakaryocytes are virtually absent. The findings are those of marrow hypoplasia. Cellularity is 10–20%.
Skin biopsy:
Interface dermatitis with hemorrhage, edema, and necrotic keratinocytes with follicular extension.
Colon biopsy:
Colonic mucosa with marked increased glandular apoptotic activity and extensive crypt dropout.
Cytomegalovirus – DNA positive
Human Herpes virus 6 (HHV6) – DNA positive

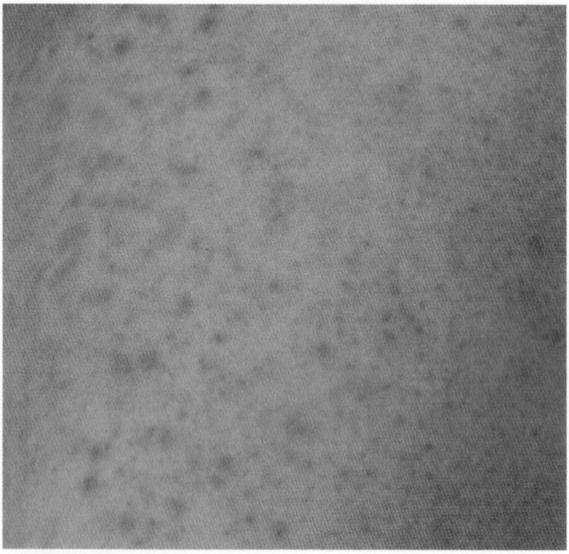

Fig. 88.1 Skin rash

Answer: Acute Graft vs. Host Disease

This middle aged man presents within 3 months of transplant (when immunosuppression is still high) with diarrhea, fever, and abdominal pain. The very low white cell count is suggestive of a bone marrow issue and hence the initial concern has to be for an infectious process such as CMV colitis or a bacterial infection, which may have been the primary problem but also may have been related to neutropenia related to medications such as mycophenolate or bactrim. Both of these medications were held, blood cultures were taken, and he was started on granulocyte colony stimulating factor (GCSF).

He also underwent a bone marrow biopsy, which showed a hypocellular marrow, and by this time he is pancytopenic and spiking fevers in the setting of a skin rash (Fig. 88.1). Both his CMV and human herpes virus 6 (HHV6) viral titers are positive so perhaps this is the diagnosis (despite the fact he was on valganciclovir which is good prophylactic therapy).

HHV6 can reactivate after transplant and is associated with several clinical syndromes and bone marrow suppression, but typically there is infection with other viral infections including CMV. In addition, circulating HHV6 DNA is not uncommon in healthy transplant recipients. CMV infection posttransplant is discussed in another case and could lead to neutropenia and colitis but the skin rash is not typical.

The colonoscopy in this case shows ulceration in the right colon with nonspecific histology. The skin biopsy is important here as it shows features that are consistent with acute graft versus host disease (GVHD).

GVHD is a common complication after hematopoietic stem cell transplant (HCT) but is rare after liver transplant. The diagnosis after HCT is based on the clinical presentation of rash, GI involvement (usually diarrhea and crampy abdominal pain) and an elevated bilirubin, and can be confirmed on skin or liver biopsy. The division into acute and chronic is based on presentation before or after 100 days post-HCT. After liver transplant the diagnosis is more difficult as liver tests can be elevated for other reasons.

GVHD is essentially due to donor (graft) immune cells recognizing recipient (host) cells as foreign and initiating a reaction to destroy them. For this to occur, there are several requirements including the following: the graft must contain immunologically competent cells; there should be transplantation antigens in the host that are lacking in the graft, thereby appearing foreign to the graft; stimulation of donor cells by host cells via these specific antigenic determinants; and the host must be incapable of mounting a reaction against the graft for a period of time sufficient to allow graft cells to attack the host.

The liver does have an immune function so these cells (mainly T cells) do get transplanted and the diagnosis of GVHD after liver transplant relies on an appropriate clinical situation and demonstration of donor cells in the bone marrow (chimerism) using a variety of techniques.

Treatment of GVHD after liver transplant is based on anecdotal reports. After HCT steroids are the first line treatment but anti-thymocyte globulin, tacrolimus, and a variety of monoclonal antibodies against T cells have been used. In this patient, we increased his immunosuppression and used steroids but, as with most patients with this condition, he did not recover and died eventually of sepsis. Interestingly, some reports have suggested that the presence of HHV6 and CMV is associated with GVHD and may initiate the recognition of non-self by donor immune cells.

References

1. de Pagter PJ, Schuurman R, Visscher H et al. Human herpes virus 6 plasma DNA positivity after hematopoietic stem cell transplantation in children: an important risk factor for clinical outcome. Biol Blood Marrow Transplant 2008;14:831–9.
2. Piton G, Larosa F, Minello A et al. Infliximab treatment for steroid-refractory acute graft-versus-host disease after orthotopic liver transplantation: a case report. Liver Transpl 2009;15:682–5.
3. Kanehira K, Riegert-Johnson DL, Chen D et al. FISH diagnosis of acute graft-versus-host disease following living-related liver transplant. J Mol Diagn 2009;11:355–8.
4. Kohler S, Pascher A, Junge G et al. Graft versus host disease after liver transplantation – a single center experience and review of literature. Transpl Int 2008;21:441–51.

Case 89

A 52-year-old lady presents for follow-up in your posttransplant clinic. She had undergone orthotopic liver transplant 9 months ago for cirrhosis secondary to hepatitis C that was complicated by HCC. She had a complicated postoperative course that included a prolonged stay in the intensive care unit and several trips back to the operating room because of bleeding. She has not yet had a biopsy to assess the degree of recurrent hepatitis C. Her immunosuppression dose has been difficult to stabilize.

Her other medical problems include hypertension and hyperlipidemia, which have been under good control. She is also depressed at having missed so much time from work and financial difficulties as a result, as well as significant weight gain.

Her current medications include tacrolimus 2 mg bid, mycophenolate mofetil 1,000 mg bid, amlodipine, atorvastatin, and acetaminophen as required. Her primary physician started her on 10 days of fluconazole for a fungal infection last week. She continues to take several herbal remedies which she states calm her down, as well dieting to try and lose weight and improve her frequent headaches, which consists of fruit at every meal.

She denies tobacco or alcohol use. She is married with grown-up children. She used to work at a local department store as a fashion consultant.

Her review of systems is significant for the headaches, which have been more frequent over the last few days, and some pins and needles in her legs, which she puts down to her weight gain. She denies fever, chills, abdominal pain, or diarrhea.

On exam she looks well and is alert and oriented.

Vital signs show BP 140/90, pulse 82, BMI 33kg/m^2, and she is afebrile. There is no scleral icterus, and heart and lungs are normal.

Abdomen is soft and nontender without ascites. She has mild ankle edema. There is no focal neurological deficit. She does have some decreased sensation in the stocking distribution.

Laboratory Studies Reveal

Hb 12.1 g/dl
Platelets 189,000/μl
WBC 6.2 × 10^3/μl
Creatinine 1.3 mg/dl (baseline 0.8 mg/dl)
Tbili 0.7 mg/dl
AST 34 iu/l
ALT 41 iu/l
Tacrolimus level 16 ng/ml

You reduce her tacrolimus level to 1.5 mg bid and tell her to get repeat laboratory tests in a week.
Repeat tacrolimus level <0.5 ng/ml

Questions

1. What are the concerns regarding her tacrolimus level?
2. What other parts of the history might contribute to the fluctuation in tacrolimus level?

Answer: Drug Interactions with Calcineurin Inhibitors (CNI)

This lady presents with an elevated tacrolimus level and a history of difficulty controlling the level in the past. Her headaches and peripheral neuropathy are likely related to the increased tacrolimus level, as may her elevated blood pressure, which was previously well-controlled.

Tacrolimus and cyclosporine are immunosuppressive drugs that share a common mechanism of action and also metabolism. Both drugs avidly bind to a family of cytoplasmic proteins present in most cells and the drug-receptor complex specifically and competitively binds to and inhibits the calcium and calmodulin-dependent phosphatase, calcineurin. This leads to decreased transcription of several cytokines including interleukin-2 (IL-2) and tumor necrosis factor alpha (TNF-alpha). Both drugs act primarily on T-helper cells, and to a lesser extent, inhibit T-suppressor and T-cytotoxic cells.

Metabolism occurs through the cytochrome P450 family enzymes in the liver and metabolites are excreted into bile. Hence, liver dysfunction prolongs the half-life of both cyclosporine and tacrolimus. Since the hepatic cytochrome P450-3A enzymes are involved in their metabolism, multiple drug interactions are possible that can increase or decrease CNI levels and action.
Increased levels are seen with the following:

Calcium channel blockers – diltiazem, nicardipine, verapamil
Antifungals – fluconazole, itraconazole, ketoconazole
Macrolides – clarithromycin, erythromycin
Acid suppressors – lansoprazole, rabeprazole, cimetidine
Miscellaneous – methylprednisolone, allopurinol, colchicine, metoclopramide, amiodarone and grapefruit juice

Decreased levels are seen with the following:

Anticonvulsants – carbamazepine, phenytoin, Phenobarbital
Antibiotics – nafcillin, rifampicin, rifabutin
Miscellaneous – ticlodipine, orlistat, St John's Wort

This lady may well be using St John's Wort in her herbal supplement and grapefruit juice as part of her fruit diet and these may be affecting the tacrolimus level. The antifungal was probably responsible for the current increase in the tacrolimus level and the very low repeat level was taken when she was off the antifungal and the tacrolimus level had been decreased. The effect of antifungals and calcium channel blockers on the tacrolimus level can be used to decrease the cyclosporine dose (and cost) in transplant patients.

Patients after transplant are given verbal and written instruction regarding these drug interactions but given their sheer number it is not surprising that drug interactions are frequently seen.

References

1. European FK506 Multicentre Liver Study Group. Randomised trial comparing tacrolimus (FK506) and cyclosporin in prevention of liver allograft rejection. Lancet 1994;344:423–8.
2. The U.S. Multicenter FK506 Liver Study Group. A comparison of tacrolimus (FK 506) and cyclosporine for immunosuppression in liver transplantation. N Engl J Med 1994;331:1110–5.

Case 90

A 33-year-old lady presents to an outside hospital with sudden onset of nausea and epigastric pain. She had undergone liver transplant 12 years earlier for fulminant hepatic failure secondary to acetaminophen and retransplant 2 years later for chronic rejection.

She had been well over the last few years and maintained on sirolimus-based immunosuppression.

She denied any change in her medications or over the counter medications. Her bowel movements were normal, but she had a low grade fever.

She had no other medical problems.

Exam demonstrated a patient in no obvious distress and a soft abdomen with minimal epigastric tenderness.

Initial workup included completely normal liver panel and normal bilirubin. Amylase and lipase were normal and the white cell count was not elevated. Ultrasound was normal.

She was empirically started on broad spectrum antibiotics and transferred to your tertiary care transplant center.

On arrival she looks comfortable and confirms that she has been taking all her immunosuppression medication as prescribed.

Over the following few days she remains febrile but otherwise asymptomatic, and her liver enzymes begin to rise in a mixed pattern but with normal bilirubin.

Repeat imaging is pretty unremarkable although the hepatic vasculature is poorly seen and there is minimal intrahepatic ductal dilation and a liver biopsy is unhelpful, showing no rejection and really no inflammation.

Laboratory Parameters

Tbili 1.4 mg/dl
AST 106 iu/l
ALT 103 iu/l
GGTP 345 iu/l
Sirolimus level normal
Creatinine 1.1 mg/dl

Questions

1. What should you do next?
2. What is the significance, if any, of sirolimus?

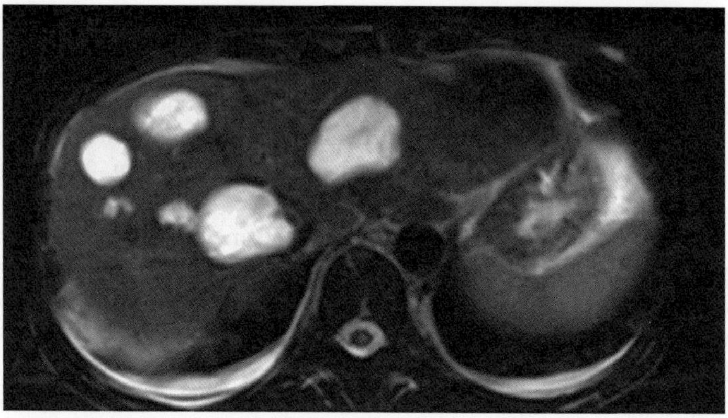

Fig. 90.1 MRI showing T2-weighted images taken 4 weeks after initial presentation

Answer: Bilomas from Hepatic Artery Thrombosis (HAT)

This case shows classic imaging characteristics of the aftermath of HAT. After transplant this most commonly occurs in the area of the arterial anastomosis. The MRI is notable for multiple lesions in both lobes of the liver that were not apparent several weeks ago suggesting these are infective or bilomas.

The patient had one of these lesions drained and dirty brown/bilious fluid was aspirated.

The clinical course of this patient was not typical of HAT since it occurred so late after transplant. On closer examination of her operative note, an interposition hepatic artery graft had been used in the second transplant for unclear reasons but presumably increased her risk for HAT. A prothrombotic workup is mandatory but was negative in this case.

When the patient first presented with nausea and epigastric pain this presumably was acute HAT since no collaterals were seen. She had a Doppler ultrasound that showed no flow in the hepatic artery and this was confirmed on angiography. ERCP was also performed because of the biliary dilation that showed a normal post-OLT cholangiogram.

The MRI (Fig. 90.1) shows bilomas that have occurred due to ischemia of the biliary tree. The liver biopsy was unremarkable either because of sampling error or because it was done early in the course of her disease.

Sirlolimus is associated with early HAT and has a black box warning from the FDA regarding this. In this particular case the patient was intolerant of tacrolimus and had been switched to sirolimus. She had been on it for many years and it was unlikely to be a contributory factor in this case.

HAT complicates up to 5% of liver transplants and is more common in pediatric recipients. It is associated with arterial reconstruction or aberrant anatomy and some studies suggest older donors are a risk factor. Endovascular intervention has been tried with limited success and unfortunately complete HAT usually leads to graft failure and the need for retransplant. Survival rates after retransplant are only 50–60% at 5 years.

References

1. Tzakis AG, Gordon RD, Shaw BW Jr et al. Clinical presentation of hepatic artery thrombosis after liver transplantation in the cyclosporine era. Transplantation 1985;40:667–71.
2. Duffy JP, Hong JC, Farmer DG et al. Vascular complications of orthotopic liver transplantation: experience in more than 4,200 patients. J Am Coll Surg 2009;208:896–903.

Index